Handbook of Neonatal Care

Handbook of Neonatal Care

Edited by Audrina Howell

STATES
ACADEMIC PRESS
www.statesacademicpress.com

States Academic Press,
109 South 5th Street,
Brooklyn, NY 11249, USA

Visit us on the World Wide Web at:
www.statesacademicpress.com

ISBN: 978-1-63989-263-1

Cataloging-in-Publication Data

Handbook of neonatal care / edited by Audrina Howell.
p. cm.
Includes bibliographical references and index.
ISBN 978-1-63989-263-1
1. Newborn infants--Care. 2. Pediatric nursing. 3. Neonatal intensive care.
4. Newborn infants--Hospital care. I. Howell, Audrina.

RJ253 .H36 2022
618.920 1--dc23

Table of Contents

Preface VII

Chapter 1 **Neonatal Osteomyelitis** 1
Lidia Decembrino, Nunzia Decembrino and Mauro Stronati

Chapter 2 **Respiratory Care Protocols in Neonatal Intensive Care** 12
Wissam Shalish and Guilherme Mendes Sant' Anna

Chapter 3 **Neonatal Hypoglycemia** 31
Adauto Dutra Moraes Barbosa, Israel Figueiredo Júnior and Gláucia Macedo de Lima

Chapter 4 **Neonatal Care in the First Hour of Life** 50
Teja Škodič Zakšek, Anita Jug Došler, Ana Polona Mivšek and Petra Petročnik

Chapter 5 **Non-Pulmonary Management of Newborns with Respiratory Distress** 67
Petja Fister and Štefan Grosek

Chapter 6 **Respiratory Care of the Neonate** 96
Štefan Grosek and Petja Fister

Chapter 7 **Fungal Infections in Neonatal Intensive Care** 113
Rejane P. Neves, Ana Maria R. de Carvalho Parahym, Carolina M. da Silva, Danielle P.C. Macêdo, André F.G. Leal, Henrique J. Neves and Reginaldo G. Lima-Neto

Chapter 8 **Hemodynamic Monitoring in Neonates** 126
Petja Fister and Štefan Grosek

Chapter 9 **Neonatal Gene Therapy for Inherited Disorders** 143
Koichi Miyake, Noriko Miyake and Takashi Shimada

Chapter 10 **Neonatal Care for Anesthesiologists** 152
Esra Caliskan

Chapter 11 **Update on Neonatal Male Circumcision: A Public Health Perspective** 170
Kriengkrai Srithanaviboonchai

Chapter 12 **Endocrine Active Compounds Actions during Neonatal Period: Effect on the Ovary** 191
Maria Slomczynska, Malgorzata Grzesiak and Katarzyna Knapczyk-Stwora

Chapter 13 **Pre- and Postnatal Surgery, Most Common Conditions, Diagnosis and Treatment** 210
Carlos Baeza Herrera, Alin Villalobos Castillejos and Ricardo Cortés García

Chapter 14 **Reducing Early Neonatal Mortality in Nigeria—The Solution** **233**
Hippolite O. Amadi and Mohammed B. Kawuwa

Permissions

List of Contributors

Index

Preface

Neonatal care is a sub-specialty of nursing that is concerned with the care for newborn infants. They can suffer from a wide range of problems such as prematurity, infections, birth defects, cardiac malformations and surgical problems. There are different levels of neonatal nursery; level 1, level 2, level 3 and level 4. Level 1 deals with the care of healthy newborns while level 2 consists of immediate care for ill or premature newborns. Level 3 provides special care for newborns that are in need of technological intervention. Level 4 treats newborns that are in complex and critical conditions, and need extensive care. This book unravels the recent studies in the field of neonatal care. It strives to provide a fair idea about this discipline and to help develop a better understanding of the latest advances within this field. This book will help new researchers by foregrounding their knowledge in this field.

All of the data presented henceforth, was collaborated in the wake of recent advancements in the field. The aim of this book is to present the diversified developments from across the globe in a comprehensible manner. The opinions expressed in each chapter belong solely to the contributing authors. Their interpretations of the topics are the integral part of this book, which I have carefully compiled for a better understanding of the readers.

At the end, I would like to thank all those who dedicated their time and efforts for the successful completion of this book. I also wish to convey my gratitude towards my friends and family who supported me at every step.

Editor

1

Neonatal Osteomyelitis

Lidia Decembrino, Nunzia Decembrino and
Mauro Stronati

Abstract

Osteomyelitis in neonates is relatively uncommon, but burdened with an increased hospital stay and possible long-term sequelae if not diagnosed on time. It differs from that of older children for etiology, clinical and radiological findings, and treatment. Due to anatomic contiguity, osteomyelitis may coexist with septic arthritis. Soft-tissue swelling or joint effusion is often associated. Our aim is to review the literature to provide the most recent data related to epidemiology, clinical presentation, diagnosis, treatment, and outcome.

Keywords: neonatal osteomyelitis, septic arthritis, antibiotics, imaging studies, micro-organisms

1. Introduction

Osteomyelitis (OM) refers to an infection of the bone that affects around 8/100,000 children [1]. For neonatal OM, an estimated incidence of 1–7/1000 hospital admissions has been reported [2, 3]. Due to their immature immune response, neonates are more susceptible than older children. Preterm infants are at a higher risk because of frequent blood withdrawal, invasive monitoring, diagnostic and treatment procedures, parent's nutrition, ventilatory support, perinatal hypoxia and prolonged NICU stay [4–7]. The long bones are the most frequently affected sites, especially of lower extremities, femur and tibia. Sites less commonly involved include the upper limbs, the pelvis, the clavicle, and the rib [8]. The presence of interosseous collateral arteries makes vertebral bodies less susceptible to infarction from septic emboli and more able to clear bacteria secondary to septic embolization. This explains the low incidence of vertebral body infection in neonates compared to older children and adults [9]. Few studies have focused on race differences. In low-risk neonates with OM, an accompanying fracture should be considered [10]. Sternal OM is extremely rare, but has been reported [11]. Neonates are most vulnerable to multifocal infection [12, 13]. **Pathophysiology.** Osteomyelitis in neonates is usually due to hematogenous spread of bacterial infections or less frequently to direct inoculation as a result of a trauma or puncture wounds or surgery, infected cephalohematoma [14–16]. In preterm infants, direct injection of bacteria can result from heel or venipuncture and artery or vein umbilical catheterization. Indirect contamination from a nearby infection, for example, cellulitis is also possible. Premature rupture of membranes, transplacental infection, and urinary tract infections has been described as risk factors too [17, 18]. A few cases of neonatal Gram-negative germ osteoarthritis have been reported, associated with a vesico-ureteral reflux (VUR) or hydronephrosis by the same microorganism [19, 20]. The most susceptible areas to haematogenous seeding of infection are metaphyseal of long bones, in particular the areas adjacent to the cartilaginous growth plate (physis) that is highly vascularized with slow intravascular flow. Abscess can result from the passage of bacteria through gaps from the sinusoidal veins to the capillaries into the tissue, where they are provided an ideal environment to grow. These abscesses frequently rupture into the joint [21]. Acute haematogenous OM and septic arthritis of the adjacent joint coexist in up to 76% of all cases as a result of a unique vascular anatomy characterized by the presence of vascular connections between the metaphysis and the epiphysis, particularly before the appearance of a secondary ossification center. Involvement of the shoulder or hip joints is noted when the intracapsular metaphyseal end of the humerus or femoral are involved from infection.

2. Symptoms

Asymmetric movement of extremities, irritability and poor feeding may be often the early and unspecific findings of OM [9, 22]. Common symptoms include bone pain, swelling, redness, guarding and failure to move the affected body part (pseudoparalysis). Fever may or may not be present because of an immature immune system. It is important to ascertain joint involvement through the detection of pseudoparalysis and pain during passive movements and signs of local inflammation [22]. Dierig et al. [23] reported a newborn with combined OM and suppurative arthritis caused by *Streptococcus pyogenes* giving rise to right brachial plexus palsy. Acute haematogenous OM is usually defined acute if the signs or symptoms are present for less than 14 days, and subacute if signs or symptoms are present for more than 14 days. In neonates, acute forms predominate [1].

3. Causative microorganisms

The causative agents of OM reflect those of neonatal sepsis, which vary from country to country and in many cases remain unknown. The most common pathogen is *Staphylococcus aureus*, found in 70–90% of culture positive cases [24, 25]. Other pathogens include *Streptococcus* mainly group B (*Streptococcus agalactiae*) and Gram-negative enteric bacteria (*Escherichia coli and Klebsiella pneumonia*) *Pseudomonas aeruginosa* [26, 27]. Multi-drug resistant *S. aureus*

(MRSA), community-acquired strains of methicillin-resistant *Staphylococcus aureus* (CA-MRSA) and *Kingella kingae* have emerged as being relevant in recent years and are responsible for serious infections [28]. *Candida albicans* OM needs to be considered in neonates, especially if preterms with specific risk factors. The presentation is more subtle and subacute, even in the absence of fever and elevated inflammatory markers. The progression is prolonged. OM from *Haemophilus influenzae* type b (Hib) has declined significantly; thanks to the introduction of the Hib vaccine.

4. Differential diagnoses

Differential diagnosis may be difficult and cellulitis, septic arthritis, subcutaneous abscess, fractures, and bone tumors should be taken into account. CNS disease (cerebral hemorrhage), trauma, scurvy, and child abuse are to be considered in the case of pseudoparalysis. Allagui et al. [29] described a case of acute OM of the clavicle in a 30-day-old newborn, with clinical symptoms simulating obstetric brachial plexus palsy. Laboratory tests are necessary to confirm a clinical diagnosis of OM. Neonates with OM may have a normal leukocyte count that is elevated in only half of the patients with or without thrombocytosis. The C-reactive protein (CRP) and erythrocyte sedimentation rate (ESR) are almost always elevated (except in small bone infections). It is important to obtain blood, bone, or joint aspirate cultures if necessary, to identify the causative organism, before any antibiotics are given. Because OM usually is a consequence of sepsis, hence lumbar puncture should be considered. Any potential source of infection should be examined, including intravascular catheter tips. Serum procalcitonin may be used as a sensitive and specific marker in the diagnosis of acute OM [30] more suitable as an aid for rule-in diagnosis rather than for exclusion. Its diagnostic performance is better for a lower cut-off value compared to a conventional cut-off of 0.5 ng/ml which is specific but less sensitive [31]. A bone biopsy is advisable if the patient does not respond to the standard therapy.

5. Imaging studies

Imaging (computed tomography (CT) scan, radiography, bone scan, US and/or MRI) is used to identify the site of an infection, the presence of liquid collections for diagnostic aspiration and/or biopsy, to differentiate a unifocal from multifocal disease and to identify present or impending complications, such as joint or extradural involvement. Montgomery et al. [32] showed that the use of advanced imaging (CT scan, bone scan, and/or MRI) in infants younger than 4 months of age may shorten hospital stays, decrease the number of operative procedures required, and possibly limit infection-related sequelae. MRI has become the gold standard to evaluate musculoskeletal infection. It has the capability of assessing the osseous, articular and muscular structures simultaneously and does not require ionizing radiation. In particular MRI plays an important role in defining the extent of soft tissue involvement, defining drainable fluid collections and bone biopsy sites pre-operatively and thereby decreasing the need for repeating the surgery. Increased marrow intensity with surrounding inflammation are the most suggestive signs of OM. MRI of the spine is useful in children not responding to therapy and/or to detect complications, such as extradural and paraspinal collections that will require surgical treatment because of causing spinal cord compression. The enhanced uptake of the radioisotope, distinguishes OM from deep cellulitis Gadolinium-enhanced fat-saturated T1-weighted sequences increase the confidence of the diagnosis of OM and may help also to distinguish edema from an abscess [33] and allows one to see the isolated involvement of the epiphyseal growth cartilage that is occult on radiographs and bone scintigraphy because of the paucity of growth cartilage ossification. The finding of hypo-enhancing foci in the growth cartilage suggests cartilage ischemia, necrosis or abscess as a consequence of infectious chondritis or septic thrombosis [34]. MRI may not be appropriate for monitoring the evolution of the lesions. Technetium bone scanning has a false-negative rate of as much as 20%, particularly in the first few days of illness. Indium-labeled leukocytes have limitations in newborns. Gallium scanning is not recommended because of lower specificity and exposure to higher levels of radiation. Ultrasonography: Although ultrasonography is an operator dependant technique with an inability to differentiate infectious fluid from traumatic ones, in able hands, it allows the detection of changes of acute OM as early as 48 h after the onset of infection. In the early stages ultrasound document deep soft tissue swelling (1–3 d), then the elevation of the periosteum by a thin layer of fluid, a definite subperiosteal collection, joint effusion and finally cortical erosion (2–4 w). In this last case it is used to guide needle drainage aspiration if necessary. Ultrasound images normalize by 4 weeks in the case of response to treatment [35]. Doppler venous ultrasonography is the first imaging study indicated in the case of clinical suspicion for deep vein thrombosis in patients with OM caused by CA-MRSA. A normal ultrasound scan does not exclude OM. Radiography is usually the first radiological investigation in a neonate with suspected OM, although it is reported that only 20% of the radiographs are abnormal at 10–14 days [36, 37]. Despite the low prevalence of abnormal features at presentation, it allows the exclusion of fractures and is useful to show long-term follow-up of complications. Initially it may reveal normal results, after 10–15 days signs of bone destruction, osteopenia, lytic lesions, and periosteal changes. Metaphyseal irregularities and periostitis (both non-specific) may be documented [37]. It has low sensitivity toward detection of a joint effusion or deep soft tissue swelling; the diagnosis of suspicion may include widening of the joint space with or without subluxation and soft tissues protruding that can be detected as early as 48 h after the onset of infection. Radiography may detect bone destruction when at least one-third of the matrix has been involved. Findings related to the spine may be limited to a loss of the normal lumbar lordosis, disc space narrowing, end plate erosions, pressure erosion of the superior and inferior margins of the adjacent vertebral body if the infection prolonged. Normally, other imaging tests are required. A bone scan is reserved for the cases in which radiographs and/or ultrasound are unclear, for suspected multifocal infection, chronic multifocal OM, and discitis. Bone scintigraphy is highly sensitive to the detection of OM in the early stages of the disease. In the first week of the disease, technetium (99mTc)-labeled bone scans revealed positive in 87% of the cases as compared with 42% diagnosed with radiography. Scintigraphy is useful for detecting multifocal diseases that are more common in neonates. A 99mTc-labeled phosphonate complex is the most used isotope. Scintigraphic study, even if non-specific, is useful to document through increased uptake of all three phases: perfusion, blood pool activity and bone metabolism. Cold spots occur as a result of decreased blood flow secondary to edema and subperiosteal or articular infection. It may be a discriminating diagnosis in secondary bone infection in the case of persisting coagulase negative staphylococcus (CONS) bacteremia [38]. Computed tomography (CT) scan use is limited in the neonate. It is superior to MRI in chronic OM with cortical destruction, air and sequestra. It may also be used to guide aspiration and biopsy, especially when the spine and paraspinal soft tissues are involved [9].

6. Procedures

If signs and symptoms do not begin to resolve within 48–72 h of initiation of appropriate antimicrobial treatment, bone aspiration may be necessary to identify the pathogen and to drain the pus in accordance with the orthopedic surgeon. Bone and/or joint fluid aspirate for culture, can be bactericidal. Bone biopsy is necessary in the suspicion of tumors.

7. Management

It is a necessary antibiotic treatment, as soon as possible, in order to prevent the potentially adverse anatomic and functional consequences, preferably after obtaining blood and bone aspirates for culture. As cultures may be negative or difficult to obtain, empirical treatment is based on the local prevalence of organisms, resistance patterns taking account of the change over the years of the spectrum of organisms causing OM. The choice of an agent is generally either a penicillinase-resistant penicillin (e.g. nafcillin, oxacillin, flucloxacillin), which will be effective against S. aureus but may be of limited value against other organisms, or a broad-spectrum cephalosporin, which could have reduced the activity against *S. aureus*. Antibiotics against methicillin-sensitive *S. aureus* (MRSA) and streptococci (a penicillinase-resistant penicillin, first generation cephalosporin or clindamycin) must be incorporated into any empiric regimen for OM because *S. aureus*, *group A Streptococci* and group B streptococcus (GBS) and *S. pneuomoniae* together account for more than 90% of the cases of osteoarthritis in neonates [39]. Immunization rates worldwide have obviated the need to use antibiotics against Hib in many countries. Cefuroxime, a second-generation cephalosporin can be used as a single agent against both methicillin-sensitive *S. aureus* (MSSA) and Hib, if they are the suspected pathogens. The increasing incidence of penicillin-resistant S pneumoniae warrants the use of a clindamycin and cefotaxime/ceftriaxone combination. When treating neonatal OM, consider nafcillin and tobramycin or vancomycin and gentamicin combinations to provide coverage of bacteria from the Enterobacteriaceae family, in addition to group B streptococci and *S. aureus*. Vancomycin is preferred for proven or suspected MRSA-related septicaemia or known multi-drug resistant MRSA infection. The suspicion of enteric organisms justify additional therapy with an aminoglycoside, such as gentamicin, tobramycin or amikacin or an extended-spectrum, a Pseudomonas-active agent, such as cefepime [40]. In the case of acquired MRSA infections should be started vancomycin, rather than a penicillin antibiotic [5]. Daptomycin, Linezolid, and Quinupristin-dalfopristin have not been fully evaluated or approved for use in neonates and should be employed when the neonate cannot tolerate vancomycin [40]. If B streptococcical infection is confirmed, combination therapy with penicillin G (or ampicillin) and gentamicin should be given for 2–5 days, after which time penicillin G (or ampicillin) alone is adequate. Monitoring serum acute-phase proteins, particularly the C-reactive protein, has been proposed as a useful way to determine resolution of infection and duration of therapy [40]. Management of *C. albicans* OM requires prolonged antifungal therapy. Society of America practices guidelines, including surgical debridement in selected cases and fluconazole therapy for 6–12 months, intravenous initially and then orally [26]. Amphotericin B is the most commonly used antifungal therapy. They are not provided clear guidelines on the optimum duration of treatment to eradicate infection. Even if by many are advocated shortened courses of antibiotic therapy because of morbidity and cost implications related to the prolonged therapy, the recommended entire duration of treatment still consists of at least 4–6 weeks until normalization of the C-reactive protein level [41]. Moreover it is typically recommended that infants under 3 months are given the full course of antibiotics parentally due to concerns over absorption and efficacy of oral antibiotics and to ensure adequate serum levels of the antibiotic. Recently some studies reported about oral therapy after a few days of intravenous therapy. Jagodzinski et al. [42] treated 70 children with intravenous therapy, converted after 3 (59%) or 5 (86%) days and continued for three weeks using temperature and C-reactive protein as parameters to response to therapy. The use of third-generation cephalosporins alone to treat OM is not recommended because they are not optimal for treating serious *S. aureus* infections. An earlier study by Vinod et al. [43] suggested that a reduced course of antibiotic therapy could be effective in the treatment of acute OM. Ecury-Goossen et al. [44] resolved clinical symptoms, microbiologic, and radiologic signs by using a short course of two weeks of intravenous antibiotics followed by 4 weeks of oral clindamycin, in selected preterm neonates with OM. The signs of continuing infection are persisting pain, fever, and rising hematologic markers that need prolonged antibiotics and repeated surgical intervention. While in children >3 months an early transition from intravenous to oral therapy (3–4 days) is suggested and a total course of 3 weeks in the treatment of acute OM, there are insufficient data on neonates to alter the current recommendation that a full course of at least 4 weeks of antibiotics be given parentally for neonatal OM due to concerns over absorption and efficacy of oral antibiotics [5]. Intraarticular administration of antibiotic is unnecessary. Some authors reported about successful treatment of newborns with oral dicloxacillin [45–47] fluclocacillin, fusidic acid and penicillin V for an additional period ranging from 14 to 42 days after an initial course of intravenous therapy. Despite everything, large, randomized controlled trials are needed to clarify the best practice in treating acute OM in children. It is important underline that OM and septic arthritis have a potential for life-long disability if treated insufficiently. Vertebral OM of the upper cervical spine requiring surgical treatment in children is rare. Glotzbecker et al. [48] described a surgery of stabilization of the upper cervical spine due to progressive instability caused by OM.

8. Consultations

The involvement of a multidisciplinary team of pediatricians, orthopaedists, and infectious disease specialists is helpful in the management of OM and results in a more efficient diagnostic workup, and improved adherence to recommendations. An orthopedic and an intervention radiologist would be very helpful in determining the surgery for diagnosis and treatment and to obtain a bone biopsy under fluoroscopic guidance. The involvement of physiotherapists allows individualized rehabilitation programs, designed to improve the anatomical and functional characteristics of the affected bones. A prompt approach to obtaining tissue and blood specimens for the culture led to a higher rate of organism identification. Additionally a multidisciplinary team led to a shorter total length of hospital stay and a lower hospital readmission rate [3].

9. Prognosis and outcome

Considerable morbidity may be associated with neonatal OM. Joint effusion may lead to subluxation or dislocation of the affected joint, accumulation of inflammatory exudate within the joint causes vascular compression and may result in avascular necrosis of the affected epiphysis. Vein thrombosis and fractures are recently reported. Osteomyelitis may become responsible for permanent sequelae in 6–50% like joint disabilities, change in bone growth due to the damage of the cartilaginous growth plate, limb length discrepancies, arthritis, pathologic fractures, and rarely complete destruction of joints. Multiple risk factors are associated with bad outcomes in the long run. A delay in diagnosis and treatment can result in complications that include: damage to the growth plate with premature and/or asymmetrical closure of the growth plate; avascular necrosis of the femoral head with or without complete dissolution of the femoral head and neck; pseudoarthrosis; limb length discrepancies, angular deformities at joints; joint dislocations; joint arthrodesis; vertebra magna (with narrowing of the spinal canal); and block vertebrae. Other factors are: late in surgical drainage and appropriate antibiotic coverage, involvement of hip or shoulder, culture positivity and *S. aureus* isolation [3]. It has been documented that as many as 40% of children with septic arthritis of the hip will develop a serious complication, and a long-term follow-up is mandatory. Especially for concomitant septic arthritis and OM, the final outcome may be not evident until 9–10 years of age. Copley et al. [49] proposed criteria for discharge based on having a CRP < 2 mg/dL prior to discharge along with clinical improvement, resolution of fever, and having two sets of negative blood cultures for at least 48 h following any initial findings of bacteremia. Given the reported peripheral inserted central catheter complications (adverse drug reaction, a return emergency department visit or rehospitalization for adverse outcome), it should be considered the practice of oral antibiotic therapy instead of prolonged intravenous antibiotics after hospital discharge [50].

10. Conclusions

Acute OM, although rare in neonates, is a condition associated with morbidity and possible functional sequelae that need a prompt diagnosis and treatment. The implementation of evidence-based, clinical practice guidelines, a lower rate of initial bone scans, a faster change to oral antibiotics, a lower rate of presumptive drainage, and a shorter length of hospital stay are challenging objectives [51].

Author details

Lidia Decembrino[1*], Nunzia Decembrino[2] and Mauro Stronati[1]

*Address all correspondence to: l.decembrino@smatteo.pv.it

1 Neonatal Intensive Care Unit, Fondazione IRCCS Policlinico San Matteo, Pavia, Italy

2 Pediatric Oncohaematologic Unit, Fondazione IRCCS Policlinico San Matteo, Pavia, Italy

References

[1] Riise ØR, Kirkhus E, Handeland KS, et al. Childhood osteomyelitis-incidence and differentiation from other acute onset musculoskeletal features in a population-based study. BMC Pediatrics. 2008;**8**:45-54

[2] Goldmann DA, Durbin WA Jr, Freeman J. Nosocomial infections in a neonatal intensive care unit. Journal of Infectious Disease. 1981;**144**(5):449-459

[3] Berberian G, Firpo V, Soto A, Lopez Mañan J, Torroija C, Castro G, Polanuer P, Espinola C, Piñeiro JL, Rosanova MT. Osteoarthritis in the neonate: Risk factors and outcome. Brazilian Journal of Infectious Disease. 2010;**14**(4):413-418

[4] Frederiksen B, Christiansen P, Knudsen FU. Acute osteomyelitis and septic arthritis in the neonate, risk factors and outcome. European Journal of Pediatrics. 1993;**152**(7):577-580

[5] Ish-Horowicz MR, McIntyre P, Nade S. Bone and joint infections caused by multiply resistant *Staphylococcus aureus* in a neonatal intensive care unit. Pediatrics Infectious Disease Journal. 1992;**11**(2):82-87

[6] Fox L, Sprunt K. Neonatal osteomyelitis. Pediatrics. 1978;**62**(4):535-542

[7] Dessì A, Crisafulli M, Accossu S, Setzu V, Fanos V. Osteo-articular infections in newborns: Diagnosis and treatment. Journal of Chemotherapy. 2008;**20**(5):542-550

[8] John SK, Payyanur Thotan S, Kumar V, Prabhu S. Neonatal osteomyelitis of the first rib causing lung abscess. BMJ Case Reports. 2016;2016

[9] Offiah AC. Acute osteomyelitis, septic arthritis and discitis: Differences between neonates and older children. European Journal of Radiology. 2006;**60**(2):221-232

[10] Ono S, Fujimoto H, Kawamoto Y. A rare full-term newborn case of rib osteomyelitis with suspected preceding fracture. AJP Reports. 2016;**6**(1):104-107

[11] Sayed S, Prabhu S, Thomas M, McBride CA, Alphonso N. Primary sternal osteomyelitis with extensive mediastinal abscess in a neonate. Annals of Thoracic Surgery. 2015;**100**(4):85-87

[12] Weichert S, Sharland M, Clarke NM, Faust SN. Acute haematogenous osteomyelitis in children: Is there any evidence for how long we should treat? Current Opinion Infectious Disease. 2008;**21**:258-262

[13] Somford MP, Huibers MHW, Schuppen J, Struijs PAA, van Lee R. Multifocal osteomyelitis in a neonate, an overview of diagnosis and treatment. Journal of Orthopedic Research and Physiotherapy. 2015;**1**(3)

[14] Vale B, Morais S, Resende C, Taborda A. Neonatal meningitis associated with osteomyelitis and epidural empyema. BMJ Case Reports. 2013. DOI: 10.1136/bcr-2013-009149

[15] Brook I. Infected neonatal cephalohematomas caused by anaerobic bacteria. Journal of Perinatal Medicine. 2005;**33**(3):255-258

[16] Staudt MD, Etarsky D, Ranger A. Infected cephalohematomas and underlying osteomyelitis: A case-based review. Child's Nervous Systems. 2016;**32**(8):1363-1369

[17] Liao SL, Lai SH, Lin TY, Chou YH, Hsu JF. Premature rupture of the membranes: A cause for neonatal osteomyelitis? American Journal of Perinatology. 2005;**22**(2):63-66

[18] Schulz U, Obladen M, Wolke S, Hauptmann K. Fetal osteomyelitis with ruptured membranes in a case of limb amputation. Pediatric and Developmental Pathology. 2009; **12**(1):77-78

[19] Ottonello G, Dessì A, Trudu ME, Porcu C, Fanos V. A case of neonatal urosepsis with multifocal osteoarthritis: Could ultrasonography change the clinical course? Iranian Journal of Radiology. 2013;**10**(3):169-171

[20] Nair S, Schoeneman MJ. Septic arthritis in an infant with vesicoureteral reflux and urinary tract infection. Pediatrics. 2003;**111**(2):195-196

[21] Bergdahl S, Ekengren K, Eriksson M. Neonatal hematogenous osteomyelitis: Risk factors for long-term sequelae. Journal of Pediatric Orthopaedics. 1985;**5**(5):564-568

[22] Berkowitz T, Young D. An infant not moving her leg. The American Journal of Emergency Medicine. 2016;**34**(4):756.e1-756.e12

[23] Dierig A, Ritz N, Tacke U, Heininger U. Group A streptococcal suppurative arthritis and osteomyelitis of the shoulder with brachial plexus palsy in a newborn. Pediatric Infectious Disease Journal. 2016;**35**(10):1151-1153

[24] Asmar BI. Osteomyelitis in the neonate. Infectious Disease Clinics of North America. 1992;**6**(1):117-132

[25] Street M, Puna R, Huang M, Crawford H. Pediatric acute hematogenous osteomyelitis. Journal of Pediatric Orthopaedics. 2015;**35**:634-639

[26] Pan N, Herzogc R, Blancob JS, Nauseefg WM, Jenkinsd S, Kovanlikayae A, Salvatoref CM, Toussif SS. *Candida albicans* osteomyelitis in an infant: A case report and literature review. Journal of Pediatric Orthopaedics B. 2013;**22**:491-497

[27] Qadir M, Ali SR, Lakhani M, Hashmi P, Amirali A. Klebsiella osteomyelitis of the right humerus involving the right shoulder joint in an infant. Journal of the Pakistan Medical Association. 2010;**60**(9):769-771

[28] Korakaki E, Aligizakis A, Manoura A, et al. Methicillin-resistant *Staphylococcus aureus* osteomyelitis and septic arthritis in neonates: Diagnosis and management. Japanese Journal of Infectious Diseases. 2007;**60**:129-131

[29] Allagui M, Bellaaj Z, Zrig M, Abid A, Koubaa M. Acute osteomyelitis of the clavicle in the newborn infant: A case report. Archives de Pédiatrie. 2014;**21**:211-213

[30] Maharajan K, Patro DK, Jagdish M, Ananthanarayanan PH, Sabhash CP, Murali P, Sreenivas T. Serum procalcitonin is a sensitive and specific marker in the diagnosis of septic arthritis and acute osteomyelitis. Journal of Orthopaedic Surgery and Research. 2013;**8**:19

[31] Shen CJ, Wu MS, Lin KH, Lin WL, Chen HC, Wu JY, Lee CC. The use of procalcitonin in the diagnosis of bone and joint infection: A systemic review and meta-analysis. European Journal of Clinical Microbiology & Infectious Diseases. 2013;**32**(6):807-814. DOI: 10.1007/s10096-012-1812-6. [Epub: 21 January 2013]

[32] Montgomery CO, Siegel E, Blasier RD, Suva LJ. Concurrent septic arthritis and osteomyelitis in children. Journal of Pediatric Orthopedics. 2013;**33**:464-467

[33] Guillerman RP. Osteomyelitis and beyond. Pediatrics Radiology. 2013;**43**(Suppl 1): S193-S203

[34] Browne LP, Guillerman RP, Orth RC, et al. Community acquired staphylococcal musculoskeletal infection in infants and young children: Necessity of contrast-enhanced MRI for the diagnosis of growth cartilage involvement. AJR: American Journal of Roentgenology. 2012;**198**:194-199

[35] Mah ET, Lequesne GW, Gent RJ, Dennis C. Ultrasound features of acute osteomyelitis in children. Journal of Bone Joint Surgery (BR). 1995;**76-B**:969-974

[36] Capitanio MA, Kirkpatrick JA. Acute roentgen observations in acute osteomyelitis. AJR: American Journal of Roentgenology. 1970;**108**:488

[37] Blickman JG, van Die CE, de Rooy JW. Current imaging concepts in pediatric osteomyelitis. European Radiology. 2004;**14**(Suppl 4):55-64

[38] Guilbert J, Meau-Petit V, De Labriolle-Vaylet C, Vu-Thien H, Renolleau S. Coagulase-negative staphylococcal osteomyelitis in preterm infants: A proposal for a diagnostic procedure. Archives de Pediatrie. 2010;**17**:1473-1476

[39] Fisher RG. Neonatal osteomyelitis. NeoReviews. 2011;**12**:374

[40] Overturf GD. Bacterial infections of the bones and joints. In: Remington JS, Klein JO, Wilson CB, Nizet V, Maldonado Y, editors. Philadelphia, PA: Elsevier/Saunders. Infectious Diseases of the Fetus and Newborn. 7th ed. Philadelphia

[41] Howard-Jones AR, Isaacs D. Systematic review of duration and choice of systemic antibiotic therapy for acute haematogenous bacterial osteomyelitis in children. Journal of Paediatrics and Child Health. 2013;**49**:760-768

[42] Jagodzinski NA, Kanwar R, Graham K, Bache CE. Prospective evaluation of a shortened regimen of treatment for acute osteomyelitis and septic arthritis in children. Journal of Pediatric Orthopedics. 2009;**29**:518-525

[43] Vinod MB, Matussek J, Curtis N, Graham HK, Carapetis JR. Duration of antibiotics in children with osteomyelitis and septic arthritis. Journal of Pediatric Child Health. 2002;**38**(4):363-367

[44] Ecury-Goossen GM, Huysman MA, Verhallen-Dantuma JCTM, Man P. Sequential intravenous-oral antibiotic therapy for neonatal osteomyelitis. The Pediatric Infectious Disease Journal. 2009;**28**(1):72-73 [Letter]

[45] Cole WG, Dalziel RE, Leitl S. Treatment of acute osteomyelitis in childhood. Journal of Bone & Joint Surgery. British Volume. 1982;**64**:218

[46] Fajardo JE, et al. Oral dicloxacillin for the treatment of neonatal osteomyelitis. American Journal of Diseases of Children. 1984;**138**:991 [Letter to the Editor]

[47] Schwards GJ, Hegyi T, Spitzer A. Sub-therapeutic dicloxacillin levels in a neonate: Possible mechanisms. Journal of Pediatrics. 1976;**89**:310

[48] Glotzbecker MP, Wasser AM, Troy MJ, Proctor M, Emans JB. Neonatal C1 to C2 osteomyelitis leading to instability and neurological decline: Novel treatment with occiput-C1-C2 fusion and occiput to thorax growing rods. A case report. Journal of Pediatric Orthopaedics. 2015;**35**(4):379-384

[49] Copley LAB, Kinsler MA, Cheen T, Shar A, Sun D, Browne R. The impact of evidence-based clinical practice guidelines applied by a multidisciplinary for the care of children with osteomyelitis. Journal of Bone & Joint Surgery. American Volume. 2013;**95**:686-693

[50] Keren R, Shah SS, Srivastava R, Rangel S, Bendel-Stenzel M, Harik N. Comparative effectiveness of intravenous vs oral antibiotics for post-discharge treatment of acute osteomyelitis in children. JAMA Pediatrics. 2015;**169**(2):120-128

[51] Kocher MS, Mandiga R, Murphy JM, Goldmann D, Harper M, Sundel R, Ecklund K, Kasser JR. A clinical practice guideline for treatment of septic arthritis in children: Efficacy in improving process of care and effect on outcome of septic arthritis of the hip. Journal of Bone & Joint Surgery. American Volume. 2003;**85**(6):994-999

2

Respiratory Care Protocols in Neonatal Intensive Care

Wissam Shalish and Guilherme Mendes Sant' Anna

Abstract

Neonatal respiratory care involves physicians with variable backgrounds treating multiple respiratory problems and populations with a number of invasive and non-invasive devices and strategies. Unfortunately, there is a lack of strong evidence to guide the most adequate management for several specific situations. Altogether, this complexity leads to significant practice variability that can affect patient and health care outcomes. Respiratory care protocols, guided by evidence and/or consensus, are an attractive solution to promote standardization of care and reduction of unnecessary practice variations. Indeed, despite the limited evidence supporting the use of respiratory protocols in neonates, a significant number of units have already developed and implemented them into clinical practice. Respiratory care protocols appear to promote evidence-based practices, discourage outdated approaches and ultimately improve patient safety.

Keywords: neonates, protocols, respiratory support, mechanical ventilation, intensive care

1. Introduction

The hallmark of neonatology relies on adequate provision of respiratory care, most commonly in the form of noninvasive respiratory support or mechanical ventilation (MV). Also, adjunctive therapies such as surfactant, caffeine, postnatal steroids and inhaled nitric oxide play important roles. In the past decade, a large number of strategies to guide respiratory care practices have been investigated in an attempt to improve neonatal short- and long-term outcomes, including length of MV, extubation failure rates, bronchopulmonary dysplasia (BPD) and neurodevelopment. Unfortunately, there is often limited or conflicting evidence to guide clinicians, leading to highly variable practices and a wide display of outcomes across neonatal intensive care units (NICUs). One way to decrease unnecessary variations in practice is through the use of clinical protocols. The objective of this chapter is to (1) describe the variability of respiratory care practices in neonatology; (2) evaluate the impact of practice variability on patient and health care outcomes; (3) review the evidence for using respiratory care protocols in neonates; and (4) provide an overview on how to develop and implement these protocols in the NICU.

2. Variability of respiratory care practices in neonatology

In the modern era of neonatology, with the introduction of many new technologies and adjunctive therapies, the provision of adequate respiratory care has become very complex and challenging. Several local, national and international surveys have been undertaken to describe how these therapies are utilized across NICUs, consistently revealing wide intra- and inter-center variability.

2.1. Respiratory care management in the delivery room

Approximately 10% of neonates require some degree of respiratory assistance after birth [1]. As an inadequate delivery of respiratory support may have serious repercussions, it is crucial for health care providers to have a solid foundation in neonatal resuscitation while staying up-to-date with recent advances in the field. A number of national and international expert consortiums regularly publish evidence-based guidelines to help providers during this critical period [1]. Despite these recommendations, surveys from around the world continue to demonstrate wide variations in many aspects of respiratory care management in the delivery room.

The most striking illustration of variability is ventilation during neonatal resuscitation. Units provide positive pressure ventilation using various methods, including the flow-inflating bag (2–63%), self-inflating bag (6–96%), T-piece/Neopuff (1–79%) and ventilator (16–49%) [2–9]. These can be delivered via face mask, binasal prongs, single nasal prong or a nasopharyngeal tube. Many institutions have more than one device at their disposal. Although positive-end-expiratory pressure (PEEP) is now commonly used during positive pressure ventilation, many centers that use the self-inflating bag do not apply it with a PEEP valve or manometer [6]. In addition, delivered peak inflation pressures vary with regard to the maximal level and duration of the inflation [5, 8]. Continuous positive airway pressure (CPAP) in the delivery room has gained popularity over the past years, particularly for the preterm population. But its use varies between 50 and 85% across countries, with units setting different gestational age thresholds (anywhere from 24–32 weeks) above which they would attempt CPAP [2, 3, 5, 9]. For those infants who get intubated, 3–45% of units have reported using CO_2 detectors [4, 6–9]. Moreover, there are variations in the preferred routes of intubation (oral vs. nasal) and types of endotracheal tubes used (straight vs. shouldered) [5].

The second most prominent source of variability in the delivery room relates to oxygenation. Despite evidence-based recommendations on the use of pulse oximetry (PO), oxygen blenders and resuscitation of term infants with room air [1], some units have not yet adopted these practices. Routine use of PO and O_2 blenders ranges from 30 to 100% and 36 to 100% across units, respectively [2, 5–10]. Although guidelines recommend preductal saturation measurements, one survey showed that only 37% of units placed their saturation probes correctly [3]. Similarly, 7–56% of units have been reported to initiate resuscitation in 100% oxygen [3, 4, 7, 10]. In the case of preterm infants, the starting concentration of oxygen varies considerably (between 21 and 100%), with some providers starting high and tapering down and others doing the contrary [8]. Oxygen is commonly titrated based on predefined oxygen saturation targets, but some units still adjust according to color and heart rate [6].

2.2. Invasive mechanical ventilation

With the rapid advent of technology, clinicians can now choose from a wide range of ventilators and modalities for invasive MV. Some surveys have reported as many as 12 different brands of ventilators for delivering conventional MV and at least 4 different types of machines for providing high-frequency oscillatory ventilation (HFOV), with many units having more than one type at their disposal [11–13]. There are currently over 10 different MV modes available, including assist control (pressure or volume controlled), intermittent mandatory ventilation (with or without synchronization, with or without pressure support), HFOV (with or without volume control), high-frequency jet ventilation and neurally adjusted ventilatory assist (NAVA). Use of all these ventilators and modalities is rarely guided by patient disease or best evidence, but rather by availability, familiarity and personal preferences [11–16].

A noticeable observation from recent surveys reveals that volume-targeted ventilation has yet to gain widespread adoption during MV, despite established evidence for its use as a lung-protective strategy [17]. There are significant geographical variations in volume-targeted ventilation use, ranging from 5 to 60% [12–14, 16, 18, 19]. With regard to the preset tidal volume (V_T), the recommended target is generally 4–7ml/kg. However, surveys have demonstrated that some units use V_T targets as low as 3–4ml/kg and as high as 10ml/kg [18, 19]. Another prospective observational study showed that as many as 18% of units used V_T levels higher than 7ml/kg [12]. These extremes of low and excessive V_T may predispose to inadequate ventilation and volutrauma, respectively.

Furthermore, tools used for monitoring and titrating MV settings are quite heterogeneous. For instance, gas exchange can be monitored using $PaCO_2$ levels in the blood, transcutaneous CO_2, end tidal CO_2 or near-infrared spectroscopy [16, 20]. There is generally no consensus on the blood gas route (venous, arterial or capillary), frequency of sampling and thresholds for titrating. Although some evidence suggests that permissive hypercapnia may be a lung-protective strategy during MV, a recent survey in the USA showed that clinicians aimed for various target PCO_2 levels, anywhere between 45 and 65 mmHg [21]. Ventilator settings are also titrated in many different ways. In one Canadian survey, PEEP could be titrated on the basis of oxygen saturation, pulse oximetry, blood gas, fraction of inspired oxygen (FiO_2) or chest x-ray findings [16]. The indications and frequency of performing chest x-rays in intubated neonates are also rarely delineated and subject to individual preferences.

There are many other aspects of MV that lend themselves to practice inconsistencies. Endotracheal tubes (ETTs) are secured using various taping methods. Infants are suctioned via the ETT at different frequencies and techniques. Practices relating to infant positioning (supine vs. prone) or the ability to do kangaroo care during MV are also nurse or clinician dependent. Most importantly, the use of sedation during MV is so controversial that it has led to very changeable practices; some clinicians always provide opiates and/or sedatives to intubated patients, while others sometimes or never use it [14, 15].

2.3. Peri-extubation practices

In order to limit complications associated with MV, infants are often extubated as early as possible. The process of extubation is quite complex and consists of three important steps: weaning from MV, assessment of extubation readiness and provision of post-extubation respiratory support. Significant variations in practice exist for all components of this process, with decisions often being physician dependent and not always evidence based. For instance, synchronized intermittent mandatory ventilation (SIMV) appears to be the most commonly used weaning mode across surveys [13, 14, 16], despite the evidence that assist control ventilation confers more homogeneous V_T and faster weaning when compared to SIMV [22]. Furthermore, in a recent international survey focused on extremely preterm infants, extubation readiness was primarily assessed based on the subjective interpretation of ventilator settings, blood gases and overall clinical stability [23]. In addition, 16% of infants were extubated infants on the basis of passing a spontaneous breathing trial, although the trial was often conducted in variable ways. The timing of extubation was extremely variable, with some units removing the ETT immediately after surfactant administration while others only after 2 weeks of MV. Finally, 10% of the centers still reported extubating extremely preterm infants to low-flow nasal cannula, oxyhood or no respiratory support despite the undisputed evidence favoring the use of noninvasive ventilation in this population [24].

2.4. Noninvasive ventilation

Continuous positive airway pressure—Since its discovery in the late 1970s, CPAP has been extensively studied in neonates. Consequently, it is by far the most widely used noninvasive mode across the world. Although CPAP has been well established and widely adopted for the treatment of apnea of prematurity and following extubation of preterm infants, its use as a primary therapy for respiratory distress syndrome (RDS) has only recently gained attraction. A recent study comparing epidemiological data from the Vermont Oxford and Italian Neonatal Networks revealed significantly high coefficients of variation in the use of CPAP as a primary therapy, ranging from 0 to 80% [25]. To provide CPAP, a variety of devices (ventilator, infant flow SiPAP or bubble) and interfaces (nasal prongs, nasal mask, nasopharyngeal tubes, nasal cannula) are used [11, 26]. There is no clear consensus on the level of CPAP to be applied as well as on how to wean and discontinue CPAP therapy. For instance, cycling off CPAP and transitioning from CPAP to high-flow nasal cannula (HFNC) therapy are common non-evidence-based practices.

Nasal intermittent positive pressure ventilation (NIPPV) —This has also gained popularity, with rates of use varying from 18 to 88% in different parts of the world [25–28]. It is most commonly applied as a rescue mode for infants who fail CPAP, to prevent intubation in infants with RDS or immediately after extubation. This variability in usage mainly stems from conflicting evidence on its effectiveness as well as limited understanding of its mechanisms of action, clinical indications and optimal means of delivering the pressures. Similar to CPAP, units may have at their disposal up to five different devices and interfaces for delivering NIPPV [26–28]. Synchronized NIPPV is still used by some units, but for the majority it is no longer commercially available [27, 28]. This is particularly important because the only studies demonstrating physiological and clinical benefits have used synchronized NIPPV [28].Furthermore, there is no consensus on what constitutes best settings (peak inflation pressure, PEEP and rate) and how to optimally wean NIPPV.

High-flow nasal cannula—Well before any clinical trials had established its safety and effectiveness, high-flow nasal cannula (HFNC) had been widely used across units. Surveys revealed that between 50 and 77% of units were using it [25, 29, 30]. The most common indication was in the immediate post-extubation period. In two surveys, 33% of extremely preterm infants (≤28 weeks) and 12% of infants with birth weight ≤1kg were extubated directly to HFNC, respectively [23, 30]. This is particularly concerning, given the lack of evidence for infants below 26 weeks and experts cautioning against its routine use in this population [31]. Another popular application for HFNC is as an alternative to CPAP or as a weaning step between CPAP and no respiratory support. However, no evidence currently exists to support any of those practices [32]. With regard to the actual delivery of HFNC, current evidence (from the literature and manufacturers) recommends using no more than 8 L of flow and a nasal cannula that allow some degree of leakage around the nares (around 50%). In spite of this, there is wide variability in HFNC delivery; one survey reported that as many as 15% use maximal flows greater than 8 L, over half of the respondents apply nasal cannula that exactly fits the nostrils and 23% apply measures to keep the mouth closed [29]. All these actions have the potential to deliver unreliable and dangerously high levels of pressure.

Other modes of noninvasive ventilation—More novel noninvasive modes have recently made their way into clinical practice despite the lack of evidence to support their use. Two such examples include noninvasive HFOV and noninvasive NAVA. A recent European survey reported that 17% were using noninvasive HFOV for diverse indications, mainly for CPAP failure or as primary therapy. There were significant variations in the types of equipment, interfaces and settings used for its delivery, with little information about its safety profile [33]. Similarly, noninvasive NAVA is increasingly applied in many NICUs across North America using evidence mainly based from animal data, retrospective clinical studies and case series [34].

2.5. Adjuvant therapies

Caffeine—A succession of animal, pharmacological and clinical evidence over the years has led to widespread caffeine use in neonates. The most influential publication of all was the large, multicenter Caffeine for Apnea of Prematurity (CAP) trial, which showed that caffeine significantly reduced incidence of bronchopulmonary dysplasia and cerebral palsy in preterm infants [35, 36]. Nonetheless, in the real world, caffeine practices continue to be highly variable and not always reflective of current evidence. For example, two recent surveys that reported 54 and 77% of units ensured that extremely preterm infants were loaded with caffeine prior to extubation [14, 23]. This is contrary to recommendations advocating for caffeine use in order to improve chances of successful extubations in preterm infants [37]. As another example, the use of prophylactic caffeine for the prevention of apnea has been heavily debated. The latest Cochrane review in 2010 [38] did not support routine use of prophylactic caffeine, but a series of recent retrospective studies have shown that early administration of caffeine (in the first 48 h of life) significantly reduced length of MV and improved short-term respiratory outcomes in preterm infants [39, 40]. As a result, the off-label use of prophylactic caffeine has risen from 22% (at the time of the CAP trial) to 60–75% [39, 41, 42]. The first dose is given anytime between days 1 to 25 of life and for a duration ranging from 2 to 119 days [42]. There are also noticeable differences in practices related to monitoring and discontinuation of caffeine. Ten percent of units still routinely measure caffeine levels [41]. The timing of caffeine cessation often depends on the unit's prespecified gestational age cutoff (anywhere from 32 weeks to greater than 35 weeks). A significant proportion of units also discontinue caffeine once the infant has become apnea-free for 5–7 days (81%), ≤4 days (11%) or ≥8 days (8%) [41].

Surfactant—The introduction of surfactant is probably one of the most important and life-saving discoveries in the history of neonatology. It improved survival and reduced important morbidities associated with MV, especially for the extremely preterm population. However, the role of surfactant in everyday practice has markedly evolved over time. Originally, surfactant was mainly recommended as prophylaxis for all extremely preterm infants and was preferably administered in the first 2 hours of life [43]. Nowadays, clinicians are trying to avoid MV all together and are therefore looking for alternative ways to administer it using less invasive routes [44]. As such, use of prophylactic surfactant varies anywhere between 0 and 90% [10, 11, 14, 25, 45]. Most units use the intubation-surfactant-extubation method, but other strategies are increasingly tried [46]. When surfactant is provided as rescue therapy, clinicians use different clinical indications (e.g., FiO_2 thresholds), number of doses and methods of administration (e.g. infant's position, rate of infusion, pressures and lung recruitment maneuvers used pre- and post-administration) [14, 45, 46].

Inhaled nitric oxide—The use of iNO for persistent pulmonary hypertension and acute hypoxic respiratory failure has been comprehensively studied in late preterm and term infants. In spite of this, there exists wide practice variations related to iNO administration in this population. Clinicians assess illness severity in a variety of ways (e.g., oxygenation index, pre-post ductal saturation difference, O_2 requirements and echocardiographic findings) and have different thresholds or indications to start iNO and use variable starting doses (5–20 ppm) and maximal doses (20–40 ppm) [47, 48]. Moreover, there is no standard approach for monitoring and weaning iNO (blood gases, oxygenation index, oxygen saturation and/or O_2 needs), especially in patients who are non-responders to the therapy. The most striking observation of all is the rising off-label use of iNO in preterm infants less than 34 weeks gestation, despite firm position statements and consensus guidelines recommending against it. In fact, a number of surveys and large epidemiological studies have documented wide regional and inter-hospital variations in iNO use, indications, age of initiation, dosage and duration of therapy for this group [48–50]. This raises great concern, especially when iNO is associated with staggering health costs and has not been demonstrated to improve short- or long-term outcomes in this population, with potential to cause harm in the subset of extremely preterm infants less than 1000 g [51].

3. The impact of respiratory care practice variability

For the many reasons explained in the first session of this chapter, variability in respiratory care practices is extremely prevalent. The NICU is a fast-paced environment where decisions are often made on the go and clinicians do not always have the time or sufficient knowledge to make the most informed decisions. In addition, units are often restrained in their ability to adopt a certain practice by its cost, ease of use or resource requirements (space, personnel, etc.). Most importantly though, despite the abundant existing literature, the evidence to justify most respiratory care practices is often limited or conflicting, leading clinicians to interpret study results in various ways, or shape their practices according to different background experiences and personal beliefs.

There are many implications of practice variability on patient outcomes (**Box 1**). In cases where high-grade evidence exists to guide respiratory care practices, it is easy to perceive how deviations (e.g., evidence-based therapies are introduced too late, too soon or are misused for certain populations and conditions) can negatively affect patients. But, even in cases where the evidence is unclear, the mere presence of variability has been linked to marked differences in pulmonary morbidities across NICUs. For example, rates of extubation failure range from 20 to 70% in preterm infants [52, 53]; this means that units with low extubation failure rates may perhaps be exposing infants to prolonged periods of MV while units with high failure rates may be disconnecting infants from the ventilator too soon. Both prolonged MV and the need for reintubation have been associated with serious, preventable morbidities [54, 55]. In a similar way, rates of unplanned extubation vary between 1 and 80% depending on unit MV practices and ETT fixation methods [56]. These accidental extubations also expose infants to unnecessary complications, including hemodynamic instability, need for reintubation and prolonged MV [56]. Moreover, several benchmarking studies have demonstrated important variations in the incidence of BPD across centers, which persist even after adjusting for variables known to affect this outcome [57, 58]. Authors of these studies have suggested that differences in clinical practice may actually be affecting this clustering effect. Similar observations have been made for non-respiratory related outcomes, including survival and neonatal sepsis [59–61].

Box 1.
Impact of respiratory care practice variability.

On patients

- Potential for using non-evidence-based practices

- Potential for increased errors and morbidities

- Unpredictable management

- Lack of continuity

- Parental distress

In workplace

- Increased costs

- Increased resources

- Confusion of health care team

- Inconsistent learning environment for trainees

- Reduced potential for quality control initiatives

Practice variability has potentially negative consequences that go even beyond patient outcomes (**Box 1**). It is not uncommon for a single patient to be exposed to several ventilation modes or therapies throughout hospitalization, or for a family to receive conflicting opinions regarding their child's respiratory management. This could be a great source of anxiety for the parents and may weaken their alliance with the health care team. Besides, this could create a lot of confusion among nurses, respiratory therapists and trainees, leading to lesser opportunities for productive teaching or learning. Finally, with little continuity or predictability of management, it becomes quasi impossible to effectively audit respiratory care practices or perform any quality control studies in the unit.

4. The role of respiratory care protocols in neonates

One way of harmonizing practices is through the use of respiratory care protocols. Protocols are a set of guidelines or rules to follow for a prespecified population with a prespecified condition. They have been extensively studied in critically ill adult and pediatric patients, namely for sepsis, sedation, hyperglycemia and MV. In these patients, MV protocols have consistently been demonstrated to improve outcomes by reducing costs, decreasing MV duration and shortening length of stay [62, 63]. They also have been shown to reduce rates of extubation failure as well as unplanned extubations [64, 65]. As such, MV protocols have been considered standard of care and have been developed and implemented by over two-thirds of adult ICUs [66, 67].

In contrast, the evidence for using respiratory care protocols in neonates is still limited. Studies are small, single center and retrospective or observational in nature. In one Canadian study, the implementation of a respiratory therapist-driven MV protocol for premature infants with birth weight <1250 g resulted in earlier extubation, greater number of successful extubations and shorter duration of MV [68]. In another study, the implementation of a standardized SBT protocol for extubation of extremely preterm infants resulted in faster weaning times with no impact on extubation failure rates [69]. In a further study, the implementation of a nurse-driven comfort protocol in ventilated preterm infants significantly reduced the amount of morphine used which translated in fewer days on MV and a shorter course of hospitalization [70]. Lastly, the use of a standardized surfactant protocol allowed clinicians to audit their practice and identify strategies to reduce adverse events associated with surfactant administration [71]. The results of this quality control initiative led to later modifications of the surfactant protocol, which has recently been published [72].

Despite the lack of strong evidence, it is interesting to observe that many units have already developed and implemented respiratory care protocols. In a recent Canadian survey, we showed that 38% of NICUs had at least one MV protocol, while 29% had a protocol for NIV [16]. In another international survey, 36% of units reported having a guideline or written protocol for ventilator weaning [23]. Protocols for CPAP and NIPPV are available in approximately 20% of units [16, 27, 28], while guidelines for HFNC are present in 25–50% of units [16, 29, 30].

The most striking trend is the increasing use of iNO protocols in practice. With the rising costs of iNO treatment, there have been many incentives from clinical managers and hospital administrators to audit iNO practices within their respective units. As a result, it is no surprise that almost two-thirds of units have developed and implemented iNO protocols [16]. To our knowledge, there have been no studies directly evaluating the impact of implementing iNO protocols in neonates, but there is some evidence from the pediatric literature that iNO protocols reduce practice variability, decrease iNO usage and thus lower costs without affecting mortality [73, 74]. As such, several local, national and international committees have published evidence-based guidelines to assist NICUs in developing their own institutional protocol.

Finally, there is a rising body of evidence recommending the development and implementation of clinical protocols for other specific neonatal practices or conditions. Some of these include pain control, sedation, feeding and delivery room management of extremely preterm infants (i.e., the golden hour) [75–77]. But the area in which protocols have been most well studied remains the respiratory management of neonates with congenital diaphragmatic hernia (CDH). In this population, implementation of a standardized, evidence-based protocol for respiratory care (e.g., using gentle ventilatory approaches, and permissive hypercapnia) has reliably led to lesser practice variations, improved survival and decreased morbidities [78–80].

5. Development and implementation of respiratory care protocols in the NICU

From the above sections, there is no doubt that respiratory care protocols confer many benefits. But, under some circumstances, they may also have some disadvantages (**Box 2**). Developing and implementing a respiratory care protocol is not an easy task. It requires mobilization of many collaborators, careful scrutiny of a large body of evidence and ongoing monitoring to ensure adequate application of the protocol in practice. This section will outline the key principles for effectively developing and implementing respiratory care protocols in clinical practice (also summarized in **Box 3**).

Box 2.

Pros and cons of respiratory care protocols.

Pros

- Reduces unnecessary variability in care
- Quick adoption of new information at the bedside
- Educational aids for trainees and allied health care team
- Improves communication
- Decreases costs
- Decreases errors
- Improves patient safety

Cons

- Inappropriately used for certain patients or conditions
- Oversimplified or too prescriptive
- Designed around low-quality evidence
- Potential loss of individualization of care
- Potential to be outdated if not kept current

Box 3.

General principles for effectively developing and implementing respiratory care protocols.

Preconception

- Obtain support from all team members

- Form a multidisciplinary working group

- Take into account that developing and implementing protocols require ample time, organization and resources

Development

- Easy to use

- Patient and disease specific

- Not too prescriptive

- Does not replace clinical judgment

Implementation

- Readily available

- Regular educational sessions

- Regular monitoring of adherence and compliance

- Periodical revision to accommodate for new evidence or clinical practice patterns

---

5.1. Preconception

Well before any protocol is drafted, it is important to take the time to get buy-in from all members of the team who will eventually be using the protocol. This includes nurses, nurse practitioners, respiratory therapists, neonatologists and their respective professional leadership. Many providers are often unaware of the negative impacts of variability on health care outcomes. Others may feel skeptical about the benefits of protocols, potentially fearing that it will take away from their ability to individualize patient care. Thus, it is of utmost importance to provide a clear rationale for using a certain protocol in the unit. Showing unit-specific data that highlight practice variations and compare outcomes with other centers may be a useful step to further justify the need for a protocol. Thus, by involving all stakeholders as early as the preconception phase, all team members will feel included and invested in the realization of the project. This will further aid in improving later rates of adherence and compliance to the protocol.

Once buy-in is obtained, the next crucial step is to create a working group that will be in charge of preparing the protocol. A member from each discipline involved in providing respiratory care (e.g., neonatologist, respiratory therapist, nurse, pharmacist and respirologist) should be encouraged to participate in this group. By using such approach, all key disciplines are represented and given the opportunity to share their perspectives. This multidisciplinary endeavor should lead to a stronger, more comprehensive and especially more inclusive protocol.

5.2. Preparation of the protocol

The development of a sound protocol depends heavily on the accuracy of its content. If a protocol is based on outdated or low quality evidence, it may actually lead to undesirable or even harmful effects. For that reason, it is essential to perform a thorough review looking for the best available evidence in the literature. Ideally, protocols should be based on results from randomized controlled trials, systematic reviews and meta-analysis. In the absence of such high-quality evidence, other studies should be carefully scrutinized with a critical mind. Additional information should be sought out from expert opinion or from other units who already have had some experience with that specific protocol. Furthermore, epidemiological databases can be a useful resource to identify centers that have better outcomes in a certain aspect of respiratory care and collaborate with them in order to identify potentially better practices responsible for these positive outcomes.

With regard to the information contained in the protocol, it should preferably be patient specific, disease specific and easy to follow. A protocol that is too flexible or unclear may lead to variable interpretations and misuses. In contrast, a protocol that is too rigid, detailed or overly specific may become inapplicable for most patients. Thus, careful attention should be placed on developing a protocol that englobes most targeted patients but that also leaves some room for individualized decision making.

5.3. Implementation and monitoring

Once the protocol is completed and approved by the necessary regulatory authorities, a number of steps need to be undertaken in order to ensure its adequate implementation. First, the protocol needs to be made readily available to all health care providers who will use it. Different channels can be used to disseminate the protocol, including the hospital intranet, monthly newsletters, posters in the unit, printed copies at the bedside and small laminated cards for staff to carry. Second, the protocol should be formally presented at educational sessions, in-services and special rounds with the aim to raise awareness, answer people's questions and clarify their concerns.

Following implementation, an effort should be made to monitor adherence to the protocol in an ongoing manner. In the absence of monitoring, it is not uncommon for protocol compliance rates to decrease with time. Thus, it is important to regularly monitor protocol usage in the unit in order to identify any major issues and promptly correct them. Regular refresher sessions may also be useful to reinforce the protocol. Finally, it is plausible that with time, new evidence-based recommendations will be made available, and hence the protocol might become outdated. As such, protocols should be revised periodically and resubmitted for approval.

6. Conclusion

Neonatal respiratory care involves prompt lung recruitment and adequate ventilation and oxygenation during the transition period immediately after birth to management of a variety of respiratory conditions. For this, a number of different technologies and adjunctive therapies are available with lack of high-level evidence for several of them. Thus, it is not surprising that practice variability is a reality. Respiratory care protocols are an attractive tool to promote practice standardization and reduce unnecessary variations and health care-related costs. Despite the limited evidence supporting their use in neonates, a significant number of NICUs have already developed and implemented clinical protocols into practice. Overall, respiratory care protocols appear to promote evidence-based practices, discourage outdated approaches and ultimately improve patient safety.

Author details

Wissam Shalish and Guilherme Mendes Sant' Anna*

*Address all correspondence to: guilherme.santanna@mcgill.ca

Department of Pediatrics, McGill University Health Center, Montreal Children's Hospital, Montreal, Canada

References

[1] Wyckoff MH, Aziz K, Escobedo MB, et al. Part 13: Neonatal resuscitation: 2015 American Heart Association guidelines update for cardiopulmonary resuscitation and emergency cardiovascular care. *Circulation* 2015;132(18 Suppl 2):S543–60.

[2] Singh Y, Oddie S. Marked variation in delivery room management in very preterm infants. *Resuscitation* 2013;84(11):1558–61.

[3] El-Naggar W, McNamara PJ. Delivery room resuscitation of preterm infants in Canada: current practice and views of neonatologists at level III centers. *J Perinatol* 2012;32(7): 491–7.

[4] O'Donnell CP, Davis PG, Morley CJ. Use of supplementary equipment for resuscitation of newborn infants at tertiary perinatal centres in Australia and New Zealand. *Acta Paediatr* 2005;94(9):1261–5.

[5] Trevisanuto D, Satariano I, Doglioni N, et al. Delivery room management of extremely low birthweight infants shows marked geographical variations in Italy. *Acta Paediatr* 2014;103(6):605–11.

[6] Leone TA, Rich W, Finer NN. A survey of delivery room resuscitation practices in the United States. *Pediatrics* 2006;117(2):e164–75.

[7] Hosono S, Tamura M, Kunikata T, et al. Survey of delivery room resuscitation practices at tertiary perinatal centers in Japan. *Pediatr Int* 2015;57(2):258–62.

[8] Roehr CC, Grobe S, Rudiger M, et al. Delivery room management of very low birth weight infants in Germany, Austria and Switzerland – a comparison of protocols. *Eur J Med Res* 2010;15(11):493–503.

[9] Iriondo M, Thio M, Buron E, et al. A survey of neonatal resuscitation in Spain: gaps between guidelines and practice. *Acta Paediatr* 2009;98(5):786–91.

[10] Mann C, Ward C, Grubb M, et al. Marked variation in newborn resuscitation practice: a national survey in the UK. *Resuscitation* 2012;83(5):607–11.

[11] Rocha G, Saldanha J, Macedo I, et al. Respiratory support strategies for the preterm newborn – National survey 2008. *Rev Port Pneumol* 2009;15(6):1043–71.

[12] van Kaam AH, Rimensberger PC, Borensztajn D, et al. Ventilation practices in the neonatal intensive care unit: a cross-sectional study. *J Pediatr* 2010;157(5):767–71.e1-3.

[13] Sharma A, Greenough A. Survey of neonatal respiratory support strategies. *Acta Paediatr* 2007;96(8):1115–7.

[14] Dani C, Bresci C, Lista G, et al. Neonatal respiratory support strategies in the intensive care unit: an Italian survey. *Eur J Pediatr* 2013;172(3):331–6.

[15] Alander M, Peltoniemi O, Saarela T, et al. Current trends in paediatric and neonatal ventilatory care – a nationwide survey. *Acta Paediatr* 2013;102(2):123–8.

[16] Shalish W, Anna GM. The use of mechanical ventilation protocols in Canadian neonatal intensive care units. *Paediatr Child Health* 2015;20(4):e13–9.

[17] Wheeler KI, Klingenberg C, Morley CJ, et al. Volume-targeted versus pressure-limited ventilation for preterm infants: a systematic review and meta-analysis. *Neonatology* 2011;100(3):219–27.

[18] Klingenberg C, Wheeler KI, Owen LS, et al. An international survey of volume-targeted neonatal ventilation. *Arch Dis Child Fetal Neonatal Ed* 2011;96(2):F146–8.

[19] Chowdhury O, Wedderburn CJ, Lee S, et al. Respiratory support practices in infants born at term in the United Kingdom. *Eur J Pediatr* 2012;171(11):1633–8.

[20] Tan RN, Mulder EE, Lopriore E, et al. Monitoring oxygenation and gas exchange in neonatal intensive care units: current practice in the Netherlands. *Front Pediatr* 2015;3:94.

[21] Mu TS ST, Jordan CP, UyeharaCFT. Permissive hypercapnia practices among neonatologists in the United States: results of a national survey. *J Neonatal-Perinat Med* 2011;4(2):111–7.

[22] Kapasi M, Fujino Y, Kirmse M, et al. Effort and work of breathing in neonates during assisted patient-triggered ventilation. *Pediatr Crit Care Med* 2001;2(1):9–16.

[23] Al-Mandari H, Shalish W, Dempsey E, et al. International survey on periextubation practices in extremely preterm infants. *Arch Dis Child Fetal Neonatal Ed* 2015;100(5):F428–31.

[24] Davis PG, Henderson-Smart DJ. Nasal continuous positive airways pressure immediately after extubation for preventing morbidity in preterm infants. *Cochrane Database Syst Rev* 2000(3):CD000143.

[25] Gagliardi L, Tagliabue P, Bellu R, et al. Survey of neonatal respiratory support use in very preterm infants in Italy. *J Matern Fetal Neonatal Med* 2012;25(Suppl 3):1–5.

[26] Kieran EA, Walsh H, O'Donnell CP. Survey of nasal continuous positive airways pressure (NCPAP) and nasal intermittent positive pressure ventilation (NIPPV) use in Irish newborn nurseries. *Arch Dis Child Fetal Neonatal Ed* 2011;96(2):F156.

[27] Owen LS, Morley CJ, Davis PG. Neonatal nasal intermittent positive pressure ventilation: a survey of practice in England. *Arch Dis Child Fetal Neonatal Ed* 2008;93(2):F148–50.

[28] Medeiros SK, Carvalho WB, Soriano CF. Practices of use of nasal intermittent positive pressure ventilation (NIPPV) in neonatology in northeastern Brazil. *J Pediatr (Rio J)* 2012;88(1):48–53.

[29] Ojha S, Gridley E, Dorling J. Use of heated humidified high-flow nasal cannula oxygen in neonates: a UK wide survey. *Acta Paediatr* 2013;102(3):249–53.

[30] Hough JL, Shearman AD, Jardine LA, et al. Humidified high flow nasal cannulae: current practice in Australasian nurseries, a survey. *J Paediatr Child Health* 2012;48(2): 106–13.

[31] Wilkinson D, Andersen C, O'Donnell CP, et al. High flow nasal cannula for respiratory support in preterm infants. *Cochrane Database Syst Rev* 2016;2:CD006405.

[32] Farley RC, Hough JL, Jardine LA. Strategies for the discontinuation of humidified high flow nasal cannula (HHFNC) in preterm infants. *Cochrane Database Syst Rev* 2015;6:CD011079.

[33] Fischer HS, Bohlin K, Buhrer C, et al. Nasal high-frequency oscillation ventilation in neonates: a survey in five European countries. *Eur J Pediatr* 2015;174(4):465–71.

[34] Stein H, Beck J, Dunn M. Non-invasive ventilation with neurally adjusted ventilatory assist in newborns. *Semin Fetal Neonatal Med* 2016.

[35] Schmidt B, Roberts RS, Davis P, et al. Caffeine therapy for apnea of prematurity. *N Engl J Med* 2006;354(20):2112–21.

[36] Schmidt B, Roberts RS, Davis P, et al. Long-term effects of caffeine therapy for apnea of prematurity. *N Engl J Med* 2007;357(19):1893–902.

[37] Henderson-Smart DJ, Davis PG. Prophylactic methylxanthines for endotracheal extubation in preterm infants. *Cochrane Database Syst Rev* 2010(12):CD000139.

[38] Henderson-Smart DJ, De Paoli AG. Prophylactic methylxanthine for prevention of apnoea in preterm infants. *Cochrane Database Syst Rev* 2010(12):CD000432.

[39] Lodha A, Seshia M, McMillan DD, et al. Association of early caffeine administration and neonatal outcomes in very preterm neonates. *JAMA Pediatr* 2015;169(1):33–8.

[40] Dobson NR, Patel RM, Smith PB, et al. Trends in caffeine use and association between clinical outcomes and timing of therapy in very low birth weight infants. *J Pediatr* 2014;164(5):992–8.e3.

[41] Abu Jawdeh EG, O'Riordan M, Limrungsikul A, et al. Methylxanthine use for apnea of prematurity among an international cohort of neonatologists. *J Neonatal Perinatal Med* 2013;6(3):251–6.

[42] Lista G, Fabbri L, Polackova R, et al. The real-world routine use of caffeine citrate in preterm infants: a European postauthorization safety study. *Neonatology* 2016;109(3): 221–7.

[43] Bahadue FL, Soll R. Early versus delayed selective surfactant treatment for neonatal respiratory distress syndrome. *Cochrane Database Syst Rev* 2012;11:CD001456.

[44] Gopel W, Kribs A, Hartel C, et al. Less invasive surfactant administration is associated with improved pulmonary outcomes in spontaneously breathing preterm infants. *Acta Paediatr* 2015;104(3):241–6.

[45] Horbar JD, Carpenter JH, Buzas J, et al. Timing of initial surfactant treatment for infants 23 to 29 weeks' gestation: is routine practice evidence based? *Pediatrics* 2004;113(6): 1593–602.

[46] Borszewska-Kornacka MK, Kostuch M, Korbal P, et al. Strategies of using surfactant: results of the first Polish national survey of daily practice. *Dev Period Med* 2015;19(3 Pt 1):271–6.

[47] Shivananda S, Ahliwahlia L, Kluckow M, et al. Variation in the management of persistent pulmonary hypertension of the newborn: a survey of physicians in Canada, Australia, and New Zealand. *Am J Perinatol* 2012;29(7):519–26.

[48] Sasi A, Sehgal A. Use of inhaled nitric oxide in preterm infants: a regional survey of practices. *Heart Lung* 2014;43(4):347–50.

[49] Ellsworth MA, Harris MN, Carey WA, et al. Off-label use of inhaled nitric oxide after release of NIH consensus statement. *Pediatrics* 2015;135(4):643–8.

[50] Stenger MR, Slaughter JL, Kelleher K, et al. Hospital variation in nitric oxide use for premature infants. *Pediatrics* 2012;129(4):e945–51.

[51] Barrington KJ, Finer N. Inhaled nitric oxide for respiratory failure in preterm infants. *Cochrane Database Syst Rev* 2010(12):CD000509.

[52] Hermeto F, Martins BM, Ramos JR, et al. Incidence and main risk factors associated with extubation failure in newborns with birth weight < 1,250 grams. *J Pediatr (Rio J)* 2009;85(5):397–402.

[53] Berger J, Mehta P, Bucholz E, et al. Impact of early extubation and reintubation on the incidence of bronchopulmonary dysplasia in neonates. *Am J Perinatol* 2014;31(12):1063–72.

[54] Walsh MC, Morris BH, Wrage LA, et al. Extremely low birthweight neonates with protracted ventilation: mortality and 18-month neurodevelopmental outcomes. *J Pediatr* 2005;146(6):798–804.

[55] Manley BJ, Doyle LW, Owen LS, et al. Extubating extremely preterm infants: predictors of success and outcomes following failure. *J Pediatr* 2016.

[56] Silva PS, Reis ME, Aguiar VE, et al. Unplanned extubation in the neonatal ICU: a systematic review, critical appraisal, and evidence-based recommendations. *Respir Care* 2013;58(7):1237–45.

[57] Lapcharoensap W, Gage SC, Kan P, et al. Hospital variation and risk factors for bronchopulmonary dysplasia in a population-based cohort. *JAMA Pediatr* 2015;169(2):e143676.

[58] Ambalavanan N, Walsh M, Bobashev G, et al. Intercenter differences in bronchopulmonary dysplasia or death among very low birth weight infants. *Pediatrics* 2011;127(1):e106–16.

[59] Alleman BW, Bell EF, Li L, et al. Individual and center-level factors affecting mortality among extremely low birth weight infants. *Pediatrics* 2013;132(1):e175–84.

[60] Lee SK, McMillan DD, Ohlsson A, et al. Variations in practice and outcomes in the Canadian NICU network: 1996–1997. *Pediatrics* 2000;106(5):1070–9.

[61] Rysavy MA, Li L, Bell EF, et al. Between-hospital variation in treatment and outcomes in extremely preterm infants. *N Engl J Med* 2015;372(19):1801–11.

[62] Blackwood B, Burns KE, Cardwell CR, et al. Protocolized versus non-protocolized weaning for reducing the duration of mechanical ventilation in critically ill adult patients. *Cochrane Database Syst Rev* 2014;11:CD006904.

[63] Blackwood B, Murray M, Chisakuta A, et al. Protocolized versus non-protocolized weaning for reducing the duration of invasive mechanical ventilation in critically ill paediatric patients. *Cochrane Database Syst Rev* 2013;7:CD009082.

[64] Bankhead S, Chong K, Kamai S. Preventing extubation failures in a pediatric intensive care unit. *Nurs Clin North Am* 2014;49(3):321–8.

[65] Jarachovic M, Mason M, Kerber K, et al. The role of standardized protocols in unplanned extubations in a medical intensive care unit. *Am J Crit Care* 2011;20(4):304–11; quiz 12.

[66] Ellis SM, Dainty KN, Munro G, et al. Use of mechanical ventilation protocols in intensive care units: a survey of current practice. *J Crit Care* 2012;27(6):556–63.

[67] MacIntyre NR, Cook DJ, Ely EW, Jr., et al. Evidence-based guidelines for weaning and discontinuing ventilatory support: a collective task force facilitated by the American College of Chest Physicians; the American Association for Respiratory Care; and the American College of Critical Care Medicine. *Chest* 2001;120(6 Suppl):375S–95S.

[68] Hermeto F, Bottino MN, Vaillancourt K, et al. Implementation of a respiratory therapist-driven protocol for neonatal ventilation: impact on the premature population. *Pediatrics* 2009;123(5):e907–16.

[69] Kamlin CO, Davis PG, Argus B, et al. A trial of spontaneous breathing to determine the readiness for extubation in very low birth weight infants: a prospective evaluation. *Arch Dis Child Fetal Neonatal Ed* 2008;93(4):F305–6.

[70] Fleishman R, Zhou C, Gleason C, et al. Standardizing morphine use for ventilated preterm neonates with a nursing-driven comfort protocol. *J Perinatol* 2015;35(1):46–51.

[71] Tarawneh A, Kaczmarek J, Bottino MN, et al. Severe airway obstruction during surfactant administration using a standardized protocol: a prospective, observational study. *J Perinatol* 2012;32(4):270–5.

[72] Nouraeyan N, Lambrinakos-Raymond A, Leone M, et al. Surfactant administration in neonates: a review of delivery methods. *Can J Respir Ther* 2014;50(3):91–5.

[73] Simsic JM, Harrison S, Evans L, et al. Reducing variation in the use of inhaled nitric oxide. *Pediatrics* 2014;133(6):e1753–8.

[74] Todd Tzanetos DR, Housley JJ, Barr FE, et al. Implementation of an inhaled nitric oxide protocol decreases direct cost associated with its use. *Respir Care* 2015;60(5):644–50.

[75] Deindl P, Unterasinger L, Kappler G, et al. Successful implementation of a neonatal pain and sedation protocol at 2 NICUs. *Pediatrics* 2013;132(1):e211–8.

[76] Kish MZ. Improving preterm infant outcomes: implementing an evidence-based oral feeding advancement protocol in the neonatal intensive care unit. *Adv Neonatal Care* 2014;14(5):346–53.

[77] Reuter S, Messier S, Steven D. The neonatal Golden Hour – intervention to improve quality of care of the extremely low birth weight infant. *S D Med* 2014;67(10):397–403, 5.

[78] Tracy ET, Mears SE, Smith PB, et al. Protocolized approach to the management of congenital diaphragmatic hernia: benefits of reducing variability in care. *J Pediatr Surg* 2010;45(6):1343–8.

[79] Antonoff MB, Hustead VA, Groth SS, et al. Protocolized management of infants with congenital diaphragmatic hernia: effect on survival. *J Pediatr Surg* 2011;46(1):39–46.

[80] Kimura O, Furukawa T, Higuchi K, et al. Impact of our new protocol on the outcome of the neonates with congenital diaphragmatic hernia. *Pediatr Surg Int* 2013;29(4):335–9.

3

Neonatal Hypoglycemia

Adauto Dutra Moraes Barbosa,
Israel Figueiredo Júnior and
Gláucia Macedo de Lima

Abstract

Hypoglycemia is the most frequent metabolic abnormality in the newborn, but no consensus exists on what level of blood glucose is able to protect the brain and influence the child's neural development and which is the best course of management in cases labeled as hypoglycemia. Early diagnosis, urgent treatment, and prevention of future episodes of hypoglycemia are the cornerstones of management, now supported by recent advances in molecular genetics and in our understanding of the pathophysiology of neonatal hypoglycemia, particularly the pathogenesis of congenital hyperinsulinemic hypoglycemia.

Keywords: hypoglycemia, newborn, molecular mechanisms, hyperinsulinemia, actual treatment

1. Introduction

Hypoglycemia is the most frequent metabolic abnormality in the newborn, and although it is the most common biochemical disorder in this age group [30], it is still a source of clinical concern and controversy, as no consensus exists on what level of blood glucose is able to protect the brain and influence the child's neural development [6, 22, 53] and which is the best course of management in cases labeled as hypoglycemia. Early diagnosis, urgent treatment, and prevention of future episodes of hypoglycemia are the cornerstones of management, now supported by recent advances in molecular genetics [48] and in our understanding of the pathophysiology of neonatal hypoglycemia, particularly the pathogenesis of congenital hyperinsulinemic hypoglycemia [12].

Hypoglycemia occurs in 1.3–4.4 per 1000 full-term newborns and 15–55 per 1000 preterm newborns. This suggests that gestational age has enormous influence on its onset; in certain groups, adaptive mechanisms are not adequately developed, which predisposes them to increased risk of hypoglycemia. According to current evidence, the prevalence of hypoglycemia is approximately 10% in full-term neonates [45]; 6.5% in appropriate for gestational age (AGA), 8% in large for gestational age (LGA), and 15% in small for gestational age (SGA) newborns; and 15.5% in late-preterm infants [7].

2. Metabolic aspects

The maintenance of physiological concentrations of glucose in newborns plays important roles, including protecting the brain from damage caused by insufficient glucose intake and preventing the consequences of hyperosmolarity caused by high glucose concentrations. Although glucose is the preferred energy source of neurons, other sources, such as lactate and ketone bodies [23], seem to exert a neuroprotective effect. However, in hypoketotic states, such as hyperinsulinism or fatty acid oxidation disorders, ketone and lactate concentrations are not high enough to replace glucose, and the risk of a cerebral energy deficit is greater [60, 61].

It is known that, during fasting, several metabolic systems are activated to prevent hypoglycemia, which may be seen as a failure in one of these systems or as an abnormality affecting one or more of the hormones that control these systems [24].

As the brain mass of newborn infants in relation to body size is larger than that of adults, the rate of glucose utilization per kg body weight in newborns is two- to threefold than that of adults (4–6 mg/kg/min) [61].

2.1. Maternal provision of glucose to the fetus

The first half of pregnancy is characterized by marked anabolism. In early pregnancy, increased caloric intake not only supports fetal development but also facilitates fat deposition in the mother in preparation for the second half of pregnancy, a period of accelerated fetal growth in which maternal stores are mobilized to meet the needs of the fetus. To this end, increased insulin secretion also occurs in early pregnancy, as a way to store energy.

From the midpoint of pregnancy onward, high levels of circulating maternal insulin are also observed, but high levels of anti-insulin factors override this effect, ensuring the provision of nutrients to the fetus during the postprandial period. Thus, in pregnant women with preexisting diabetes, the effects of these anti-insulin factors are potentiated, causing excess provision of glucose and other energy sources to the fetus and thus triggering the abnormalities observed in infants born to diabetic mothers.

In the expectant mother, glucose is found at levels 25–30% higher than in the fetus, and it is transported to the fetus by concentration gradients and simple diffusion and through the action of transporters. In the fetus, the predominant transporter is GLUT-1, which has a high affinity for glucose and facilitates its passage through tissues [28].

Most glucose in the fetus undergoes oxidation to supply its energy needs, while another part contributes significantly to a buildup of glycogen, protein, and fat in triglyceride form. Glucose is the most important source of energy for the fetus and the major substrate for brain metabolism.

2.2. Glucose uptake in the newborn

At birth, the fetus becomes dependent on itself to obtain energy and meet the metabolic needs of its vital organs, particularly the central nervous system (CNS). Each mole of oxidized glucose provides 38 moles of adenosine triphosphate (ATP) [54].

Cerebral glucose transport takes place through a facilitated diffusion process, which is dependent on glycemia and is not regulated by insulin. Protection against hypoglycemia is coordinated by the autonomic nervous system by means of hormones that stimulate the production of glucose (through glycogenolysis and gluconeogenesis) and limit peripheral glucose utilization [54].

Glycogen is the only glucose storage medium in the body. Its deposits are found in the liver, striated muscle tissue (including cardiac muscle), kidneys, bowel, brain, and placenta.

The fetal liver contains a complete enzyme system for the synthesis and breakdown of glycogen, levels of which are low in early pregnancy but rise slowly and steadily from gestational weeks 15–20, before peaking in the third trimester. At this time, fat deposition also increases. Thus, part of the energy and substrates used for fetal growth is redirected for storage, which will play an important role in the peripartum and postpartum periods.

Hepatic glycogenolysis is the major mechanism of glucose release in the immediate neonatal period, which leads to depletion of glycogen stores. It is induced by an increase in glucagon and catecholamines and a reduction in insulin. This exhaustion of glycogen stores promotes activation of gluconeogenesis, which occurs largely as a result of free fatty acid oxidation in the liver.

Glucose homeostasis will thus depend on glucose intake; gluconeogenesis; glycogen, protein, and fat stores; and hormonal and neural factors.

Glucose produced from the breakdown of dietary lactose into galactose and glucose, for instance, is not taken up by the liver in the neonatal period; the newborn is thus dependent on hepatic gluconeogenesis to sustain glucose production.

Once glycogen stores are low, gluconeogenesis induced by glucagon, catecholamines, cortisol, and growth hormone mobilizes fat and protein substrates. Insulin, thyroid hormone, cortisol, and glucagon systematically promote induction of specific enzymes, thus adapting the neonate to the abrupt cessation of the supply glucose that was provided continuously before birth.

Upon clamping the umbilical cord, the maternal glucose supply, which was 54 mg/dL during pregnancy, ceases abruptly, and the neonate's blood glucose levels decline rapidly and precipitously—from a concentration similar to that of the mother to approximately 41 mg/dL within the first 6 h of life. Physiologically, glucose concentration decreases to approximately 30 mg/dL in the first 2 h after birth, subsequently rises, and plateaus at approximately 45 mg/dL 12 h after birth.

3. Definition

Current evidence is still unable to define a specific glucose concentration that is safe to prevent acute neurological damage or chronic, irreversible neurological injury in the neonate. Weight and gestational age, as well as the age at onset, severity, duration, and number of episodes of hypoglycemia, are all determinants of the blood glucose level most appropriate for protection of the neonatal brain [54]; thus, doubts persist as to whether any single level may represent a red flag for neurological safety.

A plasma glucose level below 30 mg/dL (1.65 mmol/L) in the first 2 h of life or below 45 mg/dL (2.5 mmol/L) after these first 2 h has been considered diagnostic of hypoglycemia [54].

Various situations can influence the appropriateness of a blood glucose level for use as a cutoff point for treatment initiation, including nutritional timing and the presence and absence of symptoms [64]. Thus, in 2011, the American Academy of Pediatrics proposed that neonatal hypoglycemia be defined as a blood glucose level of 2.5 mmol/L before routine feeding [1, 20]. Other studies suggest a limit of 2 mmol/L in asymptomatic newborns and 2.5 mmol/L in symptomatic neonates [42]. Although cutoff values below 2.6 mmol/L have been cited in various studies as defining of neonatal hypoglycemia, there is no guarantee that such a concentration is the most appropriate choice for establishing a diagnosis of this disorder and prompting initiation of treatment. An important finding reported by McKinlay et al. [34] has encouraged neonatologists to consider a glucose concentration >47 mg/dL as the level at which no impairment of appropriate neurological development was observed at age 2 years.

These proposed levels serve to provide a margin of safety until additional data are available to support a more accurate definition. However, the potential risk of neurologic sequelae has led many authors to consider blood glucose values <50 mg/dL in infants as the limit beyond which treatment should be instituted [61].

In practice, blood glucose levels below 50 mg/dL as measured by a glucometer should warrant careful monitoring, and plasma glucose levels below 45 mg/dL should prompt initiation of diagnostic measures and immediate treatment.

4. Etiology and pathogenesis

Overall, neonatal hypoglycemia is caused by one of the three main mechanisms: situations associated with hyperinsulinemia, situations associated with low or depleted glycogen stores, and situations associated with excessive glucose consumption. These mechanisms may also be compounded by the effects of certain drugs used in pregnancy.

4.1. Situations associated with hyperinsulinemia

4.1.1. Infant born to a mother with diabetes

Offspring of diabetic mothers may be abnormally large at birth (LGA), even when the mother was able to keep blood glucose within normal or near-normal range throughout pregnancy.

The risk of birth defects is two to four times higher in fetuses of pregnant women with diabetes, particularly when the disorder is poorly controlled during the period of fetal organ development (i.e., gestational weeks 6–7), and the neonatal mortality rate is fivefold than that of infants born to women without diabetes.

Intermittent maternal hyperglycemia causes fetal hyperglycemia, which, in turn, stimulates excess insulin production by the fetal pancreas. On the one hand, this increased fetal insulin synthesis stimulates excess organ growth (except of the brain and liver, which are not dependent on insulin supply for growth), thus causing fetal macrosomia. On the other hand, it is associated with a high incidence of neonatal hypoglycemia and marked lipolysis during the first few hours after birth. Hyperinsulinism and hyperglycemia may also cause fetal acidosis, which results in an increased rate of stillbirths. Although hyperinsulinemia is probably the leading cause of hypoglycemia, reduced epinephrine and glucagon responses can also be contributing factors. Levels of cortisol and growth hormone are normal [11].

Increased levels of glycated hemoglobin in fetal blood appear to precipitate tissue hypoxia, as this form of hemoglobin has high affinity for oxygen molecules.

Furthermore, chronic fetal hyperinsulinemia increases metabolic rates, thus increasing oxygen consumption and inducing relative hypoxemia; this, in turn, boosts red blood cell production, causing polycythemia and, consequently, hemolysis and neonatal hyperbilirubinemia. Severe hypoxemia can ultimately lead to fetal death.

After birth, the supply of glucose to the fetus is cut off, but hyperinsulinemia persists, speeding both exogenous glucose utilization and endogenous glucose production; this phenomenon may last approximately 3 days, until normal insulin secretion is established. Hypoglycemia may manifest in the intervening period.

4.1.2. Large for gestational age status

LGA neonates may also develop hypoglycemia [44], through the same mechanism observed in infants born to diabetic mothers; however, in these infants, blood glucose reaches normal levels within the first few hours of life [32].

4.1.3. Congenital hyperinsulinemic hypoglycemia

Hypoglycemia associated with congenital hyperinsulinism (CHH), also known as persistent hyperinsulinemic hypoglycemia of infancy (PHHI), is the result of inappropriate insulin secretion or hyperinsulinism. In infants with this disease, hypoglycemia is triggered by fasting and is always accompanied by an increase in plasma insulin concentrations, which are usually inappropriately high for the concomitant low blood glucose concentration. The disease appears to be more closely related to an increase in global endocrine functional activity of the pancreas rather than an increase in the number of pancreatic beta cells.

CHH is an important etiology that should be considered in cases of persistent and difficult-to-control hypoglycemia. It is a medical emergency that requires precise etiological diagnosis and represents a serious therapeutic challenge. The term PHHI was first proposed by Glaser in 1989 [19] and has since come to replace the now-outdated terms nesidioblastosis and islet-cell dysmaturity syndrome to describe pancreatic abnormalities associated with hypoglycemia and hyperinsulinism.

Most cases of CHH are sporadic (1:40,000–50,000 live births), but a higher prevalence has been described in communities with a high degree of consanguinity. This familial form associated with inbreeding may occur in up to 1:2500 live births. Thus, an autosomal recessive inheritance pattern has been posited to explain it. There is no evidence of sex predominance, and the maternal history is generally negative; however, a careful history may reveal prior neonatal deaths or unexplained seizures or mental retardation in other siblings.

Patients with CHH are mostly LGA, as a consequence of hyperinsulinism, but without significant hepatomegaly. They exhibit persistent symptoms of hypoglycemia, including hypotonia, cyanosis, apnea, and difficult-to-control seizures, as early as the neonatal period. Sudden infant death is also seen in patients with CHH. Although the condition is rare, the high frequency of brain damage and developmental delay as a result of severe, treatment-refractory hypoglycemia in these patients justifies the need for early etiologic diagnosis and immediate treatment.

Currently, the most accepted etiogenic hypothesis for the dysfunction of CHH is inappropriate insulin secretion by pancreatic beta cells. The molecular basis of congenital hyperinsulinism involves defects in key genes that regulate the complex mechanism of insulin secretion control [12]. Nine genes have been identified and classified within the potassium channelopathies (ABCC8, KCNJ11) and metabolic disorders (GLUD1, GCK, HNF4A, HNF1A, SLC16A1, UCP2, HADH) [47, 52]. Genetic defect mutations involving the ABCC8/KCNJ11 genes, which encode the SUR1/Kir 6.2 components of the ATP-sensitive potassium channels (K_{ATP}) in pancreatic beta cells, are the most common [13, 27]. In normal cells, the K_{ATP} channels remain open or closed in response to variation in blood glucose levels, which leads to changes in the action potential of the cell membrane. An increase in blood glucose raises the rate of glucose metabolism in beta cells, resulting in increased adenosine triphosphate (ATP) and decreased adenosine diphosphate (ADP) within the cell, triggering closure of K_{ATP} channels and subsequent depolarization of the beta-cell membrane. This change in potential opens voltage-dependent calcium channels and leads to calcium influx. The subsequent increase in the cytosolic calcium concentration stimulates exostosis of insulin secretory granules; thus, insulin is released continuously.

The potassium channel is a complex of two proteins: SUR1, a receptor with high affinity for sulfonylureas, and Kir 6.2, which forms the inner pore of the channel and maintains its alignment [39, 58, 59]. The regulatory genes of the sulfonylurea receptor and potassium channels were recently mapped to region 11p15.1 of chromosome 11. Individually; none of these proteins has the ability to act as a potassium channel. Depending on the type of mutation affecting the genes that regulate these proteins, CHH may manifest with three distinct phenotypes. The first represents the familial form, with truncation of SUR1 and the absence of K_{ATP}. These patients have the most severe form of CHH and, in most cases, respond poorly or not at all to clinical treatment. In the second type, which accounts for sporadic cases, there is loss of K_{ATP} function but partial response to clinical treatment, due to formation of new potassium ion channels. In the third type, onset is delayed and severity is mild, as these patients have functional K_{ATPs} and respond to clinical treatment.

A diagnosis of CHH is usually considered when hypoglycemia develops shortly after birth and requires glucose infusion at high rates, usually exceeding 10 mg/kg/min and occasionally up to 15–20 mg/kg/min. Typically, these infants have high blood levels of insulin, sometimes exceeding 10 μU/mL, and the insulin (μU/mL)-to-glucose (mg/dL) ratio is 1:4 or higher.

Beta-cell adenomas are characterized by marked, early onset hyperinsulinemia. These tumors require surgical removal or partial pancreatectomy. They are uncommon in the neonatal period. Definitive diagnosis can only be established through histopathology, and immunohistochemical study may be required.

4.1.3.1. Beckwith-Wiedemann syndrome

Beckwith-Wiedemann syndrome is one of the most common overgrowth disorders and can be identified in more than 75% of neonates above the 90th percentile for weight and length. It is estimated to occur in 1 in 13,700 births, but mild cases may lead to underestimation of its true frequency [31]. There is no gender predominance. The syndrome is characterized by gigantism, omphalocele, and macroglossia, a triad that occurs in over 80% of cases. Other abnormalities that occur less frequently include earlobe creases and posterior helical ear pits, microcephaly, wide fontanels, a prominent occipital protuberance, facial nevus flammeus, nonspecific cardiac defects, abdominal wall defects (umbilical hernia, diastasis recti), visceromegaly, and hyperplasia of the kidneys, pancreas, adrenal cortices, gonadal interstitial cells, and pituitary [50].

Neonatal hypoglycemia occurs in at least 50% of cases of Beckwith-Wiedemann syndrome. It is generally serious and may be associated with future mental retardation. Thus, early diagnosis is important for proper treatment of low serum glucose levels, to prevent neurological damage. It is believed that hypoglycemia in this syndrome is secondary to hyperinsulinism caused by beta-cell hyperplasia and hypertrophy, but glucagon deficiency and a reduction in somatostatin-producing delta cells have also been documented.

There is a clear evidence of genomic influence in the development of Beckwith-Wiedemann syndrome. A mutation in 11p15.5, a region that encompasses multiple gene loci, has been implicated [37].

4.1.3.2. Congenital hyperinsulinemic hypoglycemia and other syndromes

CHH has been described in other diseases and syndromes, including congenital hypothyroidism [29], Sotos syndrome [4], Costello syndrome [21], Donohue syndrome [63], and Kabuki syndrome [62].

4.2. Situations associated with low or depleted glycogen stores

Prematurity and intrauterine growth restriction are among the situations that can influence neonatal blood glucose levels [35].

4.2.1. Prematurity

As very low-birth-weight preterm infants have limited glycogen stores, gluconeogenesis is their main source of glucose production. Gluconeogenesis is induced by decreased glucose intake, as well as by high cortisol, catecholamine, and glucagon levels.

Increased neurologic morbidity is particularly common in children with severe, recurrent hypoglycemia. Experimental observations have stressed the resistance of the immature brain to damage caused by hypoglycemia. This resistance is a consequence of compensatory increase in blood flow to the brain, reduced energy needs, increased endogenous carbohydrate stores, and ability to take up and consume alternative organic substrates while saving glucose for energy production [36].

4.2.2. Intrauterine growth restriction

As a result of intrauterine growth restriction, SGA neonates may exhibit several abnormalities shortly after birth, including increased susceptibility to infections, pulmonary hemorrhage, hyperbilirubinemia, and hypoglycemia. The widely varying incidence of the latter may reflect the different etiologies of intrauterine growth restriction (e.g., poor maternal nutrition, mothers with advanced age, uteroplacental insufficiency, derangements in maternal metabolism, or fetal infection). Furthermore, polycythemia and fetal and neonatal hypoxemia, which are often seen in SGA infants, can themselves contribute to development of hypoglycemia [49].

SGA infants are most at risk of hypoglycemia. Of those who do develop it, 65% are premature and 25% are post-term. Hypoglycemia can be asymptomatic or symptomatic and is generally observed in the first 24 h of life.

The factors contributing to low blood glucose levels include inadequate hepatic glycogen stores due to the high brain-to-body-mass ratio of SGA infants, the glucose-dependent nature of cerebral oxidative metabolism, and high overall metabolic rates. Furthermore, a reduction in rates of gluconeogenesis is probably responsible for 1% of episodes of prolonged hypoglycemia in SGA infants, as these infants exhibit high concentrations of gluconeogenesis precursors (such as alanine); this suggests an inability to convert these exogenous precursors into glucose.

Hypoglycemia combined with asphyxia is more damaging to the immature brain than either condition alone.

4.3. Situations associated with increased glucose consumption

Various situations can increase glucose consumption in the neonate. These include severe birth asphyxia [9], severe respiratory distress, and sepsis.

Perinatal asphyxia may initially feature hyperglycemia secondary to cortisol and catecholamine release; this is followed by hypoglycemia secondary to depletion of hepatic glycogen stores, mobilized in response to this excess glucose consumption. The association of hypoglycemia with transient hyperinsulinism has been described [18].

The association of severe respiratory distress, from various causes, and hypoglycemia caused by increased glucose consumption has often been described.

Neonatal sepsis is defined as a clinical syndrome characterized by systemic signs of infection and bacteremia (detected by positive blood cultures) during the first month of life. It is becoming increasingly important due to the reduction of neonatal mortality among the most premature newborns and to the prolonged care of these infants in neonatal units.

Decreased glycogen stores, impaired gluconeogenesis, and increased peripheral glucose utilization appear to be the factors responsible for hypoglycemia associated with sepsis, although the usual response to sepsis observed in animal models has been an increase in the rates of glucose *turnover* and gluconeogenesis, as the result of a counter-regulatory hormonal response [33]. Blunting of this process is observed only during the final stage of illness and serves as a marker of fulminant sepsis [38].

4.4. Drugs used in pregnancy

Drugs such as beta-adrenergic agonists [57], corticosteroids, thiazide diuretics, oral antidiabetics, propranolol, labetalol [3], valproic acid [10], antidepressants (SSRIs) [40], phenytoin, and terbutaline [55], among others, can cause hypoglycemia in infants.

B. Zhu et al. (2016) [67] reported an association between metformin use by diabetic patients during pregnancy and a reduction in incidence of neonatal hypoglycemia when compared to mothers who used insulin. Metformin has proven an effective alternative for use in this patient population, although it can cross the placenta.

5. Manifestations and clinical diagnosis

In most cases, infants—even those at risk—are asymptomatic. Nevertheless, an infant who is apathetic and refusing feeds and has a feeble cry should heighten suspicion of hypoglycemia. In high-risk infants, major findings include fine tremors, acrocyanosis, seizures, and apnea; if left untreated, coma and death may follow.

After birth, neonates born to mothers with diabetes develop complications related to their hyperinsulinemic state. In the first 3 days of life, these infants may exhibit episodes of irritability, tremor, and hyperexcitability or may present with hypotonia, lethargy, and weak suckling—manifestations consistent with early development of hypoglycemia and late onset of hypocalcemia. However, one must bear in mind that these infants are sometimes asymptomatic and the absence of symptoms should not delay testing for hypoglycemia.

The presence of tachypnea in the first days of life may be a transient manifestation of hypoglycemia, hypothermia, polycythemia, heart failure, cerebral edema secondary to traumatic delivery (particularly in macrosomic infants), or asphyxiation. The incidence of respiratory distress syndrome is high in these infants, since hyperinsulinemia may alter fetal lung maturation, inhibiting the development of enzymes required for the synthesis of pulmonary surfactant.

6. Laboratory diagnosis

Glucometry is the method of choice for initial screening of glucose levels, due to its use and minimal blood sample required; however, levels should be confirmed through laboratory measurement in plasma, especially when the glucometer reading is very low, as this method is rather imprecise at the lower limit of detection. Several factors can affect the values obtained by glucometry, such as the expiration date of the test strip, ambient temperature and humidity in the storage environment, the presence of sugars other than glucose, metabolic acidosis, high PO_2, hyperbilirubinemia, high hematocrit, and edema, among others [25, 66]. Several devices have been tested with the aim of demonstrating that their results may be unreliable and influence the management indicated by a reading [14].

7. Diagnostic imaging

A particular vulnerability of the occipital lobe to hypoglycemia has been observed on MRI [16], with no plausible explanation. Other authors have raised the possibility that variant anatomy of the circle of Willis and occipital lobe infarct may be implicated in these cases [2].

8. Treatment

As mentioned previously, there are still no clearly set values to define hypoglycemia in the first 2 h of life. It is known that, in the healthy, full-term neonate, blood glucose levels are lowest between 30 and 60 min of life and rise thereafter to normal baseline values of 60–90 mg/dL between 90 and 180 min of life. This threshold should be considered the physiological goal or therapeutic target at which blood glucose levels should be maintained.

Although one may consider a diagnosis of hypoglycemia when plasma glucose levels are below 45 mg/dL, this is not an absolute cutoff. Depending on the etiology of hypoglycemia and, consequently, on the availability of alternative pathways for gluconeogenesis, patients may be symptomatic in the 45–60 mg/dL range, as in cases of fatty acid oxidation defects.

SGA and late-preterm infants should be fed every 2–3 h and screened before each feeding in the first 24 h. After 24 h, screening needs only be continued in those whose glucose levels remain below 50 mg/dL.

8.1. Newborns asymptomatic in the first 2 h of life

The need for treatment in these children has been called into question, as hypoglycemia may be transient and may resolve spontaneously through stimulant counter-regulatory mechanisms. In general, if the infant is asymptomatic, to start early breastfeeding without the need to draw blood for glucose measurement, formula feeding, or other special care.

However, in some newborns, this physiological process may fail, which may facilitate the development of hypoglycemia; therefore, the American Academy of Pediatrics suggests that in the first hour of life, asymptomatic at-risk infants should have a glucose check 30 min after feeding; if the blood glucose level remains below 25 mg/dL and the infant is asymptomatic, it should be fed again and blood glucose reassessed 1 h after the first check [67].

8.2. Asymptomatic high-risk newborns

Late-preterm, LGA, SGA, and intrauterine growth restriction (IUGR) infants, as well as those born to diabetic mothers, are at particular risk of hypoglycemia. However, they are often asymptomatic. Breastfeeding followed by repeated glucose measurement has been the standard of care. However, if hypoglycemia persists despite frequent feedings, continuous intravenous infusion of glucose may be indicated.

A dextrose infusion rate of 3–5 mg/kg/min may be used in infants born to diabetic mothers, both to prevent overstimulation of glucose secretion and because of the greater fat mass of these infants. A dextrose infusion rate of 4–7 mg/kg/min may be used in most full-term and late-preterm neonates. In IUGR neonates, a glucose infusion rate of 6–8 mg/kg/min is often necessary. A study in an animal model of IUGR revealed increased peripheral insulin sensitivity, which may be associated with increased glucose infusion requirements. However, some children with IUGR should be followed closely, especially preterm infants, who may develop hyperglycemia due to reduced insulin secretion and less muscle mass for glucose utilization. Continuous intravenous glucose infusion, usually preceded by an IV bolus of dextrose (200 mg/kg over 5 min), is also indicated if these newborns develop symptomatic hypoglycemia. However, the need for such massive glucose administration is hotly contested due to the risk of undesirable effects, particularly in very-low-birth-weight preterm infants. Complete or partial resolution of symptoms once glucose concentration is corrected is considered definitive proof that symptoms were caused by hypoglycemia. Nevertheless, IV dextrose infusions are not an entirely appropriate treatment; they cause discomfort to the infant, which is made worse by the need for placement of a deep IV catheter, the need for NICU admission, and physical separation of the newborn from the mother, which hinders timely initiation of breastfeeding. However, when administered safely so as to prevent these complications, IV infusion of dextrose at low concentrations can be beneficial even in asymptomatic high-risk neonates.

8.2.1. Dextrose gel

Oral administration of glucose in gel form has been considered appropriate and should be part of any protocol to prevent episodes of hypoglycemia in asymptomatic newborns [41]. Current studies have shown that oral administration of 40% dextrose gel may reduce the occurrence of neonatal hypoglycemia by up to 70% [5] and should thus be considered as the first-line treatment in these patients [65].

8.3. Symptomatic newborns

8.3.1. Glucose

Symptomatic neonates should be treated with glucose intravenously, not orally. A 200 mg/kg bolus of glucose should be administered over 1 min (10% dextrose at 2 mL/kg). This should be followed by IV infusion at 6–8 mg/kg/min. Glucose levels should be monitored after 30–60 min, with a therapeutic target of >45 mg/dL. Control measurements should be obtained every 1–2 h. Once levels are stable, they can be reassessed every 4–6 h. If values do not reach a normal range, the rate of glucose infusion is increased by 1–2 mg/kg/min every 3–4 h. In cases of hyperinsulinism, a rate of 15–30 mg/kg/min may be necessary. Oral feedings should only resume once blood glucose levels have been stable for 6 h.

High glucose concentrations (20–25%) may be necessary to maintain a rate of infusion of 15–30 mg/kg/min; concentrations above 12.5% will require a central venous catheter [56].

8.3.2. Glucocorticoids

Physiologically, glucocorticoids promote increased resistance to insulin action, reduce the secretion of insulin, and activate enzymes involved in gluconeogenesis, mobilizing amino acids for this purpose. Thus, although such effects should theoretically induce an increase in blood glucose, there is no evidence to support glucocorticoid therapy in the treatment of hypoglycemia other than that caused by primary or secondary adrenal insufficiency.

Except in cases of hypoglycemia of self-limiting etiology (e.g., infants born to diabetic mothers), blood and urine samples should be drawn at the time of hypoglycemia for investigation of possible changes in energy and hormone metabolism (lactate, free fatty acids, ketones, insulin, cortisol, growth hormone, urinary organic acids) before any specific medications are administered.

8.3.3. Glucagon

Endogenous glucagon is the counter-regulatory hormone of insulin, secreted by pancreatic beta cells. Physiologically, hypoglycemia induces glucagon secretion to raise glucose levels [43]. The administration of glucagon has proven to be quite effective in full-term and preterm neonates without hyperinsulinism. Serum sodium levels should be monitored during glucagon infusion. Hyponatremia, thrombocytopenia, and a rare paraneoplastic phenomenon, called necrolytic migratory erythema, have been associated with continuous infusion of glucagon. Hypertonic saline solution (3% sodium chloride) may be indicated to treat glucagon-associated hyponatremia.

A dose of 0.02 mg/kg/dose has been recommended [43]. A 24-h continuous infusion has been used at doses of 20–40 μg/kg/h up to a maximum of 1 mg/day. A 50% rise in blood glucose is expected in normal infants. The effect is transient. Long-acting preparations are employed in patients with glucagon deficiency and, in combination with somatostatin, in the treatment of congenital hyperinsulinism. When the expected rise in blood glucose does not occur, the diagnosis of hepatic glycogen storage disease should be suspected.

8.3.4. Diazoxide

This agent is indicated in cases of hypoglycemia associated with hyperinsulinism.

Diazoxide is a benzothiazine derivative that acts by opening ATP-sensitive potassium channels, causing inhibition of insulin secretion by pancreatic beta cells. Therefore, patients with genetic defects that affect SUR1 and Kir 6.2, the constituent proteins that form the ATP-sensitive potassium channel, may not benefit from administration of this drug. The recommended dose ranges from 10 to 15 mg/kg/day, divided in two or three oral doses, up to a maximum dose of 30 mg/kg/day. It promotes an increase in hepatic glucose production and decreases peripheral glucose utilization. Most of the drug is eliminated by glomerular filtration, and 90% of diazoxide is bound to albumin. Sodium and water retention, plasma volume expansion, edema, thrombocytopenia, anorexia, vomiting, ketoacidosis, and hyperuricemia are possible complications of the use of this drug [17].

When the drug is effective, blood glucose levels will return to normal range within 2–4 days. Any trial of diazoxide therapy should last at least 1 week before the possibility of treatment failure is considered. Onset of action occurs within 1 h of administration, and the duration of action is approximately 8 h, as long as renal function is normal.

Failure of diazoxide therapy suggests an abnormality in ATP-sensitive potassium channels. In these cases, a course of octreotide therapy, which acts further downstream on the insulin secretion pathway, is advised.

8.3.5. Octreotide

Octreotide was the first somatostatin analogue approved for clinical use, due to its more prolonged effect. This substance inhibits the secretion of glucagon, insulin, growth hormone, and thyrotropin, as well as the exocrine secretions of the bowel. Due to its ability to inhibit hormones, this drug can be used in infants with congenital hyperinsulinemic hypoglycemia [19]. A dose of 5–35 mcg/kg/day via subcutaneous injection has been recommended.

8.3.6. Sirolimus (rapamycin)

The management of diffuse hyperinsulinemic hypoglycemia, which does not respond to diazoxide, is a major therapeutic challenge. The successful use of sirolimus, both alone and as adjunctive therapy with octreotide, appears to be a potential alternative to subtotal pancreatectomy. Sirolimus is an immunosuppressant that inhibits the activation and proliferation of T lymphocytes, with effects *downstream* of the IL-2 receptor and other T-cell growth factor receptors.

In a study involving four patients with diffuse hyperinsulinemic hypoglycemia [46], therapy with sirolimus allowed discontinuation of intravenous infusions of dextrose and glucagon in all for patients and maintenance treatment with octreotide alone. At the end of the first year of life, the four patients continued to receive sirolimus and were normoglycemic, without any apparent major adverse events. Sevim Ünal et al. [63] reported the use of sirolimus in a neonate with CHH due to a KCNJ11 gene mutation who had already failed treatment with continuous infusions of glucose (14 mg/kg/min) and prednisone (2 mg/kg/day). Addition of intensive therapy with multiple medications (diazoxide, chlorothiazide, octreotide, glucagon, and nifedipine) also failed to produce an adequate response. However, before partial pancreatectomy was attempted, at age 30 days, sirolimus therapy was instituted at a dose of 0.5 mg/m^2/day.

Improvements in glycemic control were achieved, enabling progressive dosage reduction of the other drugs. At the time of publication, at age 5 months, the infant was on minimal doses of hyperglycemic agents and continued to receive twice-daily sirolimus at a dose of 0.3 $mg/m^2/day$, without any complications.

8.3.7. Exendin

Recently, exendin-(9-39), a GLP-1 receptor antagonist that raises blood glucose levels in adults, has been introduced as a possible novel therapy for management of hypoglycemia in patients with CHH. However, further studies on its effectiveness and safety are needed [8].

8.3.8. Other drugs

Growth hormone is used in cases of hypoglycemia associated with deficiency of this hormone or with hypopituitarism.

In cases of hypoglycemia due to persistent hyperinsulinemic hypoglycemia that does not respond to treatment with diazoxide, glucose, and sirolimus, partial pancreatectomy may be indicated.

9. Consequences

Recurrent or sustained hypoglycemia can cause neurological damage, mental retardation, epilepsy, and personality disorders [54]. Transient episodes of hypoglycemia are also associated with deficits in math learning around age 10 years [26].

Severe hypoglycemia can lead to impairment of cardiovascular function and is associated with high rates of neonatal mortality in very low-birth-weight infants [15].

Permanent brain damage is found in 25–50% of patients with recurrent severe symptomatic hypoglycemia under age 6 months. Furthermore, hypoxemia and ischemia may potentiate the permanent damage caused by hypoglycemia. The pathological changes described include gyral atrophy, reduced white-matter myelination, and cerebral cortical atrophy. It bears noting that the cerebral infarctions characteristic of hypoxic-ischemic processes are absent in hypoglycemia-associated brain injury [51].

10. Final considerations

Newborns with risk factors for neonatal hypoglycemia or those which, although not considered at risk, exhibit poor suckling or inadequate breast milk intake should receive follow-up monitoring and care after hospital discharge, so as to prevent possible undetected hypoglycemia.

Author details

Adauto Dutra Moraes Barbosa*, Israel Figueiredo Júnior and Gláucia Macedo de Lima

*Address all correspondence to: adutra@globo.com

Fondazione IRCCS Policlinico San Matteo, Pavia, Italy

References

[1] Adamkin DH. Postnatal glucose homeostasis in late pre-term and term infants. Pediatrics. 2011;**127**(3):575-579

[2] Alfonso I, Rerecich A. Neonatal hypoglycemia and occipital cerebral injury (letter). The Journal of Pediatrics. 2007;**151**(1):e1-2

[3] Bateman B, Patorno E, Desai RJ, et al. Late pregnancy beta-blocker exposure and risks of neonatal hypoglycemia and bradycardia. Pediatrics. 2016;**138**(3):e20160731

[4] Baujat G, Cormier-Daire V. Sotos syndrome. Orphanet Journal of Rare Diseases. 2007;**2**:36

[5] Bennett C, Fagan E, Chaharbakhshi E, Zamfirova I, Flicker J. Implementing a protocol using glucose gel to treat neonatal hypoglycemia. Nursing for Women's Health. 2016;**20**(1):64-74

[6] Brand PL. What is the normal range of blood glucose concentration in healthy term newborns? Archives of Disease in Childhood: Fetal and Neonatal Edition. 2004;**89**(4):F375

[7] Bulut C, Gürsoy T, Ovalı F. Short-term outcomes and mortality of late preterm infants. Balkan Medical Journal. 2016;**33**:198-203

[8] Calabria AC, Li C, Gallagher PR, Stanley CA, De Leon DD. GLP-1 receptor antagonist exendin-(9-39) elevates fasting blood glucose levels in congenital hyperinsulinism owing to inactivating mutations in the ATP-sensitive K^+ channel. Diabetes. 2012;**61**:2585-2591

[9] Clark W, O'Donovan D. Transient hyperinsulinism in an asphyxiated newborn infant with hypoglycemia. American Journal of Perinatology. 2001;**18**(4):175-8

[10] Çoban D, Kurtoğlu S, Akın MA, Akçakuş M, Güneş T. Neonatal episodic hypoglycemia: a finding of valproic acid withdrawal. Journal of Clinical Research in Pediatric Endocrinology. 2010;**2**(2):92-4

[11] Cowett RM, Farrag HM. Selected principles of perinatal-neonatal glucose metabolism. Seminars in Neonatology. 2004;**9**(1):37-47

[12] De Leon DD, Stanley CA. Mechanisms of disease: Advances in diagnosis and treatment of hyperinsulinism in neonates. Nature Clinical Practice. Endocrinology & Metabolism. 2007;**3**(1):57-68

[13] Del Roio Liberatore R Jr, Ramos PM, Guerra G Jr, Manna TD, Silva IN, Martinelli CE Jr. Clinical and molecular data from 61 Brazilian cases of congenital hyperinsulinemic hypoglycemia. Diabetology & Metabolic Syndrome. 2015 Feb 18;**7**:5. DOI: 10.1186/1758-5996-7-5. eCollection 2015

[14] Diaw CS, Piol N, Urfer J, Werner D, Roth-Kleiner M. Prospective evaluation of three point of care devices for glycemia measurement in a neonatal intensive care unit. Clinica Chimica Acta. 2013;**425**:104-108

[15] Fendler W, Walenciak J, Mlynarski W, Piotrowski A. Higher glycemic variability in very low birth weight newborns is associated with greater early neonatal mortality. Journal of Maternal-Fetal and Neonatal Medicine. 2012;**25**(7):1122-1126

[16] Filan PM, Inder TE, Cameron FJ, Kean MJ, Hunt RW. Neonatal hypoglycemia and occipital cerebral injury. Journal of Pediatrics. 2006;**148**:552-555

[17] Gillies DR. Complications of diazoxide in the treatment of nesidioblastosis. Archives of Disease in Childhood. 1985;**60**(5):500-501

[18] Giroux JD, Vernotte E, Gagneur A, Metz C, Collet M, De Parscau L. Transitory hyperinsulinism with hypoglycemia in asphyxia neonatorum. Archives of Pediatrics. 1997;**4**(12): 1213-1216

[19] Glaser B, Landau H, Smilovici A, Nesher R. Persistent hyperinsulinaemic hypoglycaemia of infancy: long-term treatment with the somatostatin analogue Sandostatin. Clin Endocrinol (Oxf). 1989;**31**(1):71-80

[20] Greenhill C. Paediatric endocrinology: Defining treatment thresholds for neonatal hypoglycaemia-how low is too low? Nature Reviews Endocrinology. 2015;**11**(12):687

[21] Alexander S, Ramadan D, Alkhayyat H, Al-Sharkawi I, Backer KC, El-Sabban F, et al. Costello syndrome and hyperinsulinemic hypoglycemia. American Journal of Medical Genetics. 2005;**139**(3):227-230

[22] Harding JE, Harris DL, Hegarty JE, Alsweiler JM, McKinlay CJ. An emerging evidence base for the management of neonatal hypoglycaemia. Early Human Development. 2016. DOI: http://dx.doi.org/10.1016/j.earlhumdev.2016.12

[23] Harris DL, Weston PJ, Harding JE. Lactate, rather than ketones, may provide alternative cerebral fuel in hypoglycaemic newborns. Archives of Disease in Childhood: Fetal and Neonatal Edition. 2014;**100**(2):F161-F164

[24] Hoe FM, Thornton PS, Wanner LA, Steinkrauss L, Simmons RA, Stanley CA. Clinical features and insulin regulation in infants with a syndrome of prolonged neonatal hyperinsulinism. Journal of Pediatrics. 2006;**148**(2):207-12

[25] Hussain K, Sharief N. The inaccuracy of venous and capillary blood glucose measurement using reagent strips in the newborn period and the effect of haematocrit. Early Human Development. 2000;**57**:111-121 DOI: 10.1016/S0378-3782(99)00060-2)

[26] Kaiser JR, Bai S, Gibson N, Holland G, Lin TM, Swearingen CJ et al. Association between transient newborn hypoglycemia and fourth-grade achievement test proficiency: A population-based study. JAMA Pediatrics. 2015;**169**(10):913. DOI: 10.1001/jamapediatrics.2015.1631

[27] Khoriati D, Arya VB, Flanagan SE, Ellard S, Hussain K. Prematurity, macrosomia, hyperinsulinaemic hypoglycaemia and a dominant ABCC8 gene mutation. BMJ Case Reports. 22013;**2013**:1-3 doi:10.1136/bcr-2013-008767

[28] Klepper J. Glucide metabolism disorders (excluding glycogen myopathies). Handbook of Clinical Neurology. 2013;**113**:1689-1694

[29] Kurtoglu S, Tutus A, Aydin K, Genc E, Caksen H. Persistent neonatal hypoglycemia: an unusual finding of congenital hypothyroidism. Journal of Pediatric Endocrinology and Metabolism. 1998;**11**(2):277-279

[30] Lang, T. Neonatal hypoglycemia. Clinical Biochemistry. 2014;**47**(9):718-719

[31] Le Vaillant C, Beneteau C, Chan-Leconte N, David A, Riteau AS. Beckwith-Wiedemann syndrome: What do you search in prenatal diagnosis? About 14 cases. Gynécologie Obstétrique & Fertilité. 2015;**43**(11):705-711

[32] Linder N, Lahat Y, Kogan A, Fridman E, Kouadio F, Melamed N, et al. Macrosomic newborns of non-diabetic mothers: Anthropometric measurements and neonatal complications. Archives of Disease in Childhood: Fetal and Neonatal Edition. 2014;**99**(5):F353-8

[33] Martin, Richard J, Fanaroff AA, Walsh MC. Metabolic and endocrine disorders. In Fanaroff and Martin's Neonatal-Perinatal Medicine. St. Louis. Elsevier; 2011

[34] McKinlay CJ, Alsweiler JM, Ansell JM, Anstice NS, Chase JG, Gamble GD, et al. Neonatal glycemia and neurodevelopmental outcomes at 2 years. New England Journal of Medicine. 2015;**373**(16):1507-1518

[35] Mericq V. Prematurity and insulin sensitivity. Hormone Research. 2006;**65**(Suppl 3): 131-136

[36] Mitanchez D. Ontogenesis of glucose regulation in neonate and consequences in neonatal management. Archives de Pédiatrie. 2008;**15**(1):64-74

[37] Mussa A, Russo S, De Crescenzo A, Freschi A, Calzari L, Maitz S, et al. (Epi)genotype-phenotype correlations in Beckwith-Wiedemann syndrome. European Journal of Human Genetics. 2016;**24**(2):183-190

[38] Najati N, Saboktakin L. Prevalence and underlying etiologies of neonatal hypoglycemia. Pakistan Journal of Biological Sciences. 2010;**13**(15):753-756

[39] Nestorowicz A, Glaser B, Wilson BA, Shyng SL, Nichols CG, Stanley CA, et al. Genetic heterogeneity in familial hyperinsulinism. Human Molecular Genetics.1998;**7**:1119-1128

[40] Norby U, Forsberg L, Wide K, Sjors G, Winbladh B, Kallen K. Neonatal morbidity after maternal use of antidepressant drugs during pregnancy. Pediatrics. 2016;**138**(5):e20160181

[41] Rawat M, Chandrasekharan P, Turkovich S, Barclay N, Perry K, Schroeder E, et al. Oral dextrose gel reduces the need for intravenous dextrose therapy in neonatal hypoglycemia. Biomed Hub. 2016;**1**:448511 DOI: 10.1159/000448511

[42] Rozance PJ, Hay WW Jr. Hypoglycemia in newborn infants: Features associated with adverse outcomes. Biology of the Neonate. 2006;**90**:74-86

[43] Roženkova K, Maria Guemes M, Shah P, Khalid HK. The diagnosis and management of hyperinsulinaemichypoglycaemia. Clinical Research in Pediatric Endocrinology. 2015;**7**(2):86-97

[44] Said AS, Manji KP. Risk factors and outcomes of fetal macrosomia in a tertiary centre in Tanzania: A case-control study. BMC Pregnancy Childbirth. 2016;**16**:243

[45] Samayam P, Ranganathan PK, Kotari UD, Balasundaram R. Study of asymptomatic hypoglycemia in full term exclusively breastfed neonates in first 48 hours of life. Journal of Clinical and Diagnostic Research. 2015;**9**(9):SC07-10

[46] Senniappan S, Alexandrescu S, Tatevian N, Shah P, Arya V, Flanagan S, Ellard S, Rampling D, Ashworth M, Brown RE, Hussain. Sirolimus therapy in infants with severe hyperinsulinemic hypoglycemia. The New England Journal of Medicine. 2014;**370**:1131-1137

[47] Senniappan S, Shanti B, James C,Hussain K. Hyperinsulinaemic hypoglycaemia: genetic mechanisms, diagnosis and management. Journal of Inherited Metabolic Disease. 2012;**35**:589-601

[48] Shah P, Rahman SA, Demirbilek H, Guemes M, Hussain K. Hyperinsulinaemic hypoglycaemia in children and adults. Lancet Diabetes & Endocrinology. Nov 30, 2016. pii: S2213-8587(16)30323-0. DOI: 10.1016/S2213-8587(16)30323-0

[49] Sharma et al. Intrauterine growth restriction: Antenatal and postnatal aspects. Clinical Medicine Insights: Pediatrics. 2016;**10**:67-83. DOI: 10.4137/CMPed.S40070

[50] Shuman C, Beckwith JB, Weksberg R. Beckwith-Wiedemann syndrome. In: Pagon RA, Adam MP, Ardinger HH, Wallace SE, Amemiya A, Bean LJH, et al., editors. Gene Reviews [Internet]. Seattle (WA): University of Washington, Seattle; 1993-2017

[51] Sperling M. Hypoglycaemia. In: Nelson Textbook of Pediatrics, 18th ed. Philadelphia: Saunders; 2007. pp. 655-669

[52] Stanescu DE, Hughes N, Kaplan B, Stanley CA, De León DD. Novel presentations of congenital hyperinsulinism due to mutations in the MODY genes: HNF1A and HNF4A. Journal of Clinical Endocrinology and Metabolism. 2012;**97**(10):E2026-E2030

[53] Steinkrauss L, Lipman TH, Hendell CD, Gerdes M, Thornton PS, Stanley CA. Effects of hypoglycemia on developmental outcomes in children with congenital hyperinsulinism. Journal of Pediatric Nursing. 2005;**20**(2):109-118

[54] Stomnaroska-Damcevski O, Petkovska E, Jancevska S, Danilovski D. Neonatal hypoglycemia: A continuing debate in definition and management. Pril (Makedon Akad Nauk Umet Odd Med Nauki). 2015;**36**(3):91-97

[55] Svenningsen NW, Holmquist P, Ingemarsson I. Antenatal management of terbutaline—Effects on infants born preterm. Journal of the Singapore Paediatric Society. 1985;**27**(3-4):208-214

[56] Sweet CB, Grayson S, Polak M. Management strategies for neonatal hypoglycemia. Journal of Pediatric Pharmacology and Therapeutics. 2013;**18**(3):199-208

[57] Synnes A. Screening for neonatal hypoglycemia after fetal exposure to β-blockers. Pediatrics. 2016;**138**(3):e20161691

[58] Thomas P, Ye Y, Lightner E. Mutation of the pancreatic islet inward rectifier Kir6.2 also leads to familial persistent hyperinsulinemic hypoglycemia of infancy. Human Molecular Genetics. 1996;**5**:1809-1812

[59] Thomas PM, Cote GJ, Wohllk N, Haddad B, Mathew PM, Rabl W, et al. Mutations in the sulfonylurea receptor gene in familial persistent hyperinsulinemic hypoglycemia of infancy. Science. 1995;**268**:426-9

[60] Thornton PS, Stanley CA, De Leon D, Harris DL, Haymond M, Hussain K, et al. Recommendations from the pediatric endocrine society for evaluation and management of persistent hypoglycemia in neonates, infants, and children. Journal of Pediatrics. 2015;**166**:1520-1525

[61] Thornton PS. Neonates at risk for hypoglycemia: associated neurological outcomes. Journal of Pediatrics. 2016;**170**:343-344

[62] Toda N, Ihara K, Kojima-Ishii K, Ochiai M, Ohkubo K, Kawamoto Y, et al. Hyperinsulinemic hypoglycemia in Beckwith-Wiedemann, Sotos, and Kabuki syndromes: A nationwide survey in Japan. American Journal of Medical Genetics. Part A. 2017;**173**(2):360-367

[63] Unal S, Aycan Z, Halsall DJ, Kibar AE, Eker S, Ozaydin E. Donohue syndrome in a neonate with homozygous deletion of exon 3 of the insulin receptor gene. Journal of Pediatric Endocrinology and Metabolism. 2009;**22**(7):669-674

[64] Van Haltren K, Malhotra A. Characteristics of infants admitted with hypoglycemia to a neonatal unit. Journal of Pediatric Endocrinology and Metabolism. 2013;**26**(5-6):525-529

[65] Weston PJ, Harris DL, Battin M, Brown J, Hegarty JE, Harding JE. Oral dextrose gel for the treatment of hypoglycaemia in newborn infants. Cochrane Database of Systematic Reviews. 2016;**5**:CD011027

[66] Woo HC, Tolosa L, El-Metwally D, Viscardi RM. Glucose monitoring in neonates: Need for accurate and non-invasive methods. Archives of Disease in Childhood: Fetal and Neonatal Edition. 2014;**99**:F153-F157. DOI: 10.1136/archdischild-2013-304682

[67] Zhou Y, Bai S, Bornhorst JA, Elhassan NO, Kaiser JR. The effect of early feeding on initial glucose concentrations in term newborns. J Pediatr. 2017; **181**:112-115 doi: 10.1016/j.jpeds.2016.10.032

4

Neonatal Care in the First Hour of Life

Teja Škodič Zakšek, Anita Jug Došler,
Ana Polona Mivšek and Petra Petročnik

Abstract

The very first hour in a baby's life can have a significant—lifelong—impact on the health of the baby and on the bond between the mother and a baby. Keeping mothers and babies together is a safe and healthy birth practice. Childbirth and the first hour after birth is a time of many changes for both mother and child. Changes are also physiological, as well as psychological. Creating an optimal environment for birth boosts the right hormones for natural birth, which reduces the need for interventions that could cause early mother-baby separation. One of the major challenges in the birth hospital is how best to combine a midwifery care and those medical procedures that are not necessary, to right form the birth as a family intimate and privacy event, if, of course, the child and maternal health would allow this. The first hour after birth is a once-in-a-lifetime occasion for both the baby and the parents, a unique experience, and once lost, it can never be relived.

Keywords: newborn, transition, golden hour, breastfeeding, skin-to-skin contact

1. Introduction

The transition to extrauterine life is a remarkable physiological event that involves a series of modifications that depend on the degree of maturation in late gestation, the process of delivery itself and establishment of independent physiological processes for regulating homeostasis after placenta lost its function. These processes are establishment for respiration, change from parallel to serial circulation, oral feeding, thermoregulation and glucose homeostasis [1]. Respiratory and cardiovascular changes occur simultaneously and are mutually dependent. The triggers of initial first breath are complex and not fully understood yet. Many factors play role in the initiation of breathing, and some of them derive already during the birthing process [2].

We must admit that these are great and demanding changes that need to occur in a short period. However, it is not the purpose of this chapter to describe the processes that occur in the body of the newborn. The main purpose is to remind the readers how to support these natural processes and not disturb them with unnecessary interventions.

When we speak of mature healthy newborn, midwives have to be alert to observe possible complications; however, the newborn in this case does not need any special interventions. On the contrary, the most precious ingredient for the baby in this immediate postpartum period is time. Midwife has to permit natural processes to occur spontaneously and not force them.

The smooth physiological transition can be promoted already by enabling natural processes of the first and second stages of labor; however, we can claim that physiological third stage is even more directly connected to the newborn. Expectant (physiological) third stage of labor is connected to many advantages; because of the delayed cord clamping, baby gets more red blood cells and hematopoietic stem cells and 30% of additional blood volume that is important for respiratory function. At birth, this blood moves into the infant's lung; the cardiac output to the lung changes from 8–10% in utero to 45% in the immediate newborn period and demands an increased blood volume. An adequate red cell volume is necessary for oxygen delivery and consequently effective tissue functioning, normal pH and circulator integrity.

Right after the birth, remarkable changes in respiration and circulation are occurring in the newborn body. Therefore, midwife has to give the baby time for these adjustments. First minute after the birth of the baby, midwife has to observe and wait, and not overstimulate the baby and manipulate with him/her in order to provide the preconditions for these major and dramatical physiological changes. The decision for procedures of stabilization are suggested to be done after the 1st minute Apgar estimation.

When there is no need for resuscitation, the best place for the baby is by her mother. Separating mother and baby can have harmful effect on breastfeeding and their relationship [3]. Skin-to-skin prevents heat loss. Ludington-Hoe et al. [4] confirmed that mother and baby can synchronize body temperatures, when skin-to-skin is practiced; the energy saved can be used to stabilize heart and respiration rates. With kangaroo method also the initiation of breastfeeding is eased. Evidence suggests that the baby, when undisturbed, usually takes about 45–55 min to find the way to its mother's breast, using the primal reflexes [5]. With the birth environment that provides warmth, safety and intimacy, the baby is able to make essential physiological adaptations. Midwives need to follow these physiological transitional processes.

World Health Organization and United Nations Children's Fund [6] say that all mothers and babies should be kept together after the birth and should be encouraged to practice skin-to-skin in the first hour after delivery, even if mothers do not intend to breastfeed. This opportunity should be offered to all, also mothers and babies after cesarean section or vacuum extraction.

World Health Organization and United Nations Children's Fund [6] recommended that all healthy mothers and babies, regardless of feeding preference and method of birth, have uninterrupted skin-to-skin care beginning immediately after birth for at least an hour, and until after the first feeding. All other procedures of initial newborn care can wait until the end of the fourth stage of labor (3 h after the birth), when the woman and the baby are to be discharged to the postpartum ward [7]. As Gunn et al. [8, p. 765] acknowledge 'in a situation where both, mother and a child are healthy and well, any actions on the part of the midwife should be made unobtrusively and with fully informed consent of the parents.' More importance should be given to the establishment of mother-infant bond, since contact with mother and baby in the hours after the birth not only fosters attachment, but at the same time fosters child's development [8].

2. Keeping mothers and babies together beyond the moment of birth

The first hour after birth, it is extremely sensitive and important for the stabilization of vital functions (breathing, saturation, blood pressure, thermoregulation, blood sugar stability, the newborn must establish pulmonary and cardiac function, etc.) in both mother and child, as well as the process of attachment between them and father. That is why the first hour after birth some call the golden hour [9].

Family bonding and baby's first breastfeed is very important act after delivery. If mother or baby needs some help or medical advice during first breastfeed, then medical staff should help them at this essential time of birth, for both vaginal and cesarean births. If the mother has general anesthesia, we can put a newborn immediately after birth on father's chest. This increases the effectiveness of breastfeeding, the process of attachment between mother and child, and reduces stress in their child [10].

At the moment of birth time, a mother needs a quiet, dim lighting, warmth and calm environment. She is still in labor. Her uterus needs to contract down. With smooth first hour after birth and mother's skin-to-skin contact to a newborn, we allow the newborn to pass through nine instinctive phases in their behavior. These phases are innate and naturally given to every newborn (**Table 1**).

Phase	Naming	Baby's instinctive behaviors—explanation
1	Crying during the birth	Because of lungs expansion, baby starts crying
2	Relaxation	Baby shows relasxed hands without mouth movements
3	Awakening	Baby shows some movements with hands, heads and shoulders
4	Baby' activity	Baby shows mouthing, suckling and way of movements
5	Baby's rest	Phase without baby's activities
6	Baby's crawling	Baby's recognizing the breast and nipple
7	Recognizing with familiarization	Baby familiarizes the nipple and breast. He also licks, touches and massages it
8	Sucking nipples	Baby is attached and is sucking the nipples
9	Baby's sleeping	Baby's restful sleep

Table 1. Baby's instinctive behaviors during bonding and 'skin-to-skin care' after delivery.

The first stage is the birth cry. This distinctive cry occurs immediately after birth as the baby's lungs expand. The second stage is the relaxation stage. During the relaxation stage, the newborn exhibits no mouth movements and the hands are relaxed. This stage usually begins when the birth cry has stopped. The baby is skin-to-skin with the mother and covered with a warm, dry towel or blanket. The third stage is the awakening stage. During this stage, the newborn exhibits small thrusts of movement in the head and shoulders. This stage usually begins about a few minutes after birth. The newborn in the awakening stage may exhibit head movements, open his eyes, show some mouth activity and might move his shoulders. The fourth stage is the activity stage. The newborn begins to make increased mouthing and sucking movements as the rooting reflex becomes more obvious. This stage usually begins about 8 min after birth. At any stage of the phase, the baby may rest. He may have periods of resting between periods of activity throughout the first hour or so after birth. The sixth stage is the crawling stage. The baby approaches the breast during this stage with short periods of action that result in reaching the breast and nipple. This stage usually begins about 35 min after birth. The seventh stage is called familiarization. During this stage, the newborn becomes acquainted with the mother by licking the nipple and touching and massaging her breast. This stage usually begins around 45 minutes after birth and could last for 20 minutes or more. The eighth stage is suckling. During this stage, the newborn takes the nipple, self-attaches and suckles. This early experience of learning to breastfeed usually begins about an hour after birth. It may take more time with skin-to-skin for the baby to complete the stages and begin suckling, especially for mothers who gave birth by cesarean section. The final stage is sleep. The baby and sometimes the mother fall into a restful sleep. Babies usually fall asleep about 1½–2 h after birth [11].

Continuous skin contact between newborn and mother should not affect on the work of the professional staff in the birth hospital. For example, procedures as it is control postpartum bleeding or disruption of the umbilical cord should be carried out without separation of the mother and newborn. If the birth was spontaneous and the child is not under the influences of medicines, keeping mother and newborn together beyond the moment of birth enables the child to be in a state of openness and vigilance and the most susceptible to the first impressions of the outside world. In the opinion of many eminent scientists of the child to design a basic response patterns, intimacy and sociality, which are matrix for all life [9, 12], one of the major challenges in the birth hospital is how best to combine a midwifery care and those medical procedures that are not necessary, to right form the birth as a family intimate and privacy event, if, of course, the child and maternal health would allow this [9, 11, 13]. Preventing separation except for compelling medical indications is an essential safe and healthy birth practice and an ethical responsibility of health-care professionals [14].

During the first hour after birth, many of hormones are releasing: dopamine, oxytocin, prolactin and estrogen. All these hormones initiate maternal instincts. Skin-to-skin contact allows that the mother and child are more relaxed and connected to each other. Whatever promotes the attachment between mother and child: touching, dermal contact, frequent eye contact and so on also promotes the development of a child's brain. Skin contact activates the amygdala, which is a part of the limbic system in the brain that regulates emotional learning, memory processing and detection appetite. This part of the brain is the most developed in just the first two months of a child's life. Oxytocin receptors in a woman's brain increase during pregnancy. When baby is born, mother is more responsive to this hormone that promotes maternal behavior. Oxytocin is produced in large amounts when breastfeeding and holding babies are close skin-to-skin. Initial attachment has a positive effect on the formation of self-esteem of both parents, because the parents more quickly identify the child's needs and can respond on it. From the child's perspective, the separation from his mother is life-threatening. Keeping mothers and babies together beyond the moment of birth protects the child against the negative consequences of segregation. The frequency of crying and the quantity of stress hormones are lower if child is in skin contact with his mother. In this way, the mother's body heat is also transmitted to the newborn, who is better able to regulate self body temperature and respiration [15]. Skin-to-skin contact heightens response, stimulates behaviors that help to meet the newborn's basic biological needs, activates neuroprotective mechanisms and enables early neurobehavioral self-regulation. Skin-to-skin care reduced maternal physiologic stress and depressive feelings after hospital discharge, which may help to empower women in their role as mothers [16].

3. Behavioral hormonal effects

Blackburn [17] sees hormones as a chemical messengers which either in the body fluids or in blood excert a physiological effect on other cells in other places in the body. The hormones interplay in labor and birth is often compared to an orchestra where every instrument knows exactly how to play perfect notes to create a beautiful melody. If the melody is played well, it sets the stage also in a more immediate way for the postpartum process for both the mother and her baby, because all the different hormones released by mother and fetus during the first and second stages of labor are not yet eliminated during the hour following birth.

One of such hormones is already mentioned oxytocin, which is relatively well studied in relationship to behaviors after birth [18] but still not fully understood [19]. As Phillips [18] notices, it has been shown to increase relaxation, attraction, facial recognition and maternal care-giving behaviors which are all necessary to ensure infant survival. Odent [19] recognizes that oxytocin is never released in isolation. It is always part of a complex hormonal balance in our metaphor part of an orchestra. That means that in the hour following birth, in physiological conditions, the high peak of oxytocin is associated with a high level of prolactin, which is also known as the 'motherhood hormone.' It is known to affect mothering behavior in animals. In humans, oxytocin induces a state of calm and reduces stress [20]. Love and affection between the mother and a child is enhanced, and bonding is optimal. These pleasant moments stimulate the secretion of oxytocin, and also prolactin, and skin-to-skin contact between mother and baby after delivery helps both breastfeeding and emotional bonding [6]. Odent [9] sees this as the most typical situation for inducing love of babies. Oxytocin and prolactin complement each other and are released in response to stimulation by the baby's sucking at the breast. When a baby suckles at the breast, sensory impulses pass from the nipple to the brain. In response, the anterior lobe of the pituitary gland secretes prolactin and the posterior lobe secretes oxytocin [21]. If a mother is in severe pain or emotionally upset, the oxytocin reflex may become inhibited, and her milk may suddenly stop flowing well. In animals also prolactin is responsible for mothering behaviors [18]. During the first few weeks, the more a baby suckles and stimulates the nipple, the more prolactin is produced, and the more milk is produced. This effect is particularly important at the time when lactation is becoming established, right after the birth.

Oxytocin is responsible for increasingly strong and effective contractions during the labor. And when, during the labor, levels of oxytocin rise, endorphins (sometimes called natural opiates) are released. Beta-endorphin is secreted by the pituitary gland in times of pain and stress. It activates the mesocorticolimbic dopamine reward system and produces pleasure in association with sex, birth and breastfeeding. It is known by now that after birth, both mother and a baby are saturated with natural opiates if the birth is physiological. They reinforce the mother-infant bond and contribute to ecstatic feelings for both [21]. Endorphins also help make the transition to extrauterine life easier for the baby, facilitating relaxation and calm [18].

As the baby descends during the labor, in fact close to the actual birth also catecholamines are released. Sometimes they are called 'fight or flight' hormones: epinephrine (adrenaline) and norepinephrine (noradrenaline).They are secreted from the adrenal gland above the kidney in response to stresses such as fright, anxiety, hunger or cold, as well as excitement, when they activate the sympathetic nervous system for fight or flight. During birth, when women are scared or have difficulty coping with pain, they can be overproduced and can inhibit production of oxytocin. However, normal values ensure mother is alert when baby is born; also, baby is alert, with eyes wide opened and trying to make eye contact with mother [19].

To our current knowledge, many *different hormones* can *influence* several *types of behavior*, but for the purpose of getting to know the behavioral effects of different hormones involved in the birth process, four most important ones were described. It is known by now that all the different hormones released by the mother and by the baby during labor and delivery are not eliminated immediately. By knowing that, we realize it is essential to promote best practices already in labor processes.

4. First hour and maternal attachment behaviors

Maternal attachment and bonding does not start at birth; from psychological point of view, the system has been prepared during the whole pregnancy, when mother imagines her baby and when the baby gets to know the odor, voice and smell of mother [22]. However, after the birth, she encounters him/her for the first time and therefore this time is so crucial for the establishment of the relationship between the baby and the mother/parent. The space for this intimate process must be given to the family and as Gunn et al. [8, p. 765] write: 'the midwife should never undermine the role of the mother who is transitioning into her new role.'

When left undisturbed, mothers demonstrate 'species-specific behavior' [23]. Mother explores her baby with her fingertips, then strokes the child and even then cuddles him/her into her arms, facing her. She establishes eye contact, talks to her baby and then introduces him/her to partner [8]. She progresses through three major steps:

- Her first preoccupation is the survival of the baby.
- Then, she needs to know that everything is fine with the baby.
- Once reassured that the baby is healthy, mother wants to make the baby her own. She seeks physical resemblance.

These steps are crucial for every new mother; however, this is not yet a relationship [24]; attachment is much more complex and takes more time to be established. The initial emotional connection that mother establishes with her newborn baby is called bonding [25]. It was believed that bonding is one-way relationship (from parents toward child), under the strong influence of important maternal and infant oxytocin that promotes empathy. Other neurotransmitters such as opioids and dopamine also play role in the bonding process [26–28]. It can be therefore concluded that bonding is eased when the birth process is natural and all these hormones are expressed. Within the context of the results of latest research, the experts began to question whether bonding is really a one-way relationship. Feldman et al. [29] found synchronic levels of oxytocin in infants and mothers who interacted with them. These high levels of oxytocin in baby help her/him to adapt to extrauterine life [16]. Despite the fact that babies communicate nonverbal, they respond to parents.

Also, the baby responds facially to mother's voice, especially in the case of physiological birth, right after the birth, when the baby is in a quiet alert state, aware of the surrounding and uses all his/her senses. The baby has competencies to develop ties with parents [24]. Besides voice, his/her strongest sense is scent, necessary to find the mother's breast. After the first feed, baby usually gets to sleep that can last even 6 h [30].

All these (nonverbal, mostly facial) responses of the baby evoke interaction with parents that sets grounds for developing a bond among them. They were acknowledged already by Bowlby [31]. He proposed that there is an attachment system that is biologically based and promotes survival. He claimed that infants have specific behaviors that attract proximity of the caregiver in order to survive or to be emotionally connected, so-called proximity-seeking behavior. Repetitions of such interactions by the caregiver lead to 'internal working model' or internal representation of the attachment relationship [32].

The infant, despite that he/she is not verbal yet, generates these affective, sensorimotor activities from parents. He cannot self-regulate yet, but can learn this capacity through parental care-giving behaviors and his own ability to self-regulate [32]. It is therefore of crucial importance that woman is relaxed and in touch with her own feelings.

Reid and Freer [33] wrote that maternal role develops smoothly when mothers' self-esteem in mothering abilities is enhanced. Midwife can strengthen her perception with different interventions. If they make parents aware of babies' behavioral and autonomic cues, they can be more confident in caring for their newborn, taking into account the child's individual tolerance (for habituation to noise, light, etc.) [34].

Benefits of skin-to-skin for attachment, breastfeeding and thermoregulation are well known, and new insights, however, revealed even other advantages. Colonization of the baby with the mother's microbiome occurs first during vaginal delivery, later on with her skin microbes, and during initial breastfeeding, also the newborn gut is colonized with microbes that built normal gastrointestinal flora.

5. A metabolic perspective

When newborn transits to a life outside a womb, it must adapt to many new circumstances. One is metabolic transition, which is not as dramatic as, for example, changes in cardiopulmonary systems, but equally complex and essential for survival. As Colson [35] notices cardiopulmonary, immune and thermal adaptations are well documented, but most texts fail to describe the normal physiological metabolic transition from fetus to neonate.

Just after birth, as soon as the umbilical cord ceases to pulsate, placental circulation stops. This means that the constant supply of maternal nutrition especially glucose transferred via the placenta stops. Before the birth, no significant production of glucose has been demonstrated [36]. In utero insulin is being used as a growth hormone instead of being a metabolic regulator. Colson [35] explains that the processes of lipogenesis (formation and storage of fat in the form of adipose tissue) and glycogenesis (formation and storage of glucose in the form of glycogen in the liver, cardiac muscle and brain) are replaced by the metabolic pathways of neonatal life. These are glycogenolysis (breakdown of glycogen), lipolysis (breakdown of fats), gluconeogenesis (endogenous glucose production) and ketogenesis (formation of ketone bodies).These pathways imply a metabolic switch at birth from glucose to fat and therefore a diet initially lower in carbohydrate and high in fats. It is true that while neonatal blood glucose levels immediately fall in almost all healthy infants, it must adapt to intermittent feeding, digestion and intestinal absorption of nutrients (adapted from Colson, p. 13). The fetus prepares for his transition mainly by storing glycogen, producing catecholamines and depositing brown and white fat [37]. After the birth, hepatic glycogen stores are mobilized and hepatic synthesis of glucose from noncarbohydrate substrates enuses. This substrate enters the citric acid cycle and produces adenosine triphosphate, which serves as the energy source for the brain [37]. These events actually allow baby to gradually mobilize glucose to meet energy requirements. So-called transient neonatal hypoglycemia is a process of normal adaptation to extrauterine life, and it is important that we realize that in first 3–4 h healthy newborn could have low blood glucose levels.

Colson [35] exposes several practices that stand behind understanding of the normal metabolic physiology:

1. Metabolic transition is not generally taught in midwifery and medical curricula as part of normal postnatal adaptation from fetus to neonate. Descriptions of metabolic changes are absent or sparse. When present, they are usually rooted in pathology.
2. Research has shown that patterns of metabolic adaptation are different according to whether the baby is breastfed or has artificial feeds and this is largely ignored in midwifery and pediatric assessment. Mixed feeding is common in the first three days postnatal even when the mother wants to breastfeed exclusively.

3. Furthermore, in the early postnatal days, current breastfeeding definitions disregard dose. A baby is considered to be breastfed when receiving any amount of mother's milk, however small. Not knowing whether the baby is exclusively breastfed blurs the understanding of those clinical characteristics associated with a baby who is wholly breastfed.

4. Mothers are often encouraged to swaddle their babies from birth and to keep them in the cot unless they are actively feeding. This practice assumes that the continuity of maternal nutrition ends at birth as in bottle-feeding. Immediate swaddling also accentuates the discontinuity of postnatal transition, as mothers are physically separated from their babies even when they are in the same room. The early physical separation negates the continuity and postnatal effectiveness of the maternal body to maintain a homeostatic neutral/thermal environment from fetus to neonate. Keeping babies in the cot in between feeds instead of holding them during the first three days postpartum may have a negative effect upon early nurturing and breastfeeding.

5. Maternal choice rather than physiology provides the framework that underpins midwifery assessment. When there are breastfeeding problems in the first three days postnatal, a bottle-feeding solution is often offered. For example, when the baby demands breastfed and is unsettled, it is often believed that mother's early colostral milk is insufficient. Mothers are often told that they can give the baby a bottle if they want. The irony is that maternal choice then appears to motivate supplementation. One often sees written in the notes 'baby unsettled, mother requested bottle' (Colson, p. 12).

In order to optimize metabolic adaptation, babies and mothers must be kept closely together after birth. Health workers must encourage mothers to maintain close body contact with their babies as often as they want in an undisturbed environment [38].

6. Impacts on infant microbiome assembly

The human body is colonized by a vast number of microbes, collectively referred to as the human microbiota. The average human has over 100 trillion microbes in and on their body, and many of the latest discoveries are challenging previously held ideas about good and bad bacteria. Funkhouser and Bordenstein [39] say that the human microbiota comprises only 1–3% of an individual's total body mass, outnumbering human cells 10 to 1 and adding over 8 million genes to our set of 22,000. At the beginning of the twentieth century, French pediatrician Henry Tissier said that human infants develop within a sterile environment and acquire their initial bacterial inoculum while traveling through the maternal birth canal but now the sterile womb hypothesis remains dogma. The intrauterine environment during healthy pregnancy has been presumed to be free of, although recent evidence of microbes presents in the amniotic fluid, umbilical cord blood, fetal membranes and placenta of healthy term pregnancies after both vaginal and C-section delivery has challenged this belief [40]. It is known by now that human infants are colonized with maternal vaginal and fecal microbes as they exit the birth. The way how is known to have long-term consequences on mothers and child health. This is especially important considering immune-mediated diseases. For example, children born via C-section are significantly more likely to develop allergic rhinitis, asthma, celiac disease, type 1 diabetes and inflammatory bowel disease [40].

Besides mode of delivery, breastfeeding also provides a route of maternal microbial transmission. Breast milk was considered sterile at first, but in colostrum collected aseptically already harbors hundreds of bacterial species [39].

To ensure the best maternal transmission of beneficial microbes, Reed [41] has made following suggestions:

- Baby should be naked on mothers chest immediately following birth for at least an hour and a lot in following frost days.
- Avoid bathing baby for at least 24 h after birth [42]. Use own linen from home for baby if in hospital.
- Minimize the handling of baby.
- Exclusively breastfeeding. If not, probiotics should be considered.
- Avoid unnecessary antibiotics for the baby [43, 44].
- Probiotics may also be beneficial for babies suffering from colic.

The complex symbiosis between humans and microbes is important for our health, and breastfeeding benefits the health and well-being of infants. Maternal transmission is also a key factor in shaping the structure of the microbiome in animal species over evolutionary time, since microbes that promote host fitness, especially in females, will simultaneously increase their odds of being transferred to the next generation; therefore, it is essential to create optimal conditions to achieve the transmission.

7. First hour and breastfeeding

Breastfeeding has many advantages for the child, mother and the environment. The smooth first hour after birth and mother's skin-to-skin contact to newborn have positive impact on the effectiveness and duration of breastfeeding. Shorter intervals between birth and the start of skin-to-skin care and longer times spent skin-to-skin after birth improved breastfeeding exclusivity and duration. In the first month, woman has to breastfeed as often as the newborn wants or even more. With this the production of milk is assured. Many females are meeting with problem of too small amount of milk. The most frequent reasons are too little ingested liquid and disorderly diet. The problem can also be tiredness, increased amount of stress and rare short passing feeds. Relaxed and satisfied mother, who lives in a pleasant and tranquil environment, will have much better conditions for smooth milk lactation. The production and amount of milk is determining by the law of demand and offer. Birth environment and each health professional in their professional action may be more or less supportive impact on the ability and confidence of women to be born, breastfeeding and care for the baby, and baby's ability to effectively breastfeed. Full breastfeeding can of course be established successfully after a cesarean section also. The beginning of the milk secretion can be delayed after caesarean section, however, there is no rule. It is important to know that a child for successful feeds need to have a search reflexes, reflexes of swallow and sucking reflex which is instinctive. The way of the childbirth does not have influence per this. It is true that the first feed is postponed as a mother is put to sleep during an intervention. Clinical staff has to help her to add a child only after a certain time, when a mother is wake and she is aware of herself and surroundings. There are qualified professionals working in various medical institutions that hold a specific and additional knowledge about lactation and breastfeeding. With breastfeeding, the 'good bacteria' from the mother's body with a calm environment create good conditions for the development and strengthening of the child's immune system. The WHO and UNICEF are recommending three important breastfeeding activities: (1) early breastfeeding and skin-to-skin contact with mother just after the birth; (2) exclusive breastfeeding to baby's age of 6 months without other food or liquids and (3) continued breastfeeding to baby's age of 2 years or even more. Meantime, the child can get complementary foods like soft foods and liquids, etc. [45–47]. Early breastfeeding and skin-to-skin contact immediately after birth keep a baby warm and have positive influence on their immune system. Despite that breastmilk is the best food with antibodies for baby's development, it also has effects on mother's ability of continuing exclusive breastfeeding. Mothers who breastfeed also have a (1) early initiation of breastfeeding—place newborns skin-to-skin with their mother immediately after birth, and support mothers to initiate breastfeeding within the baby's first hour of life; (2) exclusive breastfeeding—provide only breastmilk to infants from birth until 6 months of age, with no other food or liquids (including water); (3) continued breastfeeding—breastfeeding until age 2 or longer, in addition to adequate and safe solid, semisolid or soft foods (also called complementary foods) [45–47]. Immediate skin-to-skin contact and starting breastfeeding early keeps a baby warm, builds his or her immune system, promotes bonding, boosts a mother's milk supply and increases the chances that she will be able to continue exclusive breastfeeding. Breastmilk is more than just food for babies—it is also a potent medicine for disease prevention that is tailored to the needs of each child. The 'first milk'—or colostrum—is rich in antibodies to protect babies from disease and death, lower risk of developing breast and ovarian cancers. Breastfeeding can also delay mother's ovulation [13, 47].

One of the important factor that contributes to good establishment of breastfeeding is adding of the newborn to the mother's chest as soon as possible after birth, advisably to first half an hour or at least in hour after childbirth. If mother needs an advice or help during this time, it is very important that she gets it. First of feeds is introducing the first food and the first immunization to a child which further encourages the production of colostrum. Baby's sucking reflex is expressed the most during the first hour after a birth. It is awaken during skin-to-skin contact and care. If the mother is breastfeeding the newborn immediately after birth, the hormonal balance during pregnancy is established for a long time, which very favorable impacts on mother's overall health being. In addition, under the influence of the hormone oxytocin, which is secreted, while a newborn stimulates mother's nipples, the uterus intensively cramps and quickly returns to its original size. And this reduces the likelihood of severe bleeding after childbirth. Oxytocin, which increases significantly during skin-to-skin care, promotes newborn attachment, reduces maternal and newborn stress and helps the newborn transition to postnatal life. With breastfeeding in first hour, the child also has a stable heart rhythm without bradycardia. The possibility of apnea is reduced by 75%, since the depth of each breath becomes more stable [9, 13, 48].

Colonization by mother's bacteria and first lactation colostrum, which creates an optimal intestinal flora, is an optimal protection of the child immunity from possible allergies which might otherwise can be developed later in child life. Breastmilk is more than just food—it is also a potent medicine. It protects the child against disease, regulates the child's immune system and helps child to digest the food [47]. This process helps to program the healthy development of the infant's gut microbiome for life. There is evidence, for example, that breastmilk can help to counteract an infant's genetic predisposition for obesity and other chronic diseases. So the first hour after birth is a critical period with irreversible consequences from the point of bacteriological view [12, 48]. More on that can be found in impacts on infant microbiome assembly chapter.

Mother's breasts are natural thermoregulator to maintain the body temperature of a child. They regulate the temperature of a child. If the child is cold, the breast temperature increases, or if the child is warm, the breast temperature falls. Mother's breasts are also natural thermoregulator for child's respiratory and heart rates [8, 10, 48].

An undisturbed first hour with skin-to-skin also reduces the risk of hypoglycemia (see chapter about metabolic adaptation). Newborn babies can produce glucose from their body stores of energy until they are breastfeeding well and are more likely to do so when they remain skin-to-skin with their mothers. Breastfeeding extended period of natural immunity against mumps, measles and polio. Colostrum has a laxative effect and helps to facilitate the elimination of the first child's stool. It is extremely easy to digest and does not cause constipation. The child has also less troubling with abdominal cramps. As long as the child is breastfed, it is protected against many infections, because breast milk receipt of child antibodies that protect against diseases that can overcome its mother. The child is also protected against ear infections, diarrhea, gastrointestinal infections and diseases of the respiratory tract. For breastfed infant, it is less likely to be diagnosed with meningitis and childhood diabetes. An active intake (compared with passive swallowing bottle) promotes the proper development of the jaw, the mouth muscles and cheek bones, resulting in a very favorable impact on the development of children's speech.

8. Conclusion

First hour following birth for mature newborn is without doubt the most critical hour in life of human beings. During this time, a lot of changes happen. When woman gives birth, all the hard work she does generate changes in the chemistry in the brains. It makes women want to nurture her child. These hormones also cause the uterus to contract, shrink and stop bleeding.

Based on decades of evidence, the World Health Organization and United Nations Children's Fund [6] recommended that all healthy mothers and babies, regardless of feeding preference and method of birth, have uninterrupted skin-to-skin care beginning immediately after birth, lasting for at least an hour.

There is still a lot of unnecessary interventions in the first hour after birth in many maternity hospitals. Routine procedures are being carried out starting from early cord clamping to vitamin K injection, eye prophylaxis antibiotic ointment, navel prophylaxis, foot and hand printing, weighing, measurements and bathing and others. All health-care providers should know that immediate skin-to-skin contact is the best way for a newborn and mother to bond. Healthy newborns should be placed in 'skin-to-skin' contact with the mother until the first round of breastfeeding is established. Skin-to-skin care means placing dried, unclothed newborns on their mother's bare chest, with warmed light blankets or towels covering the newborn's back. Women who have a planned or unplanned C-section would not be in the ideal position for intimate bonding right away. Baby could be taken to a warming table for a quick assessment first. Authors [18] claim that there is no reason why stable mothers should not have the experience of skin-to-skin contact after cesarean births, to collect the same short- and long-term benefits of it. Even from psychological point of view, it helps them mourn the loss of a normal vaginal birth.

The first hour should be focused on baby's first breastfeed and mother-baby and family bonding. The manner in which a new baby is welcomed into the world during the first hours after birth may have short- and long-term consequences.

Author details

Teja Škodič Zakšek*, Anita Jug Došler, Ana Polona Mivšek and Petra Petročnik

*Address all correspondence to: teja.zaksek@zf.uni-lj.si

Faculty of Health Sciences, University of Ljubljana, Ljubljana, Slovenia

References

[1] Coad J, Dunstall M. The transition to neonatal life. In: Anatomy and Physiology for Midwives. 3rd ed. Edinburgh: Churchill Livingstone, Elsevier; 2011. pp. 379-403

[2] Novak B. Adaptations to extrauterine life—respiration and cardiac functions. In: Stables D, Rankin J, editors. Physiology in Childbearing with Anatomy and Related Sciences. 3rd ed. London: Elsevier; 2010. pp. 641-656

[3] Crenshaw JT. Healthy birth practice #6: Keep mother and baby together—it's best for mother, baby, and breastfeeding. The Journal of Perinatal Education. 2014;**23**(4):212-219

[4] Ludington-Hoe SM, Lewis T, Cong X, Anderson L, Morgan K, Reese S. Breast and infant temperatures with twins during shared kangaroo care. Journal of Obstetric, Gynecologic & Neonatal Nursing. 2006;**35**:223-231

[5] Widström AM, Lilja G, Aaltomaa-Michalias P, Dahllöf A, Lintula M, Nissen E. Newborn behaviour to locate the breast when skin-to-skin: A possible method for enabling early self-regulation. Acta Paediatrica. 2011;**100**(1):79-85

[6] World Health Organization, United Nations Children's Fund. Baby-Friendly Hospital Initiative: Revised, Updated, and Expanded for Integrated Care. Geneva, Switzerland: World Health Organization; 2009. Available from: http://whqlibdoc.who.int/publications/2009/9789241594967_eng.pdf [Accessed: February 23, 2017]

[7] Jug Došler A, Petročnik P, Mivšek AP, Škodič Zakšek T, Skubic M. Neonatal prophylaxis: Prevention of vitamin K deficiency haemorrhage and neonatal ophthalmia. Zdravstveno Varstvo. 2015;**54**(3):184-193

[8] Gunn J, Davies L, Baddock S. Supporting the newborn. In: Pairman S, Pincombe J, Thorogood C, Tracy S, editors. Midwifery: Preparation for Practice. 3rd ed. Sydney: Churchill Livingstone, Elsevier; 2014. pp. 764-801

[9] Odent M. The First Hour Following Birth: Don't Wake the Mother! Midwifery Today [Internet]. 2002. Available from: https://www.midwiferytoday.com/articles/firsthour.asp [Accessed: February 23, 2017]

[10] Stevens J, Schmied V, Burns E, Dahlen H. Immediate or early skin-to-skin contact after a caesarean section: A review of the literature. Maternal & Child Nutrition. 2014;**10**(4):456-173. DOI: 10.1111/mcn.12128

[11] Brimdyr K. The First Hour after Birth. A Baby's 9 Instinctive Stages. East Sandwich: Healthy Children Project [Internet]. 2015. Available from: http://magicalhour.com/aboutus.html [Accessed: February 23, 2017]

[12] Newman J. The Importance of Skin to Skin Contact. Breast Feeding Inc. [Internet]. 2009. Available from: http://www.breastfeedinginc.ca/content.php?pagename=doc-ISSC [Accessed: February 23, 2017]

[13] Centers for Disease Control and Prevention. Strategies to prevent obesity and other chronic diseases: The CDC Guide to Strategies to Support Breastfeeding Mothers and Babies. Atlanta: U.S. Department of Health and Human Services. 2013. Available from: https://www.cdc.gov/breastfeeding/pdf/BF-Guide-508.PDF [Accessed: June 7, 2017].

[14] Crenshaw CT. Keep mother and baby together—it's best for mother, baby and breastfeeding. The Journal of Perinatal Education. 2014;**23**(4):211-217. DOI: 10.1891/1058-1243.23.4.211

[15] Raylene P. The sacred hour: Uninterrupted skin-to-skin contact immediately after birth. In: Browne VJ, White R, Talm A, editors. Newborn and Infant Nursing Reviews. New York: Elsevier; 2013. pp. 67-72. Available from: http://www.medscape.com/viewarticle/806325 [Accessed: February 24, 2017]

[16] Buckley SJ. The Hormonal Physiology of Childbearing. New York: Childbirth Connection; 2014

[17] Blackburn ST. Maternal, Fetal, & Neonatal Physiology: A Clinical Perspective. 3rd ed. St. Louis: Saunders Elsevier; 2007

[18] Phillips R. Uninterrupted skin-to-skin contact immediately after birth. Newborn & Infant Nursing Reviews. 2013;**13**(2):67-72

[19] Oden M, editors Davids L, MacDonald S. Examination of the Newborn and Neonatal Health. 1st ed. London: Churchill Livingstone, Elsevier; 2008. pp. 95-107

[20] Uvnas-Mobert K. The Oxytocin Factor: Tapping the Hormone of Calm, Love and Healing. Cambridge, MA: Da Capa Press; 2003

[21] WHO. Baby-Friendly Hospital Initiative [Internet]. 2009. Available from: http://www.who.int/nutrition/publications/infantfeeding/bfhi_trainingcourse/en/ [Accessed: February 23, 2017]

[22] Sullivan R, Perry R, Sloan A, Kleinhaus K, Burtchen N. Infant bonding and attachment to the caregiver: Insights from basic and clinical science. Clinics in Perinatology. 2011;**38**(4):643-655

[23] Bergman N. More than a cuddle: Skin-to-skin contact is key. Practising Midwife. 2005;**8**(9):44

[24] Bruschweiler-Stern N. The neonatal moment of meeting—building the dialogue, strengthening the bond. Child and Adolescent Psychiatric Clinics of North America. 2009;**18**(3):533-544. DOI: 0.1016/j.chc.2009.02.001

[25] McPhail M, Martin C, Redshaw M. Perinatal Mental Health: A Clinical Guide. Cumbria: M & K Publishing; 2012

[26] Levine A, Zagoory-Sharon O, Feldman R. Oxytocin during pregnancy and early postpartum: Individual patterns and maternal-fetal attachment. Peptides. 2007;**28**(6):1162-1169

[27] Gordon JI, Dewey KG, Mills DA, Medzhitov RM. The human gut microbiota and undernutrition. Science Translational Medicine. 2012;**4**:137ps12

[28] Nagasawa M, Okabe S, Mogi K, Kikusui T. Oxytocin and mutual communication in mother-infant bonding. Frontiers in Human Neuroscience. 2012;**6**:31

[29] Feldman R, Gordon I, Zagoory-Sharon O. Maternal and paternal plasma, salivary, and urinary oxytocin and parent-infant synchrony: Considering stress and affiliation components of human bonding. Developmental Science. 2011;**14**:752-761. DOI: 10.1111/j.1467-7687.2010.01021.x

[30] Colson S. What happens to breastfeeding when mothers lie back? Clinical Lactation. 2010;**1**:11-14

[31] Bowlby J. Attachment and Loss: Attachment. Vol. I. New York: Basic Books; 1969/1982

[32] Birss SA. Transition to parenthood: Promoting the parent-infant relationship. In Nugent JK, Keefer CH, Minear S, Johnson LC, Blanchard Y, editors. Understanding Newborn

Behavior and Early Relationships: The Newborn Behavioral Observations [NBO] System Handbook. Baltimore, MD: Paul H. Brookes; 2007. pp. 27-49

[33] Reid T, Freer Y. Developmentally focused nursing care. In: Boxwell G, editor. Neonatal Intensive Care Nursing. London: Routledge; 2001. pp. 14-44

[34] England C. The healthy low birth weight baby. In: Marshall J, Raynor M, editors. Myles Textbook for Midwives. 16th ed. Edinburgh: Churchill Livingstone, Elsevier; 2014. pp. 617-627

[35] Colson S. Womb to World—Adaptation from Foetus to Neonate from a Metabolic Perspective. Midwifery Today [Internet]. 2002. Available from: www.midwiferytoday.com/articles/womb.asp [Accessed: February 23, 2017]

[36] Ward Platt M, Deshpande S. Metabolic adaptation at birth. Seminars in Fetal & Neonatal Medicine. 2005;**10**(4):341-350

[37] Davies L, Richards R. Maternal and newborn transition: Adjustment to extrauterine life. In: Davies L, McDonald S, editors. Examination of the Newborn and Neonatal Health: A Multidimensional Approach. London: Elservier; 2008. pp. 107-126

[38] Colson S, DeRooy L, Hawdon J. Biological Nurturing increases duration of breastfeeding for a vulnerable cohort. MIDIRS Midwifery Digest. 2003;**13**(1):92-97

[39] Funkhouser LJ, Bordenstein SR. Mom knows best: The universality of maternal microbial transmission. PLoS Biology. 2013;**11**:e1001631. DOI: 10.1371/journal.pbio.1001631

[40] Cabrera-Rubio R, et al. The human milk microbiome changes over lactation and is shaped by maternal weight and mode of delivery. American Journal of Clinical Nutrition. 2012;**96**:544-551

[41] Reed R. The Human Microbiome: Considerations for Pregnancy, Birth and Early Mothering [Internet]. 2017. Available from: https://midwifethinking.com/2016/04/13/the-human-microbiome-considerations-for-pregnancy-birth-and-early-mothering/ [Accessed: February 23, 2017]

[42] Tollin M, et al. Vernix caseosa as a multi-component defence system based on polypeptides, lipids and their interactions. Cellular and Molecular Life Sciences. 2005;**62**:2390-2399

[43] Ajslev TA, Andersen CS, Gamborg M, Sørensen TI, Jess T. Childhood overweight after establishment of the gut microbiota: The role of delivery mode, pre-pregnancy weight and early administration of antibiotics. International Journal of Obesity. 2011;**35**:522-529

[44] Penders J, Thijs C, Vink C, Snijders B, Kummeling I, van den Brandt PA, et al. Factors influencing the composition of the intestinal microbiota in early infancy. Pediatrics. 2006;**118**:511-521. DOI: 10.1542/peds.2005-2824

[45] Moore ER, Anderson GC, Bergman N, Dowswell T. Early skin-to-skin contact for mothers and their healthy newborn infants. Cochrane Database of Systematic Reviews. 2014;**16**(5):CD003519. DOI: 10.1002/14651858.CD003519.pub3

[46] Chamberlain D. Windows to the Womb. Revealing the Conscious Baby from Conception to Birth. Berkley, CA: North Atlanta Books; 2013

[47] United Nations Children's Fund (UNICEF). From the First Hour of Life: Making the Case for Improved Infant and Young Child Feeding Everywhere. New York: UNICEF; 2016. Available from: https://data.unicef.org/wp-content/uploads/2016/10/From-the-first-hour-of-life.pdf [Accessed: June 7, 2017].

[48] Richardson H. Kangaroo care: Why does it work? Midwifery Today. 1997;**44**:50-52. Available from: http://www.midwiferytoday.com/articles/kangaroocare.asp [Accessed: February 24, 2017]

5

Non-Pulmonary Management of Newborns with Respiratory Distress

Petja Fister and Štefan Grosek

Abstract

Due to the developmental immaturity of the lungs and other organs, the premature newborns are more prone to develop respiratory distress syndrome (RDS) and other problems of prematurity. The prevention of heat and water loses improves survival. Intolerance to excessive fluids and electrolytes in the transitional period may affect urine and sodium excretion together with maladaptation of cardiovascular system, the development of heart failure, and deterioration of RDS due to patent ductus arteriosus (PDA) and further development of bronchopulmonary dysplasia (BPD). Closure of PDA is frequently needed. The "trophic feeding" and intensive nutrition as soon as possible prevent weight loss and further growth restriction. Greater sensitivity to pain, short- and long-term effects of inappropriately treated pain, use of opioids and sedatives are of concern in the short- and long-term outcomes. Cardiovascular stability and adequate perfusion of the brain both affect the neurological outcome. Delayed cord clamping and erythropoietin help maintaining adequate levels of circulating hemoglobin which might affect later cognitive outcomes. In the following sections, detailed descriptions of non-pulmonary management will be presented. We conducted electronic searches of articles on supportive (non-pulmonary) management of newborns with RDS. Consensus guidelines on newborns with respiratory distress have been reviewed.

Keywords: newborns, evidence-based therapy, antenatal steroids, transport in utero, regionalization of maternity hospitals and neonatal intensive care units, thermoregulation, fluid, nutrition, antibiotics, pain, blood pressure, perfusion, patent ductus arteriosus

1. Introduction

Non-pulmonary management of newborns with respiratory distress syndrome (RDS) is neither the last nor the least important part of the management, but it is supposed to be involved and intertwined in the whole necessary work-up integrated for the well-being of the tinny newborn. Each momentum from the prenatal care, pregnancy, and finally to the birth of the newborn should be considered when we are aiming to improve the final outcome, that is, delivery of a healthy newborn. Pulmonary management of newborns with RDS is only one, though very important and lifesaving, but not sufficient and adequate part of the whole care management of the newborns with RDS.

2. Methods

This chapter will look at the importance of prenatal care, temperature control, control of hypoglycemia, fluid and nutritional intake, the impact of perinatal infection and the use and misuse of antibiotics, frequency of unnecessary procedures, proper pain management, the impact of excessive use of opiates on ventilation duration in the management of newborns with RDS. The impact of optimal blood pressure, tissue perfusion, and patent ductus arteriosus (PDA) with hemodynamic management in newborns with RDS is going to be reviewed. Also, the short- and long-term outcomes in respect of supportive management of newborns in the intensive care unit will be addressed. We conducted electronic searches of articles on supportive (non-pulmonary) management and reviewed the consensus guidelines on management of newborns with RDS [1].

3. Prenatal care

Every newborn can develop RDS, but the likelihood among the premature infants to be affected with the RDS is the highest [2, 3]. Therefore, as neonatal RDS is a disease predominantly affecting the preterm newborns, all the measures to decrease preterm delivery encompass its management. Preconception advice starting in teenage youth to prevent pregnancy in too young teenage girls is important, and social programs should be developed and delivered among the youths. This is not only the problem in poor countries in the world but is even more problematic in wealthy countries with high-gross domestic product but also extreme social inequalities. This preconception advice is closely related to proper protection from the sexually transmitted diseases which may also affect the fetal and later newborn's life. Both, youth pregnancy and sexually transmitted diseases together with under- or malnutrition, strongly affect the development of the fetus and premature delivery. Publically available access to the proper maternity care, at least in well-developed countries, should be offered to every pregnant woman: adequate number of visits at the obstetrician's, appropriate number of obstetric ultrasounds, teaching programs and screening for infections, developmental malformations, etc. Special problems are unwanted pregnancies because any termination of unwanted pregnancy brings different problems to the mother and future wanted pregnancies, but it is worth mentioning that illegal and criminal or nonprofessional abortion endangers the health and lives of the women [4].

In well-organized health systems, ultrasound measurement of cervical length in midtrimester enables prediction of preterm labor and women with short cervix (<25 mm) should be offered vaginal progesterone treatment [5]. Women with threatening preterm labor should be transferred by "in utero" transport to tertiary level medical centers where better outcomes in regards to mothers and newborns can be provided [6]. In the case of preterm premature rupture of membranes (PPROM), after reassuring maternal and fetal wellbeing threatened preterm delivery can be delayed by antibiotics treatment for 7 days to mothers from about 23 weeks up to 34 weeks of gestation [7]. Antibiotics reduce the rate of chorioamnionitis, preterm birth, infection, and respiratory insufficiency [8]. On the contrary, antibiotics have not been proved beneficial for mothers with preterm labor and intact membranes [9]. Delaying the preterm delivery has been also proved for magnesium sulfate which also has beneficial effects for the brain of the preterm newborn [10]. Preterm labor is efficaciously postponed by tocolytics [11]. Antenatal steroids given to mothers from about 23 weeks up to 34 weeks of gestation decrease the risk of neonatal death, RDS, intraventricular hemorrhage (IVH), and necrotizing enterocolitis (NEC) [12]. Moreover, antenatal steroids given more than 24 h and <7 days before elective cesarean section at term also influence the RDS in the late-preterm or term newborn [13]. Until further studies are done, one repeated dose of antenatal steroids given a week after the first dose is recommended [14].

Chorioamnionitis describes intrauterine inflammation of maternal and fetal tissues and endangers both, the mother and the newborn. It has been recognized as the major risk factor for preterm birth, prematurity-associated mortality in morbidity of newborns: the neonatal sepsis, RDS, cystic periventricular leukomalacia (PVL), IVH, and cerebral palsy [15, 16]. Since guidelines for the prevention of perinatal group B streptococcal (GBS) disease have been published, the incidence of early-onset GBS disease in newborns has dramatically decreased. The mayor prevention key is universal antenatal GBS screening of pregnant women and intrapartum antibiotic prophylaxis (IAP) for women with high-risk of infection with penicillin, ampicillin, or cefazolin. Adequate IAP is achieved by infusion of antibiotics at least 4 h before delivery [17].

4. Interhospital, "in utero" transport, and regionalization

Interhospital air and ground transportation of critically ill neonates, regionalization, organization of "in utero" transportations, and new tertiary perinatal centers, which care for the most at risk premature newborns, have greatly decreased the perinatal mortality rate over the last 30 years all over the world [6]. As an example, we present the results from the Republic of Slovenia where we have greatly decreased the perinatal mortality rate over the last 30 years to a rate of 3.5% for neonates weighing at least 1000 g in 2006. We have organized transportation since 1976, and we have transport "in utero" in two Slovenian perinatal centers since 1985 [18].

5. Temperature management

From the neonatal history, we learned that misunderstanding the adverse effects of low body temperature in the premature infants was related to higher mortality rate in hypothermic infants. With understanding the importance of normal body temperature later together with the invention of heated air incubators, the mortality rate dropped as much as twice immediately [19–21]. After birth, the newborn baby is exposed to extrauterine environment with temperature changes in relation to the environmental temperatures which are usually lower than the body temperature. Newborns and especially preterms have increased proportion of body surface in relation to body volume, their body has low-temperature capacity, and their skin is immature with increased water permeability. They also have low supplies of skin fat. Since oxygen and energy consumption are lowest in the range of thermal neutrality, it is important to keep newborns in those limited ambient temperature ranges to enable them to have their body temperature ranging from 36.5 to 37.5°C. By acknowledging the importance of thermal neutrality, this is one of the most manageable problems of non-pulmonary management of newborns with RDS [22].

Temperature regulation enables optimal efficiency of the metabolic processes and enzyme activities with the lowest oxygen and calorie consumption. Newborns are unable to produce sufficient heat by metabolic reactions, by muscle activity during motion, and by nonshivering thermogenesis in the brown fat, which starts to evolve between 26th and 30th weeks of gestation. Loosing heath from the body is modulated by changing the vascular tone of peripheral vessels and by sweating, which is not fully developed by the 36th week of gestation.

There are four ways newborns may lose heat to the environment. Immediately after birth, they are wet from the amniotic fluid and evaporation decreases their body temperature fast so all the measures to dry their body have to be taken. Recently, to decrease evaporation from the immature water permeable skin, very premature newborns, still wet, are immediately wrapped into plastic wraps or bags and caps [23–27]. To lessen the evaporation, the air in the incubators for all the preterms beyond 31 weeks of gestation should be humidified (60–80%) and preterm newborns should not be bathed until they can maintain their body temperature. The humidity should be decreased by 5% every day if they can maintain stable body temperature, and stopped when preterms can maintain their body temperature in 40% humidity [28]. Every object radiates—it gives or receives the heat in relation to the temperature difference. Therefore, it is important to keep the air temperature in a defined range and also to take into account the external temperatures, the room walls and windows and the isolation walls of the incubators [29]. Objects can lose heat by losing or gaining heat from the object in contact by conduction. Placing the newborn baby to the mother's abdomen allows skin to skin contact besides parental bonding and enables conduction of the heat from the mother to the child [22, 30–32]. Resuscitation on wet basis can cause a huge heat loss from the newborn and should be avoided. Infusing cold fluids also causes conduction loss of heat. Moving air causes heat loss by convection.

Hypothermia may lead to hypoglycemia or acidosis and has been associated with increased mortality, increased risk of late-onset sepsis, IVH, pulmonary insufficiency, and hemorrhage

[20, 21]. The vicious cycle of cooling causes norepinephrine release with pulmonary and peripheral vasoconstriction with increased right-to-left shunting of blood and maintenance of fetal circulation postnatally. To enable thermal neutrality, preterm newborns should be nursed in preheated and humidified incubators, and in heated beds after 32nd week of gestation or >1500 g. We provide them heated and humidified gases and clothe newborns with clothes and caps [33, 34].

6. Perinatal infection management

After the initial care of the newborn in the delivery room with drying the newborn's skin, providing warmth, positioning the head, and clearing the airway, the evaluation of respiration, and consequently oxygenation of peripheral organs follows. In case transitional period is prolonged and the signs of RDS persist, we have to obtain chest radiograph, blood gas analysis and perform sepsis work-up with complete blood count and cultures and start empirical antibiotic treatment with ampicillin or penicillin and gentamicin, especially if risk factors for early-onset sepsis are present. Early-onset infection with GBS typically imitates the RDS in preterm newborns with the clinical presentation and also radiographically so usually it is difficult to differentiate pneumonia from RDS without infection. Besides GBS congenital pneumonia can be caused by *Escherichia coli* and other microorganisms [35]. A well appearing newborn to a mother with chorioamnionitis should have a limited diagnostic evaluation and receive empirical antibiotic therapy. Well-appearing term newborns, born to mothers with appropriate IAP or inappropriate IAP with rupture of membranes for <18 h, need routine care and observation. Those term newborns whose mothers had inappropriate IAP and rupture of membranes for more than 18 h and all preterm newborns with inadequate IAP need clinical and laboratory evaluation and observation [17, 36]. There is no evidence to support routine antibiotic treatment of newborns with RDS and without risk factors for early-onset sepsis [37, 38]. In those newborns with RDS which do not have laboratory signs of sepsis and have negative cultures, the antibiotics should be discontinued as early as feasible [37, 39].

Late-onset sepsis occurs in one-fifth of premature newborns and is associated with increased mortality, prolonged hospitalization, and prolonged artificial ventilation, PDA, NEC, and BPD [40]. Newborns that were treated for neonatal sepsis later are at risk of poor weight gain and adverse neurodevelopmental outcome [41].

7. Fluid and electrolyte management

After birth, water and electrolyte balance is influenced by transitional and developmental adaptations of the newborn. More preterm newborns have more total body water, and extracellular fluid volume constitutes a greater part of total body water in comparison with term newborns. Furthermore, after birth, renal function of preterm newborns is reduced in comparison with term newborns and they lose more weight with diuresis which results from an isotonic reduction of extracellular fluid. Newborns, especially more preterm ones loose water insensibly through the skin and respiratory system, especially in RDS, when respiratory rate is increased [42, 43]. Insensible water loss is increased by radiant heaters, phototherapeutic lights, and inappropriate water content of inspired air. Antenatal steroids besides the already mentioned effect on lung maturation also accelerate skin and kidney maturation. Preterm newborns whose mothers have received antenatal steroids had lower insensible water loss, less hypernatremia, earlier diuresis and natriuresis, and less nonoliguric hyperkalemia [44, 45]. In the first postnatal days, water balance is kept in a slightly negative state. Excessive fluid administration is associated with increased risk of PDA, NEC, and BPD [46]. Fluid balance and volume status can be evaluated by physical examination with signs of hydration, edema, and hemodynamic stability, body weight loss or gain, balance of fluid intake and output, and biochemistry evaluation of electrolyte concentration in plasma of the newborns. Fluid requirements therefore account for maintenance requirements, obligatory losses, and possible deficits and are gestational and postnatal age, ambient temperature and humidity, renal and respiratory function dependent. The electrolyte requirements for sodium, potassium, and chloride are approximately 1–2 mEq/kg/day except for the first day when isotonic reduction of extracellular fluid ensues. Diuretics cause electrolyte disturbances due to urinary loss of sodium and potassium and loop diuretics are associated with nephrocalcinosis so we prefer not to use them routinely [47].

8. Nutritional management

The newborn's nutritional status is influenced by his past history with genetic background, maternal body composition, and nutrition before and during pregnancy [48]. Many preterm newborns are born growth restricted because of inadequate intrauterine nutrient supply. Postnatal nutrition and metabolic capacity impact postnatal growth and development and have long-term consequences on the lung, brain, and other organ development and cognitive function [49]. The newborn's brain consumes half of all the energy provided, and too little calories mean less brain volume and worse neurocognitive outcome. Adequate volume of fluids, the protein content, and energy balance in the newborn's, and especially preterm's nutrition should cover metabolic expenditure and growth requirements, thus setting the ground for optimal outcomes.

In newborns with RDS, early enteral feeding is frequently delayed because of concomitant medical problems and fear of complications as the feeding intolerance and NEC. Therefore, the parenteral nutrition is commenced as early as possible to correct prenatal, to prevent postnatal growth failure and to improve outcomes [50, 51]. The parenteral nutrition has to provide enough calories for energy and growth, which are met by carbohydrates, proteins, and lipids. Carbohydrates provide glucose, proteins provide essential amino acids and nitrogen, and lipids provide essential fatty acids. Essential nutrients needed for growth are electrolytes, vitamins, minerals, and trace elements [52–54].

The premature newborn needs parenterally about 100 kcal/kg/day of nonprotein energy for growing, 3/5 in the form of carbohydrates and 2/5 in the form of lipids. Glucose is the form of carbohydrates that we give parenterally, and it is the primary energy supply for the newborn's brain. We start with 7 g/kg/day of glucose, which provides 4.8 mg/kg/min of glucose, and we increase the amount by 1.5–2 g/kg/day, up to 15 g/kg/day and maximum of 18 g/kg/day (12.5 mg/kg/min). Preterm newborns are prone to hypoglycemia because of higher glucose needs, decreased fat stores, and higher-energy consumption. On the other hand, for many metabolic and nutritional reasons, they are also prone to hyperglycemia. As early as feasible, we start with 2 g/kg/day of proteins and increase the amount by 0.5–1 to 3.5–4 g/kg/day of proteins, which is needed to attain the intrauterine growth rate [55, 56]. It is also important to provide the preterm 25 nonprotein kcal/1 g of proteins. Low blood urea nitrogen (BUN) is a sign of inadequate protein intake, but a high BUN does not correlate well with a high protein intake [57]. A preterm newborn daily loses 1 g of proteins through the kidneys, and a good caloric input with appropriately balanced diet accumulates 2 g of proteins. Thus, improperly balanced nutrition of a newborn can lead to a loss of 15% of protein mass in 2 days [58]. There are eight essential amino acids in parenteral nutrition and six more for the preterm newborn. Adding cysteine to the parenteral nutrition improved nitrogen balance [59], but the addition of glutamine had no clinical impact [60]. Concomitantly with proteins, we administer 20% of intravenous lipids, including essential fatty acids and long-chain n–3 polyunsaturated fatty acids and start with 1 g/kg/day and increase by 0.5 g/kg/day to a maximum of 3–4 g/kg/day [61–63]. Already 0.5 g/kg/day may provide prevention of essential fatty acid deficiency, and the tolerance is guided by triglyceride level of <200 mg/dL. The tolerance is better achieved with the use of continuous infusion of intravenous lipids over 24 h rather than intermittent dosing [64].

To maintain bone health, the newborns need 1.5–2 mmol/kg/day of calcium and the same amount of phosphorus, and 0.18–0.3 mmol/kg/day of magnesium. The optimal weight ratio of calcium and phosphorus is 1.3–1.7:1. Pediatric vitamin formulations of water- and fat-soluble vitamins and trace elements are in use, but they do not provide enough amounts of vitamin A, D and E so we add them enterally if feasible. Vitamin A affects normal eye and lung development, immunity, and cell differentiation. Supplementation of vitamin A in preterm newborns was associated with reduced risk of oxygen requirement [65]. Selenium supplementation prevented short-term morbidity in preterm newborns [66]. Although carnitine supplementation was not associated with weight gain or apnea reduction [67, 68] there are recommendations to add parenteral carnitine to preterm newborns needing parenteral nutrition for more than 2 weeks [69]. Nutritional status can be evaluated by anthropometry, body composition and biochemistry, clinical assessment and quantity, and quality dietary evaluation. Adverse effects of parenteral nutrition include line infection and sepsis, extravasation of parenteral fluid, cholestasis, and bone disease.

To correct the intrauterine growth restriction and achieve appropriate postnatal weight gain, the enteral feeding is also of great significance [70]. It is important to start enteral feeding as early as feasible; in very low birth weight (VLBW) newborns 10–20 mL/kg/day is started in the first 2–5 days, in low birth weight (LBW) newborns in first days [71]. Colostrum acts as the immune therapy for the newborn's intestine. Feeding newborns with minimal volumes of milk is known as trophic feeding, which has many beneficial effects for further feeding, increased hormone secretion, motility, and decreased permeability of the gastrointestinal tract [72]. After a few days of gastrointestinal priming, feedings are increased by 10–20 mL/kg/day. Human milk in comparison with formula resulted in earlier adequate energy intake [73, 74]. Fast advancement of milk volume has no adverse outcome in comparison with slow advancement [71]. Feeding every two hours was superior to feeding every three hours in regards to the time to reach full enteral feeds and better weight gain [75]. Tube feeding can be bolus or continuous and neither is superior [76]. Feeding intolerance can be determined by emesis, gastric residuals, distended, and tender abdomen with changed bowel sounds and stool output, but most of them have little prognostic value [77–80]. The prokinetic erythromycin has not been shown to be effective [81–83]. When the newborn tolerates 100 mL/kg/day or has been consuming mother's milk for 1 week, formula or mother's milk is fortified. The goal of enteral feeding of the preterm newborn is to gain more than 15 g/kg/day.

9. Pain management

Critically ill newborn is confronted with different, more or less painful procedures every day in the NICU. Not every procedure is painful, but the usual response from the newborn is typical —removal of the affected part of the body and crying. The more severe the pain, the more distressful situation is for the newborn. Brain not yet fully developed may receive too many painful stimulations per day, and the tinny newborn may overreact even if the next stimulus is less or even not painful. Newborn Individualized Developmental Care and Assessment Program (NIDCAP) is a method of ensuring an adequate physical environment, reducing overwhelming sensory stimulations, and increasing sensitive parent caregiving, for proper brain growth and development of preterm newborns. Despite non-convincing evidence that NIDCAP improves long-term neurodevelopmental or short-term medical outcome, there is a need for high-quality researches using different techniques to diminish high environmental stress on the premature infants during their treatment in the NICU [84].

Newborns with RDS experience different kinds of pain depending on their morbidities: skin breaking procedures and tissue injury provoke acute or physiological pain, surgery, localized inflammation, and birth trauma cause established pain and diseases like NEC, meningitis, and scalded skin syndrome give rise to prolonged or chronic pain [85]. It has been estimated that sick newborns experience 12–16 procedures each day which are increasingly painful:

1. Routine procedures (physical examination, diaper changes, nasogastric or orogastric insertion, bladder catheterization) [86];
2. Moderately invasive procedures (endotracheal suction, heel lance, venipuncture, arterial puncture, peripherally inserted central catheter placement); and
3. Severely invasive procedures (central venous line placement, chest tube insertion) [87].

Management of pain in newborns with RDS encompasses prevention with first awareness of causing pain with different painful procedures and reduction of painful management of the newborn. The second line includes objective assessment for the detection of pain in each neonate. Thirdly, controlling the pain includes cooperation with parents to diminish pain experience, delivering proper analgesia before expected painful medical care and combining nonpharmacological interventions and pharmacological therapy [88–90].

An important issue in caring for a newborn with RDS is minimal handling or "do not touch" approach. This also enables us to take in mind the possible pain we are going to cause to the newborn with our intended handling and executed procedures. On the other hand, we have to carefully plan the management not to compromise the well-being of the newborn by not performing vital examinations and investigations. By planning the handling of the newborn in limited number of sessions per day, it is possible to disrupt the newborns less times and perform the examinations, nursing care, and blood withdrawal at the same time. We should use laboratory equipment that enables us to analyze several different chemical substances from one small blood sample to reduce the volume of blood taken from the child and avoid iatrogenic anemia. All sick newborns with RDS need intravenous line for fluid, nutritional, antimicrobial, blood pressure, and pain management so a central venous line as soon as possible and for newborns who need several blood investigations per day an artery line should be placed both with appropriate analgesia. With minimally invasive approach, we can gain many data on the well-being of the newborn by noninvasive monitoring with the use of transcutaneous measuring of the oxygen saturation in peripheral arteries and in different organs by the use of near-infrared spectroscopy (NIRS), partial pressures of oxygen, and carbon dioxide in skin capillaries or bilirubin concentrations [85, 89, 91].

For the assessment of pain, different observational scales designed for special newborn population are in use, which encompass many physiological and behavioral variables. Especially with observation of behavior, there is much subjectivity in the assessment procedure. The available assessment scales have proved usable in acute pain, but there is limited applicability of the assessment scales for assessing prolonged pain, pain in extremely low birth weight (ELBW) newborns and in those receiving paralytic agents [85].

First step on the ladder of pain management constitutes the nonpharmacological measures which include sweet peroral solutions, breastfeeding, sucking, skin-to-skin contact, and swaddling with facilitated tucking and sensorial saturation [92]. Combined use of nonpharmacological measures act synergistically [93–95]. Furthermore, when used with pharmacological measures, the pharmacologic use is lesser in frequency and dosage [88, 96]. Sucrose and glucose used before skin-breaking procedures reduced total crying time, lessened changes of physiological variables, and facial expressions and pain scores of multidimensional pain assessment scales [97, 98]. Currently, it is not entirely clear how sweet solutions suppress the responses to painful stimulation; do they only diminish the response to pain or they really influence the pain perception. With repeated dosing, there is a concern on neurodevelopmental outcome in the preterm newborns [99]. Sucrose alone is used for minor procedures, and combined with other analgesics for moderately painful procedures [97]. In cases when physically possible, breastfeeding or mother's milk is at least as effective as sweet solutions [100]. Further on, engaging different body sensors with sensations, like non-nutritive sucking, swaddling, facilitated tucking, rocking, holding, kangaroo care and sensorial saturation, gives the brain other stimuli and therefore the brain has closed door for pain reception [88, 92].

Topical analgesia with the use of Eutectic Mixture of Local Anesthetics (EMLA) or lidocaine alone are used with effect in venous, arterial, and lumbar punctures and also venous, arterial catheter placement, and circumcision. With reasonable dosing, methemoglobinemia is not a significant problem [101].

Systemic analgesia can be provided by nonopioid, nonsteroidal anti-inflammatory agents, opioid analgesics, and sedatives. Paracetamol (acetaminophen) does not diminish pain perception after assisted vaginal birth, heel lance, or eye examination. Paracetamol may diminish the need for morphine after surgical procedures in newborns [102]. We use nonsteroidal anti-inflammatory agents for closing PDA in preterm newborns, but because of their serious adverse effects, like gastrointestinal bleeding, platelet dysfunction and decreased glomerular filtration rate, we do not use them as analgesics in newborns. The most powerful analgesics are opioids, and morphine is the most frequently used, either intermittently for acute pain with invasive procedures or continuously for established pain during artificial ventilation or after surgery. Morphine reduces acute pain after some invasive procedures: central line, tracheal, and chest tube insertion [103, 104], but not heelstick [105] or tracheal suctioning [106, 107]. The NEOPAIN study showed no difference in mortality rate, severe IVH and PVL between ventilated preterm newborns receiving continuous morphine or placebo. The preterm newborns treated with morphine had less pain, but more hypotension, longer duration of artificial ventilation and longer time to full volume feeds [103]. Morphine is safe and effective for treating established pain after surgery in newborns [108, 109]. In extremely preterm newborns, opioid analgesics should be used cautiously [110, 111].

More rapid analgesia with fewer hemodynamic adverse effects is achieved by fentanyl and shorter-acting derivatives, which is suitable for acute invasive procedures in controlled clinical setting like tracheal tube and central line placement [112, 113]. There was no favorable effect on established pain during artificial ventilation of premature newborns using fentanyl [114]. Furthermore, premature newborns treated with continuous fentanyl had prolonged time of artificial ventilation and of meconium passage. Fentanyl is used for treating established pain after surgery and in newborns with pulmonary hypertension.

Ketamine causes analgesia with sedation and amnesia with no effect on respiration and increasing blood pressure and heart rate [115]. It is used in newborns with hemodynamic instability for acute pain with invasive procedures and for established pain during and after surgery [116]. Among sedatives midazolam which can cause prolonged sedation in sick preterm newborns is not recommended for use in preterm newborns [117].

Painful experiences in early childhood may have unfavorable consequences for neurodevelopment [118, 119]. Although there are some data indicating that prolonged use of analgesics in newborns does not influence long-term neurodevelopmental and behavioral outcome [120–122], more recent studies have shown some adverse long-term effects on growth, neurological, and behavioral outcome [123]. A positive autonomic nervous system's stability to pain in neonates with kangaroo care or skin to skin care can be proved by measuring heart rate variability [124, 125].

10. Blood pressure and perfusion management

Systemic blood pressure is dependent on systemic blood flow with cardiac output and systemic vascular resistance. Hypotension ensues in cases of decreased cardiac output as a result of cardiac dysfunction or hypovolemia with inadequate compensation with vasomotor tone, or, decreased vasomotor tone with inadequate compensatory increase in cardiac output. Hypotension, especially in preterms, is difficult to define unequivocally; population-based normative blood pressure data show the increment of blood pressure with increasing gestational and postnatal age, but normal gestational and postnatal age dependent blood pressure range is not known [126]. The physiological principles of blood pressure define autoregulatory threshold where there is loss of autoregulation of blood flow to vital organs, functional threshold where there is loss of cellular function, and ischemic threshold where there is loss of functional integrity [127]. Blood pressure correlates poorly with systemic and cerebral blood flow; therefore, different measurement approaches combined with clinical assessment of adequate perfusion have been investigated for the purpose of better hemodynamic monitoring. Systemic blood flow can be measured by clinician performed ultrasound of the heart and blood vessels with the pressure wave-form analysis and by magnetic resonance imaging (MRI) [128, 129]. Systemic resistance is evaluated by Laser-Doppler technique and by NIRS [130]. Noninvasively, NIRS gives us information about oxygenation of organs, inferring about oxygen delivery, and oxygen demand of certain tissues. The brain activity can continuously be monitored by concomitant use of NIRS and amplitude integrated electroencephalography (EEG) [131, 132].

The blood flow is regulated by cardiac output, carbon dioxide tension, local neuronal and chemical activity, changes in cerebrospinal fluid hydrogen ion concentration, arterial oxygen content, hemoglobin, and blood glucose [133–135]. Accordingly, systemic blood flow can be improved by inotropes or volume, and systemic resistance can be improved by vasopressors and lusitropes. Treatment of neonatal hypotension improves blood pressure, cardiac output, organ blood flow, lactic acidosis, peripheral perfusion, and urine output. Neonatal hypotension endangers cerebral autoregulation and increases morbidity and mortality in preterm newborns [136, 137].

Low systemic blood pressure frequently occurs in the early stages of RDS. Therefore, blood pressure should frequently be measured, either noninvasively or invasively with intravascular line. For volume expansion, after hypovolemia crystalloid or colloid solutions are used [138, 139]. For decreased cardiac output because of cardiac dysfunction, the initial agent is dopamine, later dobutamine, and epinephrine are added [140, 141]. In newborns with refractory hypotension or high-dose inotropic therapy, glucocorticoid therapy increases blood pressure [142, 143]. Different developmental factors affect hemodynamic response to sympathomimetic amines in newborns [144]. Before deciding on a specific therapy of hypotension, potentially reversible causes have to be taken in mind and corrected if possible (measurement error, blood loss, pneumothorax, sepsis, adrenocortical insufficiency).

There is conflicting evidence on the management of hypotension improving clinically meaningful longer-term outcome measures in VLBW newborns, but there are many confounding factors influencing the outcome of management of preterm newborns and studies are weak to show the impact [145–148].

Besides cardiac output, the oxygen supply to the tissues depends also on the content of oxygen in the arteries, which is in the biggest part a function of concentration of hemoglobin. Target values of hemoglobin or hematocrit differ with regards to the gestational and postnatal age of the newborn, the rate of evolution of anemia, the presence of clinical signs of anemia, and the degree of respiratory support [149]. Targeting to lower concentrations of hemoglobin in ELBW newborns might have no effect on short-term outcomes, but may have a negative impact on the longer-tem neurodevelopmental outcome [150, 151]. Anemia can be avoided or postponed by delayed cord clamping or cord milking and also by applications of erythropoietin. Delayed cord clamping and cord milking in preterm newborns was associated with higher hematocrit, fewer transfusions, less IVH, NEC, and no increased need for phototherapy because of jaundice [152–156]. Also, preterm newborns who were receiving erythropoietin received fewer transfusions and had higher cognitive scores at 18–22 months of corrected age [157, 158].

11. PDA management

Shunting blood from the aorta to the pulmonary artery means decreased blood flow in the systemic circulation and low perfusion of peripheral organs and increased blood flow in the pulmonary circulation with RDS, pulmonary edema, BPD, IVH, NEC, and heart failure. Newborns with PDA have higher mortality rate and increased risk of pulmonary edema, hemorrhage, and BPD. The field of management of the PDA is an area in neonatal practice which has, perhaps, changed the most in the last decades and many questions still remain unanswered. The uses of antenatal steroids, postnatal surfactant, and the gentler modes of ventilation with lower oxygen saturation targets may have lowered the incidence and the impact of clinically significant PDA shunt. In VLBV newborns with RDS, PDA is present in 30% [159, 160]. Current management of the PDA generally includes three approaches. Supportive care for newborns with PDA encompasses providing thermal neutrality, using PEEP, keeping hematocrit between 35 and 40%, fluid restriction of 110–130 ml/kg/day, permissive hypercapnia, low oxygen saturation targets and, in case of diuretic need, thiazide diuretics over loop diuretics. If the newborn has poor perfusion, a large left-to-right shunt and remains artificially ventilated for a longer time a course of cyclooxygenase (COX) inhibitors is administered, favoring ibuprofen over indomethacin, because the latter is reducing blood flow to the brain, gastrointestinal tract, and kidneys [161, 162]. Ibuprofen is efficacious for closing PDA given either intravenously or orally [163]. Newborns, who remain artificially ventilated and have failed to respond to COX inhibitor, are candidates for surgical ligation, which has been associated with adverse long-term outcomes [164].

The prophylactic therapy to reduce the incidence of PDA has not been proved to be of benefit. The prophylactic indomethacin has been shown to have no impact on mortality, neurologic impairment, BPD, or NEC although it was associated with reduction of hemodynamically important PDA and severe IVH [165]. The prophylactic ibuprofen has been linked with adverse effects [166, 167].

12. Postnatal supplemental management of respiratory support

Apnea of prematurity is a developmental consequence of immature respiratory center in premature newborns. Besides mechanical ventilation with oxygen supplementation the management of apnea of prematurity encompasses supportive measures like assuring the temperature stability, proper positioning of the newborn's head and neck and ensuring the nasal patency. Methylxanthines stimulate the respiratory drive by increasing the responsiveness of respiratory center to carbon dioxide and decreasing its hypoxic depression. The medicines also have inotropic effects on respiratory muscles [168]. Caffeine is being preferred over theophylline and other agents [169]. Caffeine therapy has been proved to shorten the duration of mechanical ventilation and supplemental oxygen and also reducing the risk of BPD and PDA ligation [170, 171]. The same effects have been shown for prophylactic use of caffeine in very preterm newborns [172, 173]. There have been some positive neurodevelopmental effects of caffeine therapy proved during follow-up of children treated with caffeine during neonatal period [174–176].

The duration of mechanical ventilation can be shortened and the risk of BPD diminished by the use of postnatal tapering course of low- (<0.2 mg/kg/day) or even very low-dose dexamethasone (0.05 mg/kg/day) [177, 178]. Hydrocortisone has been proved to have the same beneficial effects on earlier extubating of mechanically ventilated preterm newborns [179].

13. Conclusion

For the best outcomes of newborns with RDS, besides optimal pulmonary management, it is of extreme importance to have optimal supportive care (**Table 1**) starting prenatally and aiming at newborns being delivered in highly specialized tertiary centers with timing of birth after completion of a course of prenatal steroids. Body temperature should be maintained between 36.5 and 37.5°C. Preterm newborns should be nursed in incubators with high relative humidity (60–80%) and started on intravenous fluids of 70–80 ml/kg/day, later managed individually, based on weight change and serum electrolyte concentrations. Both parenteral and minimal enteral nutrition should be started as early as possible—from day 1—and quickly increased to 3.5 g/kg/day of proteins and 3 g/kg/day of lipids. Proper infection control starts prenatally with administering antibiotics to women with preterm prelabor rupture of membranes, and before labor to those with risk factors for early-onset sepsis. Furthermore, antibiotics are given to newborns with RDS until early-onset sepsis is ruled out. Adequate treatment of pain may be associated with decreased complications and mortality. Sedatives do not provide pain relief and may mask newborn's response to pain. Additionally, proper management of the PDA and hemodynamic support of the circulation with good systemic perfusion and oxygenation are also of utmost importance for the best outcomes of newborns with RDS.

Prenatal care	All the measures to prevent preterm delivery should be taken (counseling, progesterone, antibiotic, magnesium sulfate, tocolysis) If possible, birth should be delayed to allow effect of antenatal steroid therapy to the mother Timely and safe transport of the expectant mother to specialized tertiary centers Appropriate intrapartum antibiotic prophylaxis
Delivery room stabilization	Delayed cord clamping or cord milking at birth Collecting cord blood for diagnostic purposes (hemogram, hemoculture, blood group, virology) Stabilization of the preterm newborn in a plastic bag under a radiant warmer Drying the newborn's skin, providing warmth, positioning the head and clearing the airway, evaluation of respiration and oxygenation of peripheral organs
Supportive care	Nursing the newborn in incubators with heated and humidified air In cases with risk factors for early-onset sepsis and/or clinical and laboratory signs of sepsis antibiotics should be started Insertion of central lines to enable blood withdrawal for diagnostic purposes and parenteral nutrition Careful fluid and electrolyte therapy Early parenteral nutrition and early trophic feeding Minimal handling with clustered care of examination, blood withdrawal and nursing care at the same time but not to overburden the neonate Regular use of appropriate pain assessment scales and proper analgesia before planned procedures Regular measurement of blood pressure and assessment of peripheral perfusion to decide on possible hemodynamic therapy Targeting hemoglobin or hematocrit values in regards to the gestational and postnatal age, the rate of evolution of anemia, the presence of clinical signs of anemia and the degree of respiratory support needed Consideration on the presence and clinical significance of patent ductus arteriosus to decide on possible therapies Caffeine therapy to minimize the need for and duration of ventilation Consideration on postnatal tapering course of low- or very low-dose dexamethasone or hydrocortisone

Adapted from Sweet et al. [1].

Table 1. Summary of recommendations for non-pulmonary management of newborns with respiratory distress.

Author details

Petja Fister[1*] and Štefan Grosek[2,3]

*Address all correspondence to: petja.fister@kclj.si and petja_fister@yahoo.com

1 Department of Neonatology, University Children's Hospital, University Medical Centre Ljubljana, Ljubljana, Slovenia

2 Department of Pediatric Surgery and Intensive Therapy, Surgical Service, University Medical Centre Ljubljana, Ljubljana, Slovenia

3 Department of Pediatrics, Medical Faculty, University of Ljubljana, Ljubljana, Slovenia

References

[1] Sweet DG, Carnielli V, Greisen G, Hallman M, Ozek E, Plavka R, et al. European consensus guidelines on the management of neonatal respiratory distress syndrome in preterm infants—2013 update. Neonatology. 2013;103(4):353–68. doi: 10.1159/000349928.

[2] Stoll BJ, Hansen NI, Bell EF, Shankaran S, Laptook AR, Walsh MC, et al. Neonatal outcomes of extremely preterm infants from the NICHD Neonatal Research Network. Pediatrics. 2010;126(3):443–56. doi:10.1542/peds.2009–2959.

[3] Costeloe KL, Hennessy EM, Haider S, Stacey F, Marlow N, Draper ES. Short term outcomes after extreme preterm birth in England: comparison of two birth cohorts in 1995 and 2006 (the EPICure studies). BMJ. 2012;345:e7976. doi:10.1136/bmj.e7976.

[4] Robbins CL, Zapata LB, Farr SL, Kroelinger CD, Morrow B, Ahluwalia I, et al. Core state preconception health indicators—pregnancy risk assessment monitoring system and behavioral risk factor surveillance system, 2009. MMWR Surveill Summ. 2014;63(3):1–62.

[5] Di Renzo GC, Roura LC, Facchinetti F, Antsaklis A, Breborowicz G, Gratacos E, et al. Guidelines for the management of spontaneous preterm labor: identification of spontaneous preterm labor, diagnosis of preterm premature rupture of membranes, and preventive tools for preterm birth. J Matern Fetal Neonatal Med. 2011;24(5):659–67. doi:10.3109/14767058.2011.553694.

[6] Rautava L, Eskelinen J, Häkkinen U, Lehtonen L, Group PPIS. 5-year morbidity among very preterm infants in relation to level of hospital care. JAMA Pediatr. 2013;167(1):40–6. doi:10.1001/jamapediatrics.2013.415.

[7] Kenyon S, Boulvain M, Neilson J. Antibiotics for preterm rupture of membranes. Cochrane Database Syst Rev. 2010(8):CD001058. doi:10.1002/14651858.CD001058.pub2.

[8] Hutzal C, Boyle E, Kenyon S, Nash J, Winsor S, Taylor D, et al. Use of antibiotics for the treatment of preterm parturition and prevention of neonatal morbidity: a metaanalysis. Am J Obstet Gynecol. 2008;199(6):620.e1–8. doi:10.1016/j.ajog.2008.07.008.

[9] ACOG Committee Opinion No. 445: antibiotics for preterm labor. Obstet Gynecol. 2009;114(5):1159–60. doi:10.1097/AOG.0b013e3181c33c86.

[10] Doyle L, Crowther C, Middleton P, Marret S, Rouse D. Magnesium sulphate for women at risk of preterm birth for neuroprotection of the fetus. Cochrane Database Syst Rev. 2009;(1):CD004661. doi:10.1002/14651858.CD004661.pub3.

[11] Haas DM, Caldwell DM, Kirkpatrick P, McIntosh JJ, Welton NJ. Tocolytic therapy for preterm delivery: systematic review and network meta-analysis. BMJ. 2012;345:e6226. doi:10.1136/bmj.e6226.

[12] Roberts D, Dalziel S. Antenatal corticosteroids for accelerating fetal lung maturation for women at risk of preterm birth. Cochrane Database Syst Rev. 2006;(3):CD004454.

[13] Sotiriadis A, Makrydimas G, Papatheodorou S, Ioannidis J. Corticosteroids for preventing neonatal respiratory morbidity after elective caesarean section at term. Cochrane Database Syst Rev. 2009;(4):CD006614. doi: 10.1002/14651858.CD006614.pub2.

[14] Crowther C, McKinlay C, Middleton P, Harding J. Repeat doses of prenatal corticosteroids for women at risk of preterm birth for improving neonatal health outcomes. Cochrane Database Syst Rev. 2011;(6):CD003935. doi: 10.1002/14651858.CD003935.pub3.

[15] Thomas W, Speer CP. Chorioamnionitis: important risk factor or innocent bystander for neonatal outcome? Neonatology. 2011;99(3):177–87. doi:10.1159/000320170.

[16] Girard S, Kadhim H, Roy M, Lavoie K, Brochu M, Larouche A, et al. Role of perinatal inflammation in cerebral palsy. Pediatr Neurol. 2009;40(3):168–74. doi:10.1016/j.pediatrneurol.2008.09.016.

[17] Baker CJ, Byington CL, Polin RA, Diseases CoI, Newborn CoFa. Policy statement—recommendations for the prevention of perinatal group B streptococcal (GBS) disease. Pediatrics. 2011;128(3):611–6. doi:10.1542/peds.2011-1466.

[18] Grosek S, Mlakar G, Vidmar I, Ihan A, Primozic J. Heart rate and leukocytes after air and ground transportation in artificially ventilated neonates: a prospective observational study. Intensive Care Med. 2009;35(1):161–5. doi:10.1007/s00134-008-1256-8.

[19] de Almeida M, Guinsburg R, Sancho G, Rosa I, Lamy Z, Martinez F, et al. Hypothermia and early neonatal mortality in preterm infants. J Pediatr. 2014;164(2):271–5.e1. doi: 10.1016/j.jpeds.2013.09.049.

[20] Miller SS, Lee HC, Gould JB. Hypothermia in very low birth weight infants: distribution, risk factors and outcomes. J Perinatol. 2011;31(Suppl 1):S49–56. doi:10.1038/jp.2010.177.

[21] Laptook AR, Salhab W, Bhaskar B, Network NR. Admission temperature of low birth weight infants: predictors and associated morbidities. Pediatrics. 2007;119(3):e643–9.

[22] McCall E, Alderdice F, Halliday H, Jenkins J, Vohra S. Interventions to prevent hypothermia at birth in preterm and/or low birthweight infants. Cochrane Database Syst Rev. 2010;(3):CD004210. doi:10.1002/14651858.CD004210.pub4.

[23] Reilly MC, Vohra S, Rac VE, Dunn M, Ferrelli K, Kiss A, et al. Randomized trial of occlusive wrap for heat loss prevention in preterm infants. J Pediatr. 2015;166(2):262–8.e2. doi:10.1016/j.jpeds.2014.09.068.

[24] Doglioni N, Cavallin F, Mardegan V, Palatron S, Filippone M, Vecchiato L, et al. Total body polyethylene wraps for preventing hypothermia in preterm infants: a randomized trial. J Pediatr. 2014;165(2):261–6.e1. doi:10.1016/j.jpeds.2014.04.010.

[25] Leadford AE, Warren JB, Manasyan A, Chomba E, Salas AA, Schelonka R, et al. Plastic bags for prevention of hypothermia in preterm and low birth weight infants. Pediatrics. 2013;132(1):e128–34. doi:10.1542/peds.2012-2030.

[26] Trevisanuto D, Doglioni N, Cavallin F, Parotto M, Micaglio M, Zanardo V. Heat loss prevention in very preterm infants in delivery rooms: a prospective, randomized, controlled trial of polyethylene caps. J Pediatr. 2010;156(6):914–7, 7.e1. doi:10.1016/j.jpeds.2009.12.021.

[27] Cramer K, Wiebe N, Hartling L, Crumley E, Vohra S. Heat loss prevention: a systematic review of occlusive skin wrap for premature neonates. J Perinatol. 2005;25(12):763–9.

[28] Deguines C, Décima P, Pelletier A, Dégrugilliers L, Ghyselen L, Tourneux P. Variations in incubator temperature and humidity management: a survey of current practice. Acta Paediatr. 2012;101(3):230–5. doi:10.1111/j.1651-2227.2011.02492.x.

[29] Jia Y, Lin Z, Lv H, Li Y, Green R, Lin J. Effect of delivery room temperature on the admission temperature of premature infants: a randomized controlled trial. J Perinatol. 2013;33(4):264–7. doi:10.1038/jp.2012.100.

[30] Russo A, McCready M, Torres L, Theuriere C, Venturini S, Spaight M, et al. Reducing hypothermia in preterm infants following delivery. Pediatrics. 2014;133(4):E1055–E62. doi:10.1542/peds.2013-2544.

[31] Moore E, Anderson G, Bergman N, Dowswell T. Early skin-to-skin contact for mothers and their healthy newborn infants. Cochrane Database Syst Rev. 2012;(5):CD003519. doi:10.1002/14651858.CD003519.pub3.

[32] Karlsson V, Heinemann A, Sjors G, Nykvist K, Agren J. Early skin-to-skin care in extremely preterm infants: thermal balance and care environment. J Pediatr. 2012;161(3):422–6. doi:10.1016/j.jpeds.2012.02.034.

[33] Meyer M, Hou D, Ishrar N, Ishrar N, te Pas A. Initial respiratory support with cold, dry gas versus heated humidified gas and admission temperature of preterm infants. J Pediatr. 2015;166(2):245–50.e1. doi:10.1016/j.jpeds.2014.09.049.

[34] Pas A, Lopriore E, Dito I, Morley C, Walther F. Humidified and heated air during stabilization at birth improves temperature in preterm infants. Pediatrics. 2010;125(6):E1427–E32. doi:10.1542/peds.2009-2656.

[35] Stoll B, Hansen N, Sanchez P, Faix R, Poindexter B, Van Meurs K, et al. Early onset neonatal sepsis: the burden of Group B *Streptococcal* and *E. coli* disease continues. Pediatrics. 2011;127(5):817–26. doi:10.1542/peds.2010-2217.

[36] Ohlsson A, Shah V. Intrapartum antibiotics for known maternal Group B streptococcal colonization. Cochrane Database Syst Rev. 2014;(6):CD007467. doi: 10.1002/14651858.CD007467.pub4.

[37] Tzialla C, Borghesi A, Perotti GF, Garofoli F, Manzoni P, Stronati M. Use and misuse of antibiotics in the neonatal intensive care unit. J Matern Fetal Neonatal Med. 2012;25(Suppl 4):35–7. doi:10.3109/14767058.2012.714987.

[38] Kuppala V, Meinzen-Derr J, Morrow A, Schibler K. Prolonged initial empirical antibiotic treatment is associated with adverse outcomes in premature infants. J Pediatr. 2011;159(5):720–5. doi:10.1016/j.jpeds.2011.05.033.

[39] Auriti C, Ravà L, Di Ciommo V, Ronchetti MP, Orzalesi M. Short antibiotic prophylaxis for bacterial infections in a neonatal intensive care unit: a randomized controlled trial. J Hosp Infect. 2005;59(4):292–8.

[40] Stoll BJ, Hansen N, Fanaroff AA, Wright LL, Carlo WA, Ehrenkranz RA, et al. Late-onset sepsis in very low birth weight neonates: the experience of the NICHD Neonatal Research Network. Pediatrics. 2002;110(2 Pt 1):285–91.

[41] Stoll BJ, Hansen NI, Adams-Chapman I, Fanaroff AA, Hintz SR, Vohr B, et al. Neurodevelopmental and growth impairment among extremely low-birth-weight infants with neonatal infection. JAMA. 2004;292(19):2357–65.

[42] Roberts KB. Fluid and electrolytes: parenteral fluid therapy. Pediatr Rev. 2001;22(11): 380–7.

[43] Baumgart S, Costarino AT. Water and electrolyte metabolism of the micropremie. Clin Perinatol. 2000;27(1):131–46, vi–vii.

[44] Omar SA, DeCristofaro JD, Agarwal BI, La Gamma EF. Effects of prenatal steroids on water and sodium homeostasis in extremely low birth weight neonates. Pediatrics. 1999;104(3 Pt 1):482–8.

[45] Omar SA, DeCristofaro JD, Agarwal BI, LaGamma EF. Effect of prenatal steroids on potassium balance in extremely low birth weight neonates. Pediatrics. 2000;106(3):561–7.

[46] Bell EF, Acarregui MJ. Restricted versus liberal water intake for preventing morbidity and mortality in preterm infants. Cochrane Database Syst Rev. 2014;12:CD000503. doi: 10.1002/14651858.CD000503.pub3.

[47] Stewart A, Brion LP, Soll R. Diuretics for respiratory distress syndrome in preterm infants. Cochrane Database Syst Rev. 2011;(12):CD001454. doi: 10.1002/14651858.CD001454.pub3.

[48] Canani RB, Costanzo MD, Leone L, Bedogni G, Brambilla P, Cianfarani S, et al. Epigenetic mechanisms elicited by nutrition in early life. Nutr Res Rev. 2011;24(2):198–205. doi:10.1017/S0954422411000102.

[49] Stephens BE, Walden RV, Gargus RA, Tucker R, McKinley L, Mance M, et al. First-week protein and energy intakes are associated with 18-month developmental outcomes in extremely low birth weight infants. Pediatrics. 2009;123(5):1337–43. doi:10.1542/peds.2008-0211.

[50] Christmann V, Visser R, Engelkes M, de Grauw AM, van Goudoever JB, van Heijst AF. The enigma to achieve normal postnatal growth in preterm infants—using parenteral or enteral nutrition? Acta Paediatr. 2013;102(5):471–9. doi:10.1111/apa.12188.

[51] Moyses HE, Johnson MJ, Leaf AA, Cornelius VR. Early parenteral nutrition and growth outcomes in preterm infants: a systematic review and meta-analysis. Am J Clin Nutr. 2013;97(4):816–26. doi:10.3945/ajcn.112.042028.

[52] Hay WW. Aggressive nutrition of the preterm infant. Curr Pediatr Rep. 2013;1(4): 229-39. doi:10.1007/s40124-013-0026-4.

[53] Parish A, Bhatia J. Early aggressive nutrition for the premature infant. Neonatology. 2008;94(3):211–4. doi:10.1159/000143724.

[54] Ehrenkranz RA. Early, aggressive nutritional management for very low birth weight infants: what is the evidence? Semin Perinatol. 2007;31(2):48–55.

[55] Trivedi A, Sinn JK. Early versus late administration of amino acids in preterm infants receiving parenteral nutrition. Cochrane Database Syst Rev. 2013;7:CD008771. doi: 10.1002/14651858.CD008771.pub2.

[56] Klein CJ. Nutrient requirements for preterm infant formulas. J Nutr. 2002;132(6 Suppl 1):1395S–577S.

[57] Burattini I, Bellagamba MP, Spagnoli C, D'Ascenzo R, Mazzoni N, Peretti A, et al. Targeting 2.5 versus 4 g/kg/day of amino acids for extremely low birth weight infants: a randomized clinical trial. J Pediatr. 2013;163(5):1278–82.e1. doi:10.1016/j.jpeds.2013.06.075.

[58] Porcelli PJ, Jr., Sisk PM. Increased parenteral amino acid administration to extremely low-birth-weight infants during early postnatal life. J Pediatr Gastroenterol Nutr. 2002;34(2):174–9.

[59] Soghier LM, Brion LP. Cysteine, cystine or N-acetylcysteine supplementation in parenterally fed neonates. Cochrane Database Syst Rev. 2006;(4):CD004869.

[60] Tubman TR, Thompson SW, McGuire W. Glutamine supplementation to prevent morbidity and mortality in preterm infants. Cochrane Database Syst Rev. 2008;(1):CD001457. doi:10.1002/14651858.CD001457.pub3.

[61] Vlaardingerbroek H, Vermeulen MJ, Rook D, van den Akker CH, Dorst K, Wattimena JL, et al. Safety and efficacy of early parenteral lipid and high-dose amino acid administration to very low birth weight infants. J Pediatr. 2013;163(3):638–44.e1–5. doi:10.1016/j.jpeds.2013.03.059.

[62] Simmer K, Rao SC. Early introduction of lipids to parenterally-fed preterm infants. Cochrane Database Syst Rev. 2005;(2):CD005256.

[63] Simmer K, Patole SK, Rao SC. Long-chain polyunsaturated fatty acid supplementation in infants born at term. Cochrane Database Syst Rev. 2011;(12):CD000376. doi:10.1002/14651858.CD000376.pub3.

[64] Drenckpohl D, McConnell C, Gaffney S, Niehaus M, Macwan KS. Randomized trial of very low birth weight infants receiving higher rates of infusion of intravenous fat emulsions during the first week of life. Pediatrics. 2008;122(4):743–51. doi:10.1542/peds.2007-2282.

[65] Darlow BA, Graham PJ. Vitamin A supplementation to prevent mortality and short- and long-term morbidity in very low birthweight infants. Cochrane Database Syst Rev. 2011;(10):CD000501. doi:10.1002/14651858.CD000501.pub3.

[66] Darlow BA, Austin NC. Selenium supplementation to prevent short-term morbidity in preterm neonates. Cochrane Database Syst Rev. 2003;(4):CD003312.

[67] Pande S, Brion LP, Campbell DE, Gayle Y, Esteban-Cruciani NV. Lack of effect of L-carnitine supplementation on weight gain in very preterm infants. J Perinatol. 2005;25(7):470–7.

[68] Kumar M, Kabra NS, Paes B. Carnitine supplementation for preterm infants with recurrent apnea. Cochrane Database Syst Rev. 2004;(4):CD004497.

[69] Martin CR, Brown YF, Ehrenkranz RA, O'Shea TM, Allred EN, Belfort MB, et al. Nutritional practices and growth velocity in the first month of life in extremely premature infants. Pediatrics. 2009;124(2):649–57. doi:10.1542/peds.2008-3258.

[70] Agostoni C, Buonocore G, Carnielli VP, De Curtis M, Darmaun D, Decsi T, et al. Enteral nutrient supply for preterm infants: commentary from the European Society of Paediatric Gastroenterology, Hepatology and Nutrition Committee on Nutrition. J Pediatr Gastroenterol Nutr. 2010;50(1):85–91. doi:10.1097/MPG.0b013e3181adaee0.

[71] Morgan J, Young L, McGuire W. Slow advancement of enteral feed volumes to prevent necrotising enterocolitis in very low birth weight infants. Cochrane Database Syst Rev. 2015;10:CD001241. doi:10.1002/14651858.CD001241.pub6.

[72] Morgan J, Bombell S, McGuire W. Early trophic feeding versus enteral fasting for very preterm or very low birth weight infants. Cochrane Database Syst Rev. 2013;3:CD000504. doi:10.1002/14651858.CD000504.pub4.

[73] Basuki F, Hadiati DR, Turner T, McDonald S, Hakimi M. Dilute versus full strength formula in exclusively formula-fed preterm or low birth weight infants. Cochrane Database Syst Rev. 2013;11:CD007263. doi:10.1002/14651858.CD007263.pub2.

[74] Sisk PM, Lovelady CA, Gruber KJ, Dillard RG, O'Shea TM. Human milk consumption and full enteral feeding among infants who weigh ≤1250 grams. Pediatrics. 2008;121(6):e1528–33. doi:10.1542/peds.2007-2110.

[75] DeMauro SB, Abbasi S, Lorch S. The impact of feeding interval on feeding outcomes in very low birth-weight infants. J Perinatol. 2011;31(7):481–6. doi:10.1038/jp.2010.153.

[76] Premji SS, Chessell L. Continuous nasogastric milk feeding versus intermittent bolus milk feeding for premature infants less than 1500 grams. Cochrane Database Syst Rev. 2011(11):CD001819. doi:10.1002/14651858.CD001819.pub2.

[77] Jadcherla SR, Kliegman RM. Studies of feeding intolerance in very low birth weight infants: definition and significance. Pediatrics. 2002;109(3):516–7.

[78] Mihatsch WA, von Schoenaich P, Fahnenstich H, Dehne N, Ebbecke H, Plath C, et al. The significance of gastric residuals in the early enteral feeding advancement of extremely low birth weight infants. Pediatrics. 2002;109(3):457–9.

[79] Mihatsch WA, Högel J, Pohlandt F. Hydrolysed protein accelerates the gastrointestinal transport of formula in preterm infants. Acta Paediatr. 2001;90(2):196–8.

[80] Moody GJ, Schanler RJ, Lau C, Shulman RJ. Feeding tolerance in premature infants fed fortified human milk. J Pediatr Gastroenterol Nutr. 2000;30(4):408–12.

[81] Aly H, Abdel-Hady H, Khashaba M, El-Badry N. Erythromycin and feeding intolerance in premature infants: a randomized trial. J Perinatol. 2007;27(1):39–43.

[82] Nuntnarumit P, Kiatchoosakun P, Tantiprapa W, Boonkasidecha S. Efficacy of oral erythromycin for treatment of feeding intolerance in preterm infants. J Pediatr. 2006;148(5):600–5.

[83] Patole S, Rao S, Doherty D. Erythromycin as a prokinetic agent in preterm neonates: a systematic review. Arch Dis Child Fetal Neonatal Ed. 2005;90(4):F301–6.

[84] Ohlsson A, Jacobs SE. NIDCAP: a systematic review and meta-analyses of randomized controlled trials. Pediatrics. 2013;131(3):e881–93. doi:10.1542/peds.2012-2121.

[85] Committee On Fetus And Newborn And Section On Anesthesiology And Pain Medicine. Prevention and management of procedural pain in the neonate: an update. Pediatrics. 2016;137(2):1–13. doi:10.1542/peds.2015-4271.

[86] Pereira-Da-Silva L, Bergmans KI, van Kerkhoven LA, Leal F, Virella D, Videira-Amaral JM. Reducing discomfort while measuring crown-heel length in neonates. Acta Paediatr. 2006;95(6):742–6.

[87] Anand KJ, Aranda JV, Berde CB, Buckman S, Capparelli EV, Carlo W, et al. Summary proceedings from the neonatal pain-control group. Pediatrics. 2006;117(3 Pt 2):S9–S22.

[88] Bellieni CV, Buonocore G. Neonatal pain treatment: ethical to be effective. J Perinatol. 2008;28(2):87–8. doi:10.1038/sj.jp.7211899.

[89] Sharek PJ, Powers R, Koehn A, Anand KJ. Evaluation and development of potentially better practices to improve pain management of neonates. Pediatrics. 2006;118(Suppl 2):S78–86.

[90] Lago P, Garetti E, Merazzi D, Pieragostini L, Ancora G, Pirelli A, et al. Guidelines for procedural pain in the newborn. Acta Paediatr. 2009;98(6):932–9.

[91] Aranda JV, Carlo W, Hummel P, Thomas R, Lehr VT, Anand KJ. Analgesia and sedation during mechanical ventilation in neonates. Clin Ther. 2005;27(6):877–99.

[92] Pillai Riddell RR, Racine NM, Gennis HG, Turcotte K, Uman LS, Horton RE, et al. Non-pharmacological management of infant and young child procedural pain. Cochrane Database Syst Rev. 2015;12:CD006275. doi:10.1002/14651858.CD006275.pub3.

[93] Marín Gabriel M, del Rey Hurtado de Mendoza B, Jiménez Figueroa L, Medina V, Iglesias Fernández B, Vázquez Rodríguez M, et al. Analgesia with breastfeeding in addition to skin-to-skin contact during heel prick. Arch Dis Child Fetal Neonatal Ed. 2013;98(6):F499–503. doi:10.1136/archdischild-2012-302921.

[94] Cignacco EL, Sellam G, Stoffel L, Gerull R, Nelle M, Anand KJ, et al. Oral sucrose and "facilitated tucking" for repeated pain relief in preterms: a randomized controlled trial. Pediatrics. 2012;129(2):299–308. doi:10.1542/peds.2011-1879.

[95] Chermont AG, Falcão LF, de Souza Silva EH, de Cássia Xavier Balda R, Guinsburg R. Skin-to-skin contact and/or oral 25% dextrose for procedural pain relief for term newborn infants. Pediatrics. 2009;124(6):e1101–7. doi:10.1542/peds.2009-0993.

[96] Golianu B, Krane E, Seybold J, Almgren C, Anand KJ. Non-pharmacological techniques for pain management in neonates. Semin Perinatol. 2007;31(5):318–22.

[97] Stevens B, Yamada J, Lee GY, Ohlsson A. Sucrose for analgesia in newborn infants undergoing painful procedures. Cochrane Database Syst Rev. 2013;1:CD001069. doi: 10.1002/14651858.CD001069.pub4.

[98] Okan F, Coban A, Ince Z, Yapici Z, Can G. Analgesia in preterm newborns: the comparative effects of sucrose and glucose. Eur J Pediatr. 2007;166(10):1017–24.

[99] Johnston CC, Filion F, Snider L, Majnemer A, Limperopoulos C, Walker CD, et al. Routine sucrose analgesia during the first week of life in neonates younger than 31 weeks' postconceptional age. Pediatrics. 2002;110(3):523–8.

[100] Shah PS, Herbozo C, Aliwalas LL, Shah VS. Breastfeeding or breast milk for procedural pain in neonates. Cochrane Database Syst Rev. 2012;12:CD004950. doi: 10.1002/14651858.CD004950.pub3.

[101] Taddio A, Ohlsson A, Ohlsson K. WITHDRAWN: Lidocaine–prilocaine cream for analgesia during circumcision in newborn boys. Cochrane Database Syst Rev. 2015;4:CD000496. doi:10.1002/14651858.CD000496.pub2.

[102] Ohlsson A, Shah P. Paracetamol (acetaminophen) for prevention or treatment of pain in newborns. Cochrane Database Syst Rev. 2015;(6):CD011219. doi: 10.1002/14651858.CD011219.pub2.

[103] Anand KJ, Hall RW, Desai N, Shephard B, Bergqvist LL, Young TE, et al. Effects of morphine analgesia in ventilated preterm neonates: primary outcomes from the NEOPAIN randomised trial. Lancet. 2004;363(9422):1673–82.

[104] Taddio A, Lee C, Yip A, Parvez B, McNamara PJ, Shah V. Intravenous morphine and topical tetracaine for treatment of pain in [corrected] neonates undergoing central line placement. JAMA. 2006;295(7):793–800.

[105] Carbajal R, Lenclen R, Jugie M, Paupe A, Barton BA, Anand KJ. Morphine does not provide adequate analgesia for acute procedural pain among preterm neonates. Pediatrics. 2005;115(6):1494–500.

[106] Anand KJ, Anderson BJ, Holford NH, Hall RW, Young T, Shephard B, et al. Morphine pharmacokinetics and pharmacodynamics in preterm and term neonates: secondary results from the NEOPAIN trial. Br J Anaesth. 2008;101(5):680–9. doi:10.1093/bja/aen248.

[107] Simons SH, van Dijk M, van Lingen RA, Roofthooft D, Duivenvoorden HJ, Jongeneel N, et al. Routine morphine infusion in preterm newborns who received ventilatory support: a randomized controlled trial. JAMA. 2003;290(18):2419–27.

[108] El Sayed MF, Taddio A, Fallah S, De Silva N, Moore AM. Safety profile of morphine following surgery in neonates. J Perinatol. 2007;27(7):444–7.

[109] Rouss K, Gerber A, Albisetti M, Hug M, Bernet V. Long-term subcutaneous morphine administration after surgery in newborns. J Perinat Med. 2007;35(1):79–81.

[110] Hall RW, Boyle E, Young T. Do ventilated neonates require pain management? Semin Perinatol. 2007;31(5):289–97.

[111] Hall RW, Kronsberg SS, Barton BA, Kaiser JR, Anand KJ, Group NTI. Morphine, hypotension, and adverse outcomes among preterm neonates: who's to blame? Secondary results from the NEOPAIN trial. Pediatrics. 2005;115(5):1351–9.

[112] Pereira e Silva Y, Gomez RS, Marcatto JeO, Maximo TA, Barbosa RF, Simões e Silva AC. Morphine versus remifentanil for intubating preterm neonates. Arch Dis Child Fetal Neonatal Ed. 2007;92(4):F293–4.

[113] Roberts KD, Leone TA, Edwards WH, Rich WD, Finer NN. Premedication for nonemergent neonatal intubations: a randomized, controlled trial comparing atropine and fentanyl to atropine, fentanyl, and mivacurium. Pediatrics. 2006;118(4):1583–91.

[114] Ancora G, Lago P, Garetti E, Pirelli A, Merazzi D, Mastrocola M, et al. Efficacy and safety of continuous infusion of fentanyl for pain control in preterm newborns on mechanical ventilation. J Pediatr. 2013;163(3):645–51.e1. doi:10.1016/j.jpeds.2013.02.039.

[115] Hall RW, Shbarou RM. Drugs of choice for sedation and analgesia in the neonatal ICU. Clin Perinatol. 2009;36(2):215–26, vii. doi:10.1016/j.clp.2009.04.001.

[116] Saarenmaa E, Neuvonen PJ, Huttunen P, Fellman V. Ketamine for procedural pain relief in newborn infants. Arch Dis Child Fetal Neonatal Ed. 2001;85(1):F53–6.

[117] Ng E, Taddio A, Ohlsson A. Intravenous midazolam infusion for sedation of infants in the neonatal intensive care unit. Cochrane Database Syst Rev. 2012;6:CD002052. doi:10.1002/14651858.CD002052.pub2.

[118] Ranger M, Chau CM, Garg A, Woodward TS, Beg MF, Bjornson B, et al. Neonatal pain-related stress predicts cortical thickness at age 7 years in children born very preterm. PLoS One. 2013;8(10):e76702. doi:10.1371/journal.pone.0076702.

[119] Anand KJ, Palmer FB, Papanicolaou AC. Repetitive neonatal pain and neurocognitive abilities in ex-preterm children. Pain. 2013;154(10):1899–901. doi:10.1016/j.pain.2013.06.027.

[120] de Graaf J, van Lingen RA, Simons SH, Anand KJ, Duivenvoorden HJ, Weisglas-Kuperus N, et al. Long-term effects of routine morphine infusion in mechanically ventilated neonates on children's functioning: five-year follow-up of a randomized controlled trial. Pain. 2011;152(6):1391–7. doi:10.1016/j.pain.2011.02.017.

[121] Bellù R, de Waal K, Zanini R. Opioids for neonates receiving mechanical ventilation: a systematic review and meta-analysis. Arch Dis Child Fetal Neonatal Ed. 2010;95(4):F241–51. doi:10.1136/adc.2008.150318.

[122] Rozé JC, Denizot S, Carbajal R, Ancel PY, Kaminski M, Arnaud C, et al. Prolonged sedation and/or analgesia and 5-year neurodevelopment outcome in very preterm infants: results from the EPIPAGE cohort. Arch Pediatr Adolesc Med. 2008;162(8):728–33. doi:10.1001/archpedi.162.8.728.

[123] Ferguson SA, Ward WL, Paule MG, Hall RW, Anand KJ. A pilot study of preemptive morphine analgesia in preterm neonates: effects on head circumference, social behavior, and response latencies in early childhood. Neurotoxicol Teratol. 2012;34(1):47–55. doi:10.1016/j.ntt.2011.10.008.

[124] Cong X, Cusson RM, Walsh S, Hussain N, Ludington-Hoe SM, Zhang D. Effects of skin-to-skin contact on autonomic pain responses in preterm infants. J Pain. 2012;13(7):636–45. doi:10.1016/j.jpain.2012.02.008.

[125] Cong X, Ludington-Hoe SM, McCain G, Fu P. Kangaroo Care modifies preterm infant heart rate variability in response to heel stick pain: pilot study. Early Hum Dev. 2009;85(9):561–7. doi:10.1016/j.earlhumdev.2009.05.012.

[126] Batton B, Li L, Newman NS, Das A, Watterberg KL, Yoder BA, et al. Evolving blood pressure dynamics for extremely preterm infants. J Perinatol. 2014;34(4):301–5. doi: 10.1038/jp.2014.6.

[127] Rhee CJ, Fraser CD, Kibler K, Easley RB, Andropoulos DB, Czosnyka M, et al. The ontogeny of cerebrovascular pressure autoregulation in premature infants. J Perinatol. 2014;34(12):926–31. doi:10.1038/jp.2014.122.

[128] Kluckow M, Evans N. Superior vena cava flow in newborn infants: a novel marker of systemic blood flow. Arch Dis Child Fetal Neonatal Ed. 2000;82(3):F182–7.

[129] Evans N, Kluckow M, Simmons M, Osborn D. Which to measure, systemic or organ blood flow? Middle cerebral artery and superior vena cava flow in very preterm infants. Arch Dis Child Fetal Neonatal Ed. 2002;87(3):F181–4.

[130] Soleymani S, Borzage M, Seri I. Hemodynamic monitoring in neonates: advances and challenges. J Perinatol. 2010;30(Suppl):S38–45. doi:10.1038/jp.2010.101.

[131] Tataranno ML, Alderliesten T, de Vries LS, Groenendaal F, Toet MC, Lemmers PM, et al. Early oxygen-utilization and brain activity in preterm infants. PLoS One. 2015;10(5):e0124623. Doi:10.1371/journal.pone.0124623.

[132] Pichler G, Avian A, Binder C, Zotter H, Schmölzer GM, Morris N, et al. aEEG and NIRS during transition and resuscitation after birth: promising additional tools; an observational study. Resuscitation. 2013;84(7):974–8. Doi:10.1016/j.resuscitation.2012.12.025.

[133] Kaiser JR, Gauss CH, Williams DK. The effects of hypercapnia on cerebral autoregulation in ventilated very low birth weight infants. Pediatr Res. 2005;58(5):931–5.

[134] Pellicer A, Valverde E, Elorza MD, Madero R, Gayá F, Quero J, et al. Cardiovascular support for low birth weight infants and cerebral hemodynamics: a randomized, blinded, clinical trial. Pediatrics. 2005;115(6):1501–12.

[135] Kusaka T, Okubo K, Nagano K, Isobe K, Itoh S. Cerebral distribution of cardiac output in newborn infants. Arch Dis Child Fetal Neonatal Ed. 2005;90(1):F77–8.

[136] Faust K, Härtel C, PreußM, Rabe H, Roll C, Emeis M, et al. Short-term outcome of very-low-birthweight infants with arterial hypotension in the first 24 h of life. Arch Dis Child Fetal Neonatal Ed. 2015;100(5):F388–92. Doi:10.1136/archdischild-2014-306483.

[137] Munro MJ, Walker AM, Barfield CP. Hypotensive extremely low birth weight infants have reduced cerebral blood flow. Pediatrics. 2004;114(6):1591–6.

[138] Lynch SK, Mullett MD, Graeber JE, Polak MJ. A comparison of albumin-bolus therapy versus normal saline-bolus therapy for hypotension in neonates. J Perinatol. 2008;28(1): 29–33.

[139] Osborn DA, Evans N. Early volume expansion for prevention of morbidity and mortality in very preterm infants. Cochrane Database Syst Rev. 2004;(2):CD002055.

[140] Subhedar NV, Shaw NJ. Dopamine versus dobutamine for hypotensive preterm infants. Cochrane Database Syst Rev. 2003;(3):CD001242.

[141] Sassano-Higgins S, Friedlich P, Seri I. A meta-analysis of dopamine use in hypotensive preterm infants: blood pressure and cerebral hemodynamics. J Perinatol. 2011;31(10): 647–55. Doi:10.1038/jp.2011.2.

[142] Ibrahim H, Sinha IP, Subhedar NV. Corticosteroids for treating hypotension in preterm infants. Cochrane Database Syst Rev. 2011;(12):CD003662. Doi: 10.1002/14651858.CD003662.pub4.

[143] Finer NN, Powers RJ, Ou CH, Durand D, Wirtschafter D, Gould JB, et al. Prospective evaluation of postnatal steroid administration: a 1-year experience from the California Perinatal Quality Care Collaborative. Pediatrics. 2006;117(3):704–13.

[144] Noori S, Seri I. Neonatal blood pressure support: the use of inotropes, lusitropes, and other vasopressor agents. Clin Perinatol. 2012;39(1):221–38. Doi:10.1016/j.clp. 2011.12.010.

[145] Alderliesten T, Lemmers PM, van Haastert IC, de Vries LS, Bonestroo HJ, Baerts W, et al. Hypotension in preterm neonates: low blood pressure alone does not affect neurodevelopmental outcome. J Pediatr. 2014;164(5):986–91. Doi:10.1016/j.jpeds.2013.12.042.

[146] Batton B, Li L, Newman NS, Das A, Watterberg KL, Yoder BA, et al. Use of antihypotensive therapies in extremely preterm infants. Pediatrics. 2013;131(6):e1865–73. Doi: 10.1542/peds.2012-2779.

[147] Batton B, Zhu X, Fanaroff J, Kirchner HL, Berlin S, Wilson-Costello D, et al. Blood pressure, anti-hypotensive therapy, and neurodevelopment in extremely preterm infants. J Pediatr. 2009;154(3):351–7, 7.e1. doi:10.1016/j.jpeds.2008.09.017.

[148] Logan JW, 'O'Shea TM, Allred EN, Laughon MM, Bose CL, Dammann O, et al. Early postnatal hypotension and developmental delay at 24 months of age among extremely low gestational age newborns. Arch Dis Child Fetal Neonatal Ed. 2011;96(5):F321–8. Doi:10.1136/adc.2010.183335.

[149] Bishara N, Ohls RK. Current controversies in the management of the anemia of prematurity. Semin Perinatol. 2009;33(1):29–34. Doi:10.1053/j.semperi.2008.10.006.

[150] Whyte RK. Neurodevelopmental outcome of extremely low-birth-weight infants randomly assigned to restrictive or liberal hemoglobin thresholds for blood transfusion. Semin Perinatol. 2012;36(4):290–3. Doi:10.1053/j.semperi.2012.04.010.

[151] Kirpalani H, Whyte RK, Andersen C, Asztalos EV, Heddle N, Blajchman MA, et al. The Premature Infants in Need of Transfusion (PINT) study: a randomized, controlled trial

of a restrictive (low) versus liberal (high) transfusion threshold for extremely low birth weight infants. J Pediatr. 2006;149(3):301–7.

[152] Backes CH, Rivera BK, Haque U, Bridge JA, Smith CV, Hutchon DJ, et al. Placental transfusion strategies in very preterm neonates: a systematic review and meta-analysis. Obstet Gynecol. 2014;124(1):47–56. Doi:10.1097/AOG.0000000000000324.

[153] Committee on Obstetric Practice, American College of Obstetricians and Gynecologists. Committee Opinion No.543: Timing of umbilical cord clamping after birth. Obstet Gynecol. 2012;120(6):1522–6. Doi:10.1097/01.AOG.0000423817.47165.48.

[154] Rabe H, Diaz-Rossello JL, Duley L, Dowswell T. Effect of timing of umbilical cord clamping and other strategies to influence placental transfusion at preterm birth on maternal and infant outcomes. Cochrane Database Syst Rev. 2012;8:CD003248. Doi: 10.1002/14651858.CD003248.pub3.

[155] Rabe H, Jewison A, Alvarez RF, Crook D, Stilton D, Bradley R, et al. Milking compared with delayed cord clamping to increase placental transfusion in preterm neonates: a randomized controlled trial. Obstet Gynecol. 2011;117(2 Pt 1):205–11. Doi:10.1097/AOG.0b013e3181fe46ff.

[156] Aladangady N, McHugh S, Aitchison TC, Wardrop CA, Holland BM. 'Infants' blood volume in a controlled trial of placental transfusion at preterm delivery. Pediatrics. 2006;117(1):93–8.

[157] Aher SM, Ohlsson A. Late erythropoietin for preventing red blood cell transfusion in preterm and/or low birth weight infants. Cochrane Database Syst Rev. 2014;4:CD004868. Doi:10.1002/14651858.CD004868.pub4.

[158] Ohls RK, Kamath-Rayne BD, Christensen RD, Wiedmeier SE, Rosenberg A, Fuller J, et al. Cognitive outcomes of preterm infants randomized to darbepoetin, erythropoietin, or placebo. Pediatrics. 2014;133(6):1023–30. Doi:10.1542/peds.2013-4307.

[159] Benitz WE, Committee on Fetus and Newborn. Patent ductus arteriosus in preterm infants. Pediatrics. 2016;137(1):1–6. Doi:10.1542/peds.2015-3730.

[160] Fanaroff AA, Stoll BJ, Wright LL, Carlo WA, Ehrenkranz RA, Stark AR, et al. Trends in neonatal morbidity and mortality for very low birthweight infants. Am J Obstet Gynecol. 2007;196(2):147.e1–8.

[161] Ohlsson A, Walia R, Shah SS. Ibuprofen for the treatment of patent ductus arteriosus in preterm or low birth weight (or both) infants. Cochrane Database Syst Rev. 2015;2:CD003481. Doi:10.1002/14651858.CD003481.pub6.

[162] Herrera C, Holberton J, Davis P. Prolonged versus short course of indomethacin for the treatment of patent ductus arteriosus in preterm infants. Cochrane Database Syst Rev. 2007;(2):CD003480.

[163] Neumann R, Schulzke SM, Bührer C. Oral ibuprofen versus intravenous ibuprofen or intravenous indomethacin for the treatment of patent ductus arteriosus in preterm

infants: a systematic review and meta-analysis. Neonatology. 2012;102(1):9–15. Doi: 10.1159/000335332.

[164] Malviya MN, Ohlsson A, Shah SS. Surgical versus medical treatment with cyclooxygenase inhibitors for symptomatic patent ductus arteriosus in preterm infants. Cochrane Database Syst Rev. 2013;3:CD003951. Doi:10.1002/14651858.CD003951.pub3.

[165] Fowlie PW, Davis PG, McGuire W. Prophylactic intravenous indomethacin for preventing mortality and morbidity in preterm infants. Cochrane Database Syst Rev. 2010;(7):CD000174. Doi:10.1002/14651858.CD000174.pub2.

[166] Gournay V, Roze JC, Kuster A, Daoud P, Cambonie G, Hascoet JM, et al. Prophylactic ibuprofen versus placebo in very premature infants: a randomised, double-blind, placebo-controlled trial. Lancet. 2004;364(9449):1939–44.

[167] Van Overmeire B, Allegaert K, Casaer A, Debauche C, Decaluwé W, Jespers A, et al. Prophylactic ibuprofen in premature infants: a multicentre, randomised, double-blind, placebo-controlled trial. Lancet. 2004;364(9449):1945–9.

[168] Abu-Shaweesh JM, Martin RJ. Neonatal apnea: 'what's new? Pediatr Pulmonol. 2008;43(10):937–44. Doi:10.1002/ppul.20832.

[169] Eichenwald EC, Committee on Fetus and Newborn. Apnea of prematurity. Pediatrics. 2016;137(1):1–7. Doi:10.1542/peds.2015-3757.

[170] Schmidt B, Roberts RS, Davis P, Doyle LW, Barrington KJ, Ohlsson A, et al. Caffeine therapy for apnea of prematurity. N Engl J Med. 2006;354(20):2112–21.

[171] Davis PG, Schmidt B, Roberts RS, Doyle LW, Asztalos E, Haslam R, et al. Caffeine for apnea of prematurity trial: benefits may vary in subgroups. J Pediatr. 2010;156(3):382–7. Doi:10.1016/j.jpeds.2009.09.069.

[172] Lodha A, Seshia M, McMillan DD, Barrington K, Yang J, Lee SK, et al. Association of early caffeine administration and neonatal outcomes in very preterm neonates. JAMA Pediatr. 2015;169(1):33–8. Doi:10.1001/jamapediatrics.2014.2223.

[173] Henderson-Smart DJ, Davis PG. Prophylactic methylxanthines for endotracheal extubation in preterm infants. Cochrane Database Syst Rev. 2010;(12):CD000139. Doi: 10.1002/14651858.CD000139.pub2.

[174] Schmidt B, Roberts RS, Davis P, Doyle LW, Barrington KJ, Ohlsson A, et al. Long-term effects of caffeine therapy for apnea of prematurity. N Engl J Med. 2007;357(19):1893–902.

[175] Schmidt B, Anderson PJ, Doyle LW, Dewey D, Grunau RE, Asztalos EV, et al. Survival without disability to age 5 years after neonatal caffeine therapy for apnea of prematurity. JAMA. 2012;307(3):275–82. Doi:10.1001/jama.2011.2024.

[176] Doyle LW, Schmidt B, Anderson PJ, Davis PG, Moddemann D, Grunau RE, et al. Reduction in developmental coordination disorder with neonatal caffeine therapy. J Pediatr. 2014;165(2):356–9.e2. doi:10.1016/j.jpeds.2014.04.016.

[177] Watterberg KL, American Academy of Pediatrics. Committee on Fetus and Newborn. Policy statement—postnatal corticosteroids to prevent or treat bronchopulmonary dysplasia. Pediatrics. 2010;126(4):800–8. Doi:10.1542/peds.2010-1534.

[178] Tanney K, Davis J, Halliday HL, Sweet DG. Extremely low-dose dexamethasone to facilitate extubation in mechanically ventilated preterm babies. Neonatology. 2011;100(3):285–9. Doi:10.1159/000326273.

[179] Hitzert MM, Benders MJ, Roescher AM, van Bel F, de Vries LS, Bos AF. Hydrocortisone vs. dexamethasone treatment for bronchopulmonary dysplasia and their effects on general movements in preterm infants. Pediatr Res. 2012;71(1):100–6. Doi:10.1038/pr.2011.15.

6

Respiratory Care of the Neonate

Štefan Grosek and Petja Fister

Abstract

The respiratory distress is a very common condition both in term and in preterm neonates and the most frequent reason for admission to the neonatal intensive care unit (NICU). The aetiology greatly depends on the maturation of neonate's organs and perinatal events. The clinical picture is sometimes scarce and very nonspecific for the etiologic determination. Treatment of neonatal RD begins first with the application of a mixture of oxygen and air, then with different modes of non-invasive respiratory support methods. Non-invasive respiratory support can be sustained with nasal continuous positive airway pressure, bi-level positive airway pressure and high-flow nasal cannula ventilation. Non-invasive ventilation with high-frequency oscillations through nasal cannula or masks is also possible with some respiratory devices. Non-invasive ventilation is usually combined with the application of natural surfactant and other therapeutic means, like methylxanthine therapy, prevention and closure of patent ductus arteriosus, and control of infection. In the case of non-invasive ventilation failure, different kinds of invasive ventilation methods are available and being practiced in NICUs. The invasive respiratory support can be maintained by controlled or intermittent mandatory ventilation combined with different supportive synchronous positive inspiratory ventilation, offered by modern respirators.

Keywords: neonate, respiration, ventilation, oxygenation, perfusion, evidence-based therapy, surfactant, respiratory distress

1. Introduction

The lung is the only organ during foetal development that remains dormant, although foetal breathing occurs; gas exchange is performed by the placenta, but the lung is completely ready for transition to extra-uterine life. Its development and maturation are precisely regulated during foetal life and needed to accomplish readiness for extra-uterine exchange of gases. During labour, different obstetric and non-obstetric factors may affect lung inflation in transitional period to extra-uterine life.

Even mature neonates have smaller diameter of the airways in comparison to infants, children and also adults; their chest wall is more compliant and the lung volume at the end of expiration is the same as the closing volume. Therefore, their lungs are prone to collapse. Besides, the neonates have fewer alveoli with ventilation perfusion mismatch, but a two–three–fold increase in oxygen demand in comparison to adults [1]. They have relatively inefficient respiratory muscles due to lack of red respiratory muscles and more white ones, which get tired faster. Their pulmonary vascular wall contains more muscle fibres and is therefore more prone to vasoconstriction. The sudden falls in partial oxygen pressure result quickly after short hyperpnoea in hypopnoea or apnoea. The foetal haemoglobin binds oxygen with greater affinity than adult haemoglobin. Neonates also have immature immune system with lack of the acquired immunity against microorganisms and are thus more prone to infection. In a premature infant, all these differences in lung development are more prominent in comparison to the term neonate and further influence the transitional period of extra-uterine life.

Because of all the above-mentioned developmental immaturity of the lungs, heart, blood vessels, circulation and immune system, neonates are more prone to develop idiopathic respiratory distress (RD) at the beginning of the life but also in later days and weeks and these differences are even more pronounced in premature and very premature neonates. The aetiology and pathophysiology of the RD differ between mature and premature infants [2]. In the most extreme prematurity, several forms of RD syndrome or hyaline membrane disease (HMD) may develop because of lack of surfactant and underdevelopment of the lung.

RD is very common in neonates, affecting about 10% of them [3]. Some of them have disorders of transition from foetal to extra-uterine life; others have RD caused by congenital or acquired infection or congenital malformations of different organs (thoracic and extra-thoracic). Regarding perinatal and labour history, gestational age and appropriateness of birth measures, the aetiology of the neonatal RD could be suspected. Clinical picture of neonatal RD is rather nonspecific in regard to the aetiology of it and also the management is quite universal. RD may develop immediately and acutely after birth or more slowly in the next few hours depending on the cause of neonatal breathing difficulties [4].

According to the situation in the delivery room, we have to decide how to approach the neonate with breathing difficulties. A well-equipped and trained neonatology team should be available during all difficult or premature deliveries which have to follow recommended resuscitation care of the neonate. The first golden minutes are the most important not only to properly recognize a neonate who needs our support but also to apply appropriate, sufficient and not too aggressive support if not needed. Appropriate inspiratory pressure and oxygen therapy during artificial ventilation in the delivery room may prevent immediate and later complications especially in the most vulnerable extreme premature infants. Prevention of hypothermia, in premature neonates with plastic bag, is also one of the important preventable methods because it may prevent severe metabolic derangements due to hypothermia, harmful for all organs [5].

2. Methods

We conducted electronic searches of articles on respiratory management and care of neonates with RD, using key terms: neonate, respiration, ventilation, oxygenation, oxygen, evidence based therapy, caffeine, surfactant, respiratory distress in the PubMed data base from the years 2000 to 2017 and reported the most relevant ones. Also, consensus guidelines on neonates with RD were reviewed [6]. The article describes transition from intra- to extra-uterine life, lists the methods for assessment of neonates with RD, describes the respiratory support in the delivery room, treatment with methylxantines, oxygen and surfactant, and the non-invasive and invasive tools for artificial ventilation.

This chapter includes the impact of optimal ventilation, tissue oxygenation and perfusion on the non-invasive and invasive respiratory management of neonates with RD. Also, the short- and long-term outcome in respect of respiratory management of neonates in the neonatal intensive care unit (NICU) is addressed.

3. Transition from foetal to extra-uterine life

The transition from foetal to extra-uterine life is a process of rapid physiologic changes in the neonate that begin in utero as the foetus prepares for transition from intrauterine placental support to extra-uterine self-maintenance. The process can last for up to 12 h after birth and depends on the gestational age, placenta, maternal health and congenital anomalies of the neonate. The foetus is preparing to the transition by foetal breathing, producing surfactant storing glycogen in the liver, producing catecholamines and depositing brown fat. After the umbilical cord is cut, placenta no longer does the work of lungs as they begin to exchange gasses. The first breath inflates the lungs and causes circulatory changes: the resistance to blood flow through lungs falls and more blood flows through pulmonary arteries to the lungs. Three foetal shunts close and this results in neonatal circulation. The three processes of the transition—(1) the replacement of amniotic fluid in the alveoli with air, (2) the onset of regular breathing and (3) the increase in pulmonary blood flow—may all be deranged soon after birth and RD ensues [7]. The failure of alveoli fluid clearance results in transient tachypnoea of the newborn (TTN) and causes in turn decreased lung compliance. The deficiency of surfactant mainly in preterm neonates or in term infants of diabetic mothers causes collapse of the alveoli and diffuse and progressive atelectasis that result in decreased lung compliance and small functional residual capacity (FRC) and cause HMD. The abnormal persistence of elevated pulmonary vascular resistance either due to underdevelopment, maldevelopment or maladaptation of pulmonary vessels results in persistent pulmonary hypertension of a newborn (PPHN). PPHN is often associated with congenital anomalies (i.e. congenital diaphragmatic hernia) or chronic intrauterine stress (meconium aspiration syndrome (MAS)).

At the time of birth, the umbilical cord is still pulsating. For term and preterm neonates, delayed cord clamping is recommended. The preterm neonates born before 32 weeks of gestation with delayed cord clamping had better neuro-developmental outcomes at the age of 18 months [8, 9]. Too early umbilical vein clamping, even before the first breath of the neonate, may lead to a prolonged period of low cardiac output, which along with the undeveloped self-regulation system leads to a reduction of brain blood flow. Delayed cord clamping allows blood to enter the neonate's circulation and by that enhances the performance of the left ventricle, which is the most important for the normal cardiac output and stable haemodynamics especially in foetal distress with compromised haemodynamics at birth [10].

4. Assessment of the respiratory distress of the neonate

The evaluation of a neonate with RD is based on clinical, laboratory and radiologic investigations. In clinical evaluation, the respiratory effort, breathing efficacy and the breathing effect on other organs are assessed (**Table 1**). Signs of respiratory effort may be less pronounced or not visible in three cases: (1) the neonate, who has had RD for a long time, eventually becomes tired and signs of respiratory effort are reduced. Tiredness is a pre-terminal sign of respiratory failure. (2) A neonate with central nervous depression because of either intoxication, or encephalopathy, brain malformation, or increased intracranial pressure, breathes insufficiently without increased respiratory effort. These neonates breathe insufficiently due to reduced breathing impulse. (3) A neonate with neuromuscular disease may have respiratory failure without a significantly seen respiratory effort.

Classic laboratory signs of respiratory failure include acidosis (pH < 7.25), hypoxia (PaO_2 < 50–60 mm Hg (6.7–8 kPa), FiO_2 0.6–0.8) and hypercapnia ($PaCO_2$ > 60 mm Hg (8 kPa)) which are late signs of RD. Radiologically, neonatal chest may be scanned by X-rays [11, 12] or, lately more in use, by ultrasound (US) waves [13–17]. In utero, routine foetal US scan following development and screening for malformations may reveal intra- or extra-thoracic malformations, better differentiated by magnetic resonance imaging (MRI). Combining the risk and etiologic factors for neonatal RD, gestational age and radiologic investigations, the pulmonary disease causing the RD may be diagnosed (**Table 2**), since the clinical picture and laboratory signs are almost not of any help in defining the aetiology of neonatal RD.

	Respiratory effort	Breathing efficacy	Effect on other organs
1.	Breathing rate	Chest movement	Heart rate
2.	Intercostal, jugular, supraclavicular or subcostal retractions	Chest auscultation	Skin colour: cyanosis, paleness, mottled skin
3.	Auscultatory phenomena	Arterial blood oxygen saturation	Disturbance of consciousness
4.	Feeding difficulties		
5.	Expiratory grunting		
6.	Use of auxiliary respiratory muscles		
7.	Nasal flaring, head nodding		
8.	Gasping		

Table 1. The clinical assessment of airway and breathing in a neonate.

Pulmonary disease	Gestational age, risk factors	Aetiology	Roentgenogram	Ultrasound
Hyaline membrane disease	• Preterm • Neonates of diabetic mothers	Lack of surfactant	Diffuse reticulogranular ground glass pattern with air bronchograms and small-lung volume; grading from mild (grade 1) to the most severe pattern (grade 4)	Coalescent B-lines-'white lung', thickened and irregular pleural line
Transitional tachypnoea of the newborn	• Late preterm • Elective caesarean section	Failure of adequate alveoli fluid clearance at birth	Bilateral perihilar linear streaking, patchy infiltrates	Compact B-lines in the inferior and less compact in the superior fields (double lung point) or bilateral numerous noncompact B-lines and normal pleural line and pleural sliding
Persistent pulmonary hypertension	• Term > preterm • Perinatal depression	Persistence of elevated pulmonary vascular resistance	Clear lung fields with decreased pulmonary vascularity	Echocardiography
Meconium aspiration syndrome	• Term • Perinatal depression	Meconium-stained amniotic fluid	Patchy infiltrates	Pulmonary consolidation with air bronchograms, pleural line anomalies, pleural effusion, B-lines in non-consolidation area
Pneumonia	Infection of the mother	Bacterial or viral infection	Non-symmetric bilateral patchy infiltrates	Subpleural consolidation
Pneumothorax	Preterm > term	Air entrance into the pleural space	Edge of collapsed lung	Absence of pleura sliding and B-lines, subpleural consolidation
Congenital heart defect	Term > preterm		May be diagnostic	Echocardiography diagnostic
Congenital malformation of organs	Term>preterm		Diagnostic	
Metabolic, neuromuscular diseases	Term > preterm		Normal	
Genetic defect of surfactant proteins	Term, preterm	lack of surfactant proteins	Diffuse reticulogranular ground glass pattern with air bronchograms and small lung volume; grading from mild (grade 1) to most severe (grade 4) Chronic lung disease of different patterns	

Table 2. The etiologic and radiologic assessment of respiratory state of a neonate.

5. Respiratory support in delivery room

Routine care in delivery room depends on whether we expect and take care of extreme premature neonates or near term or term neonates with breathing difficulties. In case of near term or term neonates, care starts with providing warmth, clearing airway if necessary, drying and stimulating the neonate. Care of preterm infants is different because we immediately place him/her into a heated polyethylene bag with small opening for the nose and mouth and further stabilize him/her under the heater to assure normal body temperature, prevent hypothermia and desiccation [18]. The stabilization of the neonate with RD in the delivery room comprises proper head positioning with wiping of the mouth, and rarely, in the case of more secretion, not removed by wiping, we may perform gentle suction of the neonate's mouth, then nose. We have to avoid the deep insertion of the catheter and vigorous suctioning of mouth which may cause reflex bradycardia. In the case of meconium staining and aspiration, suction of trachea under visual inspection with laryngoscopy guidance is needed first and then intubation and further washing out meconium from the trachea. In case of apnoea, gasping or bradycardia of <100 beats/minute, it is necessary to ventilate neonate's lungs with positive pressure ventilation considering the use of lowest effective inspiratory pressures and volumes to prevent damage to the lungs (barotrauma and volutrauma). Ventilation should fill neonatal lung with a gas mixture of air and oxygen. To prevent and reduce the oxidative stress, caused by excessive use of oxygen in the inspired air, it is necessary to be careful with the use of oxygen. For measuring the arterial oxygen saturation (SpO_2) in the peripheral blood, the pulse oximeter should be attached to the right wrist [19]. Latest guidelines recommend starting ventilation of term neonates with FiO_2 0.21 and later increasing the FiO_2 according to the value of the measured SpO_2. Ventilation of preterm neonates should be started with FiO_2 of 0.21, gradually rising the FiO_2 in accordance with the measured value of SpO_2. Ventilation of the extremely premature infants (born before 28 weeks gestation) should be started with FiO_2 0.30, while of very premature infants (28–31 weeks of gestation) with the FiO_2 from 0.21 to 0.30. If neonate is spontaneously breathing, the constant positive pressure is applied for the stabilization of respiration (continuous positive airway pressure) of 6 cm of H_2O through a mask, nasal tubes or endotracheal tube using neonatal respirator (neonatal resuscitator; T-piece device), intended for stabilization of the neonate in the delivery room. The maximum positive inspiratory pressure should not exceed 20–25 cm H_2O, which is used only in the case of apnoea or bradycardia [6]. No differences in mortality and morbidity of premature neonates have been demonstrated in comparing resuscitation starting with low (FiO_2 ≤0.30) or high levels of oxygen (FiO_2 ≥0.6) [20]. Currently, there is insufficient evidence of sustained lung inflation efficacy and safety in the cardiopulmonary resuscitation and stabilization of the neonate in the delivery room [21, 22].

6. Methylxanthines

Methylxanthines stimulate the respiratory centre to increase its responsiveness to the partial pressure of carbon dioxide in the blood and reduce respiratory depression by hypoxia. They also improve respiratory muscle strength. Therapy with caffeine has proven to reduce the duration of artificial ventilation and oxygen demand and decrease risk for bronchopulmonary dysplasia (BPD) and the need for patent ductus arteriosus (PDA) ligation [23, 24]. At the age of 2 years, positive effects on cognitive development were observed, but in the same group of children at the age of 5 years they were no longer detected [25]. In a premature neonate with RD, the less invasive artificial ventilation and surfactant therapy are usually combined with early prophylactic intravenous administration of caffeine to achieve the highest level of respiratory support in the least invasive form [26, 27]. Since methylxanthines affect the diaphragmatic activity and increase the tidal volume, we may use them to increase the muscle strength in floppy neonates [28].

7. Treatment with oxygen

Oxygen is necessary for aerobic metabolic processes in the body. The excess of oxygen is detrimental to neonates, particularly the premature infants with immature antioxidant, anti-inflammatory mechanisms and a greater amount of free iron. Hyperoxia affects not only the lung but also other organs, with the greatest effects to central nervous system (convulsions) and eyes (retinopathy of prematurity (ROP)). In comparison with a 'higher' level of SpO_2 (91–95%), the 'lower' level (85–89%) has been shown to diminish the risk of ROP and BPD, but unfortunately at the same time increase mortality, the incidence of necrotizing enterocolitis and poor neuro-developmental outcome [29]. Based on research, current recommendations propose the SpO_2 of preterm infants who require oxygen therapy to be between 90 and 94%, setting alarm limits to 89 and 95% [6]. The SpO_2 of term neonates who require oxygen therapy should be above 92%.

Hypercapnia is associated with acidosis and compromised cardiovascular function, while hypocapnia decreases cerebral blood flow. There is some conflicting evidence on higher $PaCO_2$ levels and the impact on mortality, severe intraventricular haemorrhage (IVH), BPD, ROP and neurodevelopmental outcome [30, 31]. Therefore, the optimal target carbon dioxide levels are not established; based on available data, it should be between 46 in 60 mm Hg (6.1–8 kPa) for ventilated neonates.

Blood gas is monitored in arterial samples, so an indwelling arterial line is necessary in taking care of a neonate with moderate or severe RD. Venous and capillary samples are not appropriate for PaO_2 measurements. They may be of use for $PaCO_2$ monitoring, although they slightly overestimate it, and pH monitoring, although they slightly underestimate it.

8. Surfactant

Pulmonary surfactant, a macromolecular lipoprotein complex, secreted by the alveolar epithelial cells type II, reduces the surface tension in the pulmonary alveoli at the end of exhalation. Sufficient amount of surfactant in the mature lungs prevents complete collapse of the lungs at the end of exhalation. A part of the inhaled air remains to be 'trapped' in the pulmonary alveoli, what is called the FRC. In each subsequent breath, it is not necessary to re-open the lungs from the total collapse, which greatly reduces the work of breathing and with that fatigue and respiratory failure. A thin layer of a surfactant in the walls of the pulmonary alveoli at the end of each inspiration is not completely waterproof, some liquid passes through the pores being in contact with the air in the lung alveoli, increasing the surface tension and preventing the overdistension of the alveoli at the end of inspiration. The lung surfactant is rapidly adsorbed and easily distributed in the form of a thin film on the surface between the liquid layer and the air in the lung alveoli [32].

Several animal surfactants of bovine or porcine origin are used in Europe (**Table 3**).

Currently, a double-blind study of a synthetic surfactant, CHF5633, with the same effect in the treatment of RD as poractant alpha, but a stronger anti-inflammatory and a more favourable effect on the cerebral haemodynamics, is being conducted [33].

Early publications recommended the application of surfactant in developed RD as a 'rescue' or therapeutic administration or prophylactically for the prevention of RD in very premature infants in the first few minutes after birth. Criticism of the prophylactic administration of surfactant was that likely 27–60% of preterm infants receive surfactant unnecessarily [34, 35]. Recommendation nowadays is to stabilize the respiration of a spontaneously breathing neonate by using CPAP and early selective surfactant administration. When an endotracheal intubation is needed due to progressive RD, the neonate should obtain surfactant as soon as possible [6, 36].

Another way of avoiding lung barotrauma and especially volutrauma, techniques to shorten the duration of artificial ventilation or even completely avoiding it, has been developed in recent years. The first of such methods of fast and non-invasive surfactant application was **IN**tubate—**SUR**factant—**E**xtubate (INSURE). The extubation was followed by non-invasive respiratory support [37, 38]. In comparing early INSURE method with CPAP without the administration of the surfactant, certain advantages were found in the INSURE group. Not enough evidence was found to conclude that one of the two methods is better than the other [39].

Type of surfactant	Company name	Origin of surfactant	Lipids (%)	Proteins (%)	Dose (body mass)
Poractant alfa	Curosurf®	Extraction from porcine lungs	99	SP-B, SP-C 1%	100–200 mg/kg (1.25–2.5 ml/kg) in suspension
Bovactant	Alveofact®	Lavage from bovine lungs	99	SP-B, SP-C 1%	50 mg/kg (1.2 ml/kg) in suspension
Beractant	Survanta®	Extraction from homogenized bovine lungs	88–90	SP-B, SP-C 1%	100 mg/kg (4 ml/kg) diluted before use

Table 3. Surfactants, registered for therapy of RD in Europe.

Less **I**nvasive **S**urfactant **A**dministration (LISA) and **M**inimally **I**nvasive **S**urfactant **T**reatment (MIST) are other two less invasive methods of surfactant application. With LISA, the preterm neonate who is supported by CPAP via nasal prongs, the larynx is opened by laryngoscope and by the Magill forceps a thin and soft aspiration tube is inserted below the level of the vocal cords, and then the surfactant is applied in two to four aliquots while the neonate is spontaneously breathing. With MIST, the tube for surfactant application is somewhat stiffer and bent so it can be inserted into the larynx without the Magill forceps. According to the authors, MIST is an easier method for less skilled doctors [40]. To confirm the hypothesis that less invasive surfactant administration combined with the respiratory support by CPAP is more successful in neonates who have some natural surfactant and not effective in those who have too little of their own surfactant, a blind, multicentre, randomized study in premature neonates between 25 and ≤28 weeks gestation, requiring CPAP and a low percentage of oxygen in the inhaled air (FiO_2 from 0.30 to 0.45) during the first 6 h after birth, is currently underway. The research group is being treated with poractant alpha at a dose of 200 mg/kg body weight, and the control group receives placebo [41]. None of the above-described methods can avoid laryngoscopy.

The methods of surfactant aerosolization have up to date been more or less unsuccessful. With the **C**atheter **A**nd **L**aryngeal **M**ask **E**ndotracheal **S**urfactant **T**herapy (CALMEST) the surfactant is administered by a catheter and the laryngeal mask [42].

The oxygen requirement higher than the $FiO_2>0.3$ after 2 h of breathing with CPAP has a high positive-predictive value of a respiratory failure at 6 h after birth. Therefore, the recent recommendations suggest an early less invasive surfactant administration before the neonate requires high proportions of oxygen in the inspired air [43]. If no improvement is seen after the first dose, the surfactant application is repeated for the second or third time. In this case, the poractant alpha at a dose of 200 mg/kg body weight is supposed to have better effect as a lower dose of poractant alpha or beractant (100 mg/kg body weight).

Late-preterm and term neonates besides rarely having a primary surfactant deficiency due to genetic defect of surfactant proteins, they more often suffer from secondary surfactant deficiency in conjunction with MAS, pneumonia and pulmonary haemorrhage. In those cases small studies have shown improved oxygenation, gas exchange and a reduced need for extracorporeal membrane oxygenation (ECMO) [44].

9. Non-invasive respiratory support

The best and most frequently used treatment of neonatal RD nowadays is CPAP through nasal spouts (nasal mask, nasal cannula and nasal tube) with the addition of the interfaces by using various physical processes to insufflate and exhale the mixture of air and oxygen into and out of the respiratory tract of a neonate [45]. It has been proven to reduce side effects that neonates could suffer if they were ventilated by the invasive methods of artificial ventilation. Until now, a variety of techniques applying positive pressure of constant pressure

(CPAP), the intermittent insufflation of positive pressure (nasal intermittent positive pressure ventilation, NIPPV), which can be time determined or synchronous triggered by inhalation (synchronous nasal intermittent positive pressure ventilation (SNIPPV)) and ventilation at two levels of positive pressure (bi-level positive pressure ventilation, Bi-Level) or even with high-frequency oscillations (high-frequency oscillation ventilation (HFOV)) have been developed. Different randomized studies have explored the advantages or disadvantages of one method of non-invasive ventilatory support over the other. In comparing the non-invasive ventilation with NIPPV to the nasal CPAP, fewer respiratory failures and the need for intubation in the NIPPV group were found [46]. Meta-analysis of the use of different devices and interfaces for CPAP has elucidated differences in outcome depending on the use of nasal adapters or interfaces, requiring further research [47]. Similarly, there is an open question whether breathing with the help of bi-level CPAP is better than breathing with CPAP alone and does it pose an advantage of better exhaling CO_2, better oxygenation or other physiological indicators [48].

If higher mean inspiratory pressures are required for the lungs to remain inflated, the potential non-invasive ventilation using HFO via nasal tubes or cannulas may be used since even long-term studies have confirmed advantages of HFO non-invasive ventilation over other invasive ventilation methods.

Ventilation of neonates using high-flow rates (high-flow nasal cannula (HFNC)) has some advantages over CPAP due to less damage to the nose and nasal septa and less pneumothorax (PTX) [49]. A multicentre study being conducted in nine centres in Australia and Norway might give answers as to which breathing support is better in very preterm infants, CPAP or HFNC [50].

Nose requires special attention because the prolonged nasal respiratory therapy may cause decubitus and malformations of the nose. Regular changes of devices and protection of the nose skin and mucosa with skin-protective strips and/or creams prevent those problems. Gastric distension has to be prevented by an opened nasogastric tube and regular checking of gastric over distension which decrease compromise of diaphragm contractions. Neonatal care in term neutral environment incubators or warm beds and preventive positions like Cocoonababy® Nest or similar home-made products besides frequent changes of neonate's positions improve ventilation during the period of acute respiratory problems. Kangaroo care is a useful method to improve bonding between the neonate and the mother or father but has to be carried out cautiously during non-invasive ventilation [51]. During kangaroo care, observations have to be made whether apnoeic spells are more frequent and whether bradycardia occurs.

Non-invasive respiratory ventilation enables non-aggressive approaches, without sedation, analgesia, tracheal intubation and mechanical ventilation. Complications of non-invasive ventilation are mainly pressure sores of skin around the nose, ulceration and necrosis of the septum, much less likely hyperinflation of the lungs, restlessness, PTX, stomach distension or food intolerance. Non-invasive ventilation failure may be predicted by the use of neonatal chest US [52].

10. Invasive artificial ventilation of the neonate

Nowadays, the invasive artificial ventilation of the neonate represents a continuation of treatment in cases where non-invasive ventilation with or without the use of surfactant is not possible or successful. In invasive mechanical support ventilation with a respirator, CPAP is usually supplied in combination with intermittent mandatory or synchronized artificial ventilation (i.e. intermittent mandatory ventilation (IMV); synchronized intermittent mandatory ventilation (SIMV)). Ventilation can be sustained at two different positive pressure levels (variable/bi-level positive airway pressure, bi-level (BiPAP)). Other forms of artificial ventilation include ventilation by releasing the pressure (airway pressure release ventilation (APRV)), neuronal-mediated respiratory support (neurally adjusted ventilatory assist (NAVA)), and so on. In the case of the artificial ventilation, one should always set the concentration of a mixture of the inspired oxygen and air, the frequency of the ventilation, the ratio of duration of the inspiration and expiration or time of inspiration, the end-inspiratory pressure or the tidal volume and the end-expiratory pressure. Each respirator is equipped with the heater and humidifier in order that neonates breathe moist and warm mixture of air and oxygen. In cases of severe pulmonary disease with severe RD, high-frequency oscillating ventilators, which use very low inspiratory volumes that do not damage the lung tissue, may be used.

High-frequency oscillation ventilation is a method of artificial ventilation, which in cases of severe RD can be the least harmful way of ensuring good oxygenation and due to the active exhalation wash out carbon dioxide as well. High-frequency oscillation ventilation will only be successful if the pulmonary alveoli are optimally opened prior to the start of oscillations. In HFO, the optimization of lung volume is achieved by small increments of continuous positive distending airway pressure and the pressure in lung alveoli. Gradually, the increase of continuous positive distending airway pressure leads to opening of the small, collapsed non-ventilated lung and by that to the increment of the FRC of the lungs that ensure good ventilation and oxygenation. Consequently, the optimally opened lung tissue is then oscillated with very small tidal gas volume (order of the neonate's dead space of the lungs), which regulates the exhalation of carbon dioxide from the lungs. Oscillations with small volumes are less harmful for the delicate lung parenchyma and do not damage it, thereby preventing the secondary injury such as barotrauma and volutrauma. When lung function improves, the neonate's ventilation can be switched to conventional artificial ventilation again [53].

The most important factor in invasive artificial ventilation of the neonate is to prevent the lung over-distension, because it injures the delicate lung tissue and causes air leakage outside the airway with the development of pulmonary interstitial emphysema (PIE), PTX or pneumomediastinum (PM) and other even more severe forms the air leakage into the chest. When lungs become more compliant, the pressure-guided artificial ventilation may lead to lung over-distension, therefore many of the neonatal respirators are programmed to the restriction of tidal volume (volume-targeted ventilation; volume-guaranteed ventilation (VGV)). Care should be taken not to cause hypocapnia during ventilation since it decreases the brain blood flow and causes periventricular leukomalacia (PVL) and IVH which jeopardize the neurological development. The volume-targeted artificial ventilation was shown to shorten the duration of artificial ventilation and hypocapnia, lessen the incidence of BPD, IVH grade III/IV, PTX and PVL in comparison to the pressure-controlled ventilation in preterm neonates. The mortality rate was unaffected by the mode of artificial ventilation [54].

During intubation and invasive ventilation, neonates are prone to cardio- and cerebrovascular instability. The intensive invasive therapy subjects neonates to more infections and the invasive ventilation to volu-, barotrauma and shear stress. Common complications due to intubations and invasive ventilation are hoarseness, aphonia, tracheal stenosis, and feeding and perioral sensation disorders.

11. Additional supportive therapies for neonatal respiratory distress

For treating pulmonary hypertension in different pulmonary diseases of the neonate the inhaled nitric oxide, pulmonary artery dilator, has been shown to have some beneficial effects [55]. On the other hand it has not been shown to be beneficial in preterm neonates with RD in reducing BPD or mortality [56]; though most NICUs are using it nowadays when hypoxic respiratory failure in extreme premature cannot be solved by other means [57].

The ECMO pumps the blood through an artificial lung back into the bloodstream, providing heart-lung bypass support outside of the neonatal body. ECMO is applied in neonates with severe RD due to congenital diaphragmatic hernia (CDH), meconium aspiration syndrome (MAS), pneumonia, air leak problems or PPHN [58]. Veno-venous ECMO is preferred to be used in infants with hypoxic respiratory failure unless an arterio-venous ECMO is needed due to combined cardio-respiratory failure. ECMO support should be used only in neonates weighing ≥2 kg of body mass.

General supportive care of a neonate with RD encompasses optimization of thermal neutral environment, fluid and nutritional management and a stable hemodynamic state ensuring adequate oxygenation and perfusion of neonatal organs.

12. Conclusion

RD of a neonate has almost identical clinical picture irrespective of many etiologic entities it originates from. The perinatal history, labour course, the gestational age and appropriateness of birth measures for the gestational age should all be taken into account in diagnosing the aetiology of the RD.

The modern management of neonatal RD is minimally invasive. In the delivery room, neonates are being stabilized. The respiratory support is primarily non-invasive ventilation as well as the surfactant is applied with less invasive methods not involving intubation and artificial ventilation. If intubation is required, the time of artificial ventilation should be as short as possible. Hyperoxia and hypocapnia should be avoided. Further studies will show whether such non-invasive treatment is also going to affect the incidence of BPD, neurodevelopmental outcome and other long-term consequences of intensive neonatal therapies.

Author details

Štefan Grosek[1,2]* and Petja Fister[3]

*Address all correspondence to: stefan.grosek@kclj.si

1 Department of Pediatric Surgery and Intensive Therapy, Surgical Service, University Medical Centre Ljubljana, Ljubljana, Slovenia

2 Department of Pediatrics, Medical Faculty, University of Ljubljana, Ljubljana, Slovenia

3 Department of Neonatology, University Children's Hospital, University Medical Centre Ljubljana, Ljubljana, Slovenia

References

[1] Keszler M, Kabir Abubakar M. Physiologic principles. In: Goldsmith JP, Karotkin EH, editors. Assisted Ventilation of the Neonate. 5th ed. St. Louis: Missouri Elsevier Saunders; 2011. pp. 19-46

[2] Mehrabadi A, Lisonkova S, Joseph KS. Heterogeneity of respiratory distress syndrome: Risk factors and morbidity associated with early and late gestation disease. BMC Pregnancy Childbirth. 2016;**16**(1):281

[3] Reuter S, Moser C, Baack M. Respiratory distress in the newborn. Pediatric Review. 2014;**35**(10):417-428; quiz 29

[4] Hermansen CL, Lorah KN. Respiratory distress in the newborn. American Family Physician. 2007;**76**(7):987-994

[5] Vento M, Lista G. Managing preterm infants in the first minutes of life. Paediatric Respiratory Review. 2015;**16**(3):151-156

[6] Sweet DG, Carnielli V, Greisen G, Hallman M, Ozek E, Plavka R, et al. European Consensus Guidelines on the Management of Respiratory Distress Syndrome - 2016 Update. Neonatology. 2017;**111**(2):107-125

[7] Hooper SB, Te Pas AB, Kitchen MJ. Respiratory transition in the newborn: A three-phase process. Archives of Disease in Childhood—Fetal and Neonatal Edition. 2016; **101**(3):F266-F271

[8] Backes CH, Rivera BK, Haque U, Bridge JA, Smith CV, Hutchon DJ, et al. Placental transfusion strategies in very preterm neonates: A systematic review and meta-analysis. Obstetrics & Gynecology. 2014;**124**(1):47-56

[9] Mercer JS, Erickson-Owens DA, Vohr BR, Tucker RJ, Parker AB, Oh W, et al. Effects of placental transfusion on neonatal and 18 month outcomes in preterm infants: A randomized controlled trial. Journal of Pediatrics. 2016;**168**:50-5.e1

[10] Kluckow M, Hooper SB. Using physiology to guide time to cord clamping. Seminars in Fetal & Neonatal Medicine. 2015;**20**(4):225-231

[11] Wolfson SL, Frech R, Hewitt C, Shanklin DR. Radiographic diagnosis of hyaline membrane disease. Radiology. 1969;**93**(2):339-343

[12] Giedion A, Haefliger H, Dangel P. Acute pulmonary X-ray changes in hyaline membrane disease treated with artificial ventilation and positive end-expiratory pressure (PEP). Pediatric Radiology. 1973;**1**(3):145-152

[13] Copetti R, Cattarossi L, Macagno F, Violino M, Furlan R. Lung ultrasound in respiratory distress syndrome: A useful tool for early diagnosis. Neonatology. 2008;**94**(1):52-59

[14] Vergine M, Copetti R, Brusa G, Cattarossi L. Lung ultrasound accuracy in respiratory distress syndrome and transient tachypnea of the newborn. Neonatology. 2014;**106**(2):87-93

[15] Lovrenski J. Lung ultrasonography of pulmonary complications in preterm infants with respiratory distress syndrome. Upsala Journal of Medical Sciences. 2012;**117**(1):10-17

[16] Raimondi F, Rodriguez Fanjul J, Aversa S, Chirico G, Yousef N, De Luca D, et al. Lung ultrasound for diagnosing pneumothorax in the critically Ill neonate. Journal of Pediatrics. 2016;**175**:74-8.e1

[17] Liu J, Cao HY, Fu W. Lung ultrasonography to diagnose meconium aspiration syndrome of the newborn. Journal of International Medical Research. 2016;**44**(6):1534-1542

[18] McCall E, Alderdice F, Halliday H, Jenkins J, Vohra S. Interventions to prevent hypothermia at birth in preterm and/or low birthweight infants. Cochrane Database of Systematic Reviews. 2010;(3):CD004210. DOI: 10.1002/14651858.CD004210.pub4

[19] Mariani G, Dik PB, Ezquer A, Aguirre A, Esteban ML, Perez C, et al. Pre-ductal and post-ductal O2 saturation in healthy term neonates after birth. Journal of Pediatrics. 2007;**150**(4):418-421

[20] Oei JL, Vento M, Rabi Y, Wright I, Finer N, Rich W, et al. Higher or lower oxygen for delivery room resuscitation of preterm infants below 28 completed weeks gestation: A meta-analysis. Archives of Disease in Childhood—Fetal and Neonatal Edition. 2017;**102**(1):F24–F30

[21] McCall KE, Davis PG, Owen LS, Tingay DG. Sustained lung inflation at birth: What do we know, and what do we need to know? Archives of Disease in Childhood—Fetal and Neonatal Edition. 2016;**101**(2):F175-F180

[22] O'Donnell CP, Bruschettini M, Davis PG, Morley CJ, Moja L, Calevo MG, et al. Sustained versus standard inflations during neonatal resuscitation to prevent mortality and improve respiratory outcomes. Cochrane Database of Systematic Review. 2015;(7):CD004953. DOI: 10.1002/14651858.CD004953.pub2

[23] Schmidt B, Roberts RS, Davis P, Doyle LW, Barrington KJ, Ohlsson A, et al. Caffeine therapy for apnea of prematurity. New England Journal of Medicine. 2006;**354**(20):2112-2121

[24] Davis PG, Schmidt B, Roberts RS, Doyle LW, Asztalos E, Haslam R, et al. Caffeine for apnea of prematurity trial: Benefits may vary in subgroups. Journal of Pediatrics. 2010;**156**(3):382-387

[25] Schmidt B, Anderson PJ, Doyle LW, Dewey D, Grunau RE, Asztalos EV, et al. Survival without disability to age 5 years after neonatal caffeine therapy for apnea of prematurity. Journal of American Medical Association. 2012;**307**(3):275-282

[26] Henderson-Smart DJ, Davis PG. Prophylactic methylxanthines for endotracheal extubation in preterm infants. Cochrane Database of Systematic Review. 2010;(12):CD000139. DOI: 10.1002/14651858.CD000139.pub2

[27] Kreutzer K, Bassler D. Caffeine for apnea of prematurity: A neonatal success story. Neonatology. 2014;**105**(4):332-336

[28] Kraaijenga JV, Hutten GJ, de Jongh FH, van Kaam AH. The effect of caffeine on diaphragmatic activity and tidal volume in preterm infants. Journal of Pediatrics. 2015;**167**(1):70-75

[29] Tarnow-Mordi W, Stenson B, Kirby A, Juszczak E, Donoghoe M, Deshpande S, et al. Outcomes of two trials of oxygen-saturation targets in preterm infants. New England Journal of Medicine. 2016;**374**(8):749-760

[30] Ambalavanan N, Carlo WA, Wrage LA, Das A, Laughon M, Cotten CM, et al. PaCO2 in surfactant, positive pressure, and oxygenation randomised trial (SUPPORT). Archives of Disease in Childhood—Fetal and Neonatal Edition. 2015;**100**(2):F145-F149

[31] Thome UH, Genzel-Boroviczeny O, Bohnhorst B, Schmid M, Fuchs H, Rohde O, et al. Permissive hypercapnia in extremely low birthweight infants (PHELBI): A randomised controlled multicentre trial. The Lancet Respiratory Medicine. 2015;**3**(7):534-543

[32] Rugonyi S, Biswas SC, Hall SB. The biophysical function of pulmonary surfactant. Respiratory Physiology & Neurobiology. 2008;**163**(1-3):244-255

[33] Rey-Santano C, Mielgo VE, Murgia X, Gomez-Solaetxe MA, Salomone F, Bianco F, et al. Cerebral and lung effects of a new generation synthetic surfactant with SP-B and SP-C analogs in preterm lambs. Pediatric Pulmonology. 2017: DOI: 10.1002/ppul.23685. [Epub ahead of print

[34] Robertson B, Speer CP. OSIRIS trial. Lancet. 1993;**341**(8838):172; author reply 3-4

[35] Kattwinkel J, Bloom BT, Delmore P, Davis CL, Farrell E, Friss H, et al. Prophylactic administration of calf lung surfactant extract is more effective than early treatment of respiratory distress syndrome in neonates of 29 through 32 weeks' gestation. Pediatrics. 1993;**92**(1):90-98

[36] Bahadue FL, Soll R. Early versus delayed selective surfactant treatment for neonatal respiratory distress syndrome. Cochrane Database of Systematic Review. 2012;**11**:CD001456

[37] Bohlin K, Gudmundsdottir T, Katz-Salamon M, Jonsson B, Blennow M. Implementation of surfactant treatment during continuous positive airway pressure. Journal of Perinatology. 2007;**27**(7):422-427

[38] Verder H, Bohlin K, Kamper J, Lindwall R, Jonsson B. Nasal CPAP and surfactant for treatment of respiratory distress syndrome and prevention of bronchopulmonary dysplasia. Acta Paediatrica. 2009;**98**(9):1400-1408

[39] Isayama T, Chai-Adisaksopha C, McDonald SD. Noninvasive ventilation with vs without early surfactant to prevent chronic lung disease in preterm infants: A systematic review and meta-analysis. Journal of American Medical Association Pediatrics. 2015; **169**(8):731-739

[40] Dargaville PA, Aiyappan A, De Paoli AG, Kuschel CA, Kamlin CO, Carlin JB, et al. Minimally-invasive surfactant therapy in preterm infants on continuous positive airway pressure. Archives of Diseases in Childhood—Fetal and Neonatal Edition. 2013; **98**(2):F122–F126

[41] Dargaville PA, Kamlin CO, De Paoli AG, Carlin JB, Orsini F, Soll RF, et al. The OPTIMIST-A trial: Evaluation of minimally-invasive surfactant therapy in preterm infants 25-28 weeks gestation. BMC Pediatrics. 2014;**14**:213

[42] Vannozzi I, Ciantelli M, Moscuzza F, Scaramuzzo RT, Panizza D, Sigali E, et al. Catheter and laryngeal mask endotracheal surfactant therapy: The CALMEST approach as a novel MIST technique. The Journal of Maternal-Fetal & Neonatal Medicine. 2016:1-3. DOI: 10.1080/14767058.2016.1248938. [Epub ahead of print]

[43] Dargaville PA, Aiyappan A, De Paoli AG, Dalton RG, Kuschel CA, Kamlin CO, et al. Continuous positive airway pressure failure in preterm infants: incidence, predictors and consequences. Neonatology. 2013;**104**(1):8-14

[44] Polin RA, Carlo WA, Newborn CoFa, Pediatrics AAo. Surfactant replacement therapy for preterm and term neonates with respiratory distress. Pediatrics. 2014;**133**(1):156-163

[45] Gregory GA, Kitterman JA, Phibbs RH, Tooley WH, Hamilton WK. Treatment of the idiopathic respiratory-distress syndrome with continuous positive airway pressure. New England Journal of Medicine. 1971;**284**(24):1333-1340

[46] Lemyre B, Laughon M, Bose C, Davis PG. Early nasal intermittent positive pressure ventilation (NIPPV) versus early nasal continuous positive airway pressure (NCPAP) for preterm infants. Cochrane Database of Systematic Review. 2016;**12**:CD005384

[47] De Paoli AG, Davis PG, Faber B, Morley CJ. Devices and pressure sources for administration of nasal continuous positive airway pressure (NCPAP) in preterm neonates. Cochrane Database of Systematic Review. 2008;(1):CD002977. DOI: 10.1002/14651858. CD002977.pub2

[48] Lampland AL, Plumm B, Worwa C, Meyers P, Mammel MC. Bi-level CPAP does not improve gas exchange when compared with conventional CPAP for the treatment of neonates recovering from respiratory distress syndrome. Archives of Diseases in Childhood—Fetal and Neonatal Edition. 2015;**100**(1):F31-F34

[49] Wilkinson D, Andersen C, O'Donnell CP, De Paoli AG, Manley BJ. High flow nasal cannula for respiratory support in preterm infants. Cochrane Database of Systematic Review. 2016;**2**:CD006405

[50] Roberts CT, Owen LS, Manley BJ, Donath SM, Davis PG. A multicentre, randomised controlled, non-inferiority trial, comparing high flow therapy with nasal continuous positive airway pressure as primary support for preterm infants with respiratory distress (the HIPSTER trial): Study protocol. British Medical Journal Open. 2015;**5**(6):e008483

[51] Bloch-Salisbury E, Zuzarte I, Indic P, Bednarek F, Paydarfar D. Kangaroo care: Cardio-respiratory relationships between the infant and caregiver. Early Human Development. 2014;**90**(12):843-850

[52] Raimondi F, Migliaro F, Sodano A, Ferrara T, Lama S, Vallone G, et al. Use of neonatal chest ultrasound to predict noninvasive ventilation failure. Pediatrics. 2014;**134**(4):e1089-e1094

[53] Keszler M, Sant'Anna G. Mechanical ventilation and bronchopulmonary dysplasia. Clinical Perinatology. 2015;**42**(4):781-796

[54] Peng W, Zhu H, Shi H, Liu E. Volume-targeted ventilation is more suitable than pressure-limited ventilation for preterm infants: A systematic review and meta-analysis. Archives of Diseases in Childhood—Fetal and Neonatal Edition. 2014;**99**(2):F158-F165

[55] Kumar P, Newborn CoFa, Pediatrics AAo. Use of inhaled nitric oxide in preterm infants. Pediatrics. 2014;**133**(1):164-170

[56] Sakonidou S, Dhaliwal J. The management of neonatal respiratory distress syndrome in preterm infants (European Consensus Guidelines--2013 update). Archives of Diseases in Childhood Education and Practice Edition. 2015;**100**(5):257-259

[57] Chandrasekharan P, Kozielski R, Kumar VH, Rawat M, Manja V, Ma C, et al. Early use of inhaled nitric oxide in preterm infants: Is there a rationale for selective approach? American Journal of Perinatology. 2017;**34**(5):428-440

[58] Prodhan P, Stroud M, El-Hassan N, Peeples S, Rycus P, Brogan TV, et al. Prolonged extracorporeal membrane oxygenator support among neonates with acute respiratory failure: A review of the Extracorporeal Life Support Organization registry. American Society for Artificial Internal Organs Journal. 2014;**60**(1):63-69

7

Fungal Infections in Neonatal Intensive Care

Rejane P. Neves, Ana Maria R. de Carvalho Parahym,
Carolina M. da Silva, Danielle P.C. Macêdo,
André F.G. Leal, Henrique J. Neves and
Reginaldo G. Lima-Neto

Abstract

Neonates represent a unique and highly vulnerable patient population. Advances in medical technology have improved the survival and quality of life of newborns, particularly those with extreme prematurity or with congenital defects. Furthermore, immunologic immaturity and altered cutaneous barriers play some role in the vulnerability of neonates to nosocomial infections. In this context, the incidence of invasive fungal infections has increased significantly worldwide, representing an important infective complication in patients hospitalized in intensive care units. Invasive fungal infections in Neonatal Intensive Care Unit (NICUs) show high mortality; being species of *Candida,* the most isolates etiologic agents. The better prognosis of the patient is associated with the early diagnosis and fast treatment. However, guidelines to facilitate the optimal therapy choice for the treatment of neonatal fungal disease do not exist. The current antifungal agents that are available to treat fungemia among newborns and children are based on clinical trials in adults, since there are few comparative studies of antifungal agents in infants. The most commonly used drugs for the treatment of invasive fungal infections in neonates are classified in four different classes: polyene, azoles, analogs of pyrimidines and echinocandins.

Keywords: antifungal therapy, fungal infections, intensive care, neonates, sepsis

1. Introduction

During the last two decades, invasive fungal infections in preterm infants have become an increasing problem, mainly when hospitalized in a Neonatal Intensive Care Unit (NICU). Thus, for the last years, 6.3 million children under the age of 5 died each year are estimated, and more than 40% of these deaths occur in the neonatal period [1, 2]. These data have several causes and particularly the neonates are at high risk due to fungal infections, mainly by yeasts of the genus *Candida* [3, 4].

In addition, species of the genus *Candida* have the capacity to inhabit several niches, thus, as part of the skin, mucosa and gastrointestinal tract [5]. Therefore, is considered that there is an association between colonization and systemic candidiasis mainly in seriously ill patients [6].

Although *Candida albicans* are more frequent, species of *Candida* non-*albicans* are also cause of diverse clinical pictures important in neonates, especially those that are in NICUs. The main Candida non-albicans species included are *Candida parapsilosis* complex, *Candida glabrata* and *Candida krusei*. However, uncommon species as *Pichia fabianii* and *Kodamaea ohmeri* may occur [7–10].

The newborns clinical course in the Intensive Care Units usually complicates after the onset of fungal infections [11]. In this hospital environment, adverse events may occur due to the complexity of the patients [12]. In this sense, the treatments and procedures instituted for primary disease may be an important factor for the onset of fungal infections; birth weight between 1000 and 1500 g is also a predictive factor and a way for the clinical worsening [13].

The predisposing factors to fungal infections include prolonged use of antibacterial and use of medical devices, among other conditions that lead to fungal disease. In addition, biofilms are frequent on the surface of medical devices, being consider a negative event, since it characterizes greater pathogenicity and antifungal resistance of fungi.

Commonly, amphotericin B, azoles and echinocandins are used for the treatment of various invasive fungal infections. However, antifungal therapeutic failures contribute to a higher mortality rate and may occur due to intrinsic resistance, so it is important to perform antifungal sensitivity tests. These tests can predict the ideal antifungal or contribute in the choice according to the use of other medicines and the condition of the neonate [9].

2. Epidemiology and incidence of neonatal invasive fungal infections

Neonates represent a unique and highly vulnerable patient population. Advances in medical technology have improved the survival and quality of life of newborns, particularly those with extreme prematurity or with congenital defects. Immunologic immaturity and altered cutaneous barriers play some role in increasing the vulnerability of neonates to infections. In this context, neonatal infection is a major cause of mortality and morbidity in newborns. Estimates suggest that >1.4 million neonatal deaths worldwide annually are due to invasive infections [14, 15].

The occurrence of invasive fungal infections has increased significantly worldwide, representing an important infective complication in patients hospitalized in intensive care units. Premature infants in NICUs are at particular risk of these invasive fungal infections, and unfortunately, the incidence of fungal septicemia appears to be increasing [16, 17]. In this context, *Candida* and *Malassezia* species are the most prevalent pathogen involved in fungal infections in NICU [18].

The incidence of bloodstream infections due to *Candida* species in the overall population ranges from 1.7 to 10 episodes per 100,000 inhabitants. An estimated 33–55% of all episodes of candidemia occur in intensive care units and are associated with mortality rates ranging from 5 to 71% [16].

Invasive candidiasis is an important cause of sepsis in the NICU. Candida infections in infants are associated with significant mortality and morbidity, including neurodevelopmental impairment. The incidence of invasive candidiasis in NICU ranges from 2.6 to 13.2% in very low birth weight infants (1500–1000 g) and from 6.6 to 26.0% in extremely low birth weight infants (<1000 g) [19].

C. albicans has been the most frequently isolated species; however, infections caused by others species have been diagnosed with increased frequency. In the NICU in the 1990s, the overall incidence of candidemia increased because of the increased survival and intensive care of extremely preterm infants. During that time period, the proportion of candidemia decreased because of *C. albicans*, whereas increased because of *C. parapsilosis* [20, 21].

Invasive infections associated with *C. parapsilosis* cause fewer acute lethal events in premature newborns than systemic infections with *C. albicans*; nevertheless, *C. parapsilosis* fungemia significantly increases the morbidity and mortality of severely ill infants who require care in a NICU [22].

Laboratory studies have documented that *C. parapsilosis* is less virulent than *C. albicans*. However, the capability to adhere tenaciously to prosthetic materials forming biofilm and to proliferate rapidly in high concentrations of glucose are factors that facilitate the infection in the hospital environment. This trait may contribute to its ability to adhere to plastic catheters and cause systemic infections in premature newborns receiving total parenteral nutrition, blood pressure transducers or other invasive devices. Such a route of transmission may account for the occurrence of epidemic outbreaks of *C. parapsilosis* bloodstream infections [21].

Other emerging *Candida* species such as *C. haemuloniii*, *C. pelliculosa* and *C. tropicalis* have also been associated with infections in NICU. *C. pelliculosa* and *C. haemuloniii* caused clonal infection in NICU [11]. An outbreak of *C. tropicalis* fungemia in a NICU was traced to receipt of total parenteral nutrition and antimicrobial agents [23].

Malassezia species in immunocompromised patients may be associated with several skin conditions and systemic diseases, including folliculitis, seborrhoeic dermatitis, catheter-related fungemia and sepsis. However, this yeast may also cause invasive infections in critically ill low birth weight infants. *Malassezia* fungemia is predominantly caused by *Malassezia furfur* and *Malassezia pachydermatis*. *M. furfur* has been described predominantly in conjunction with nosocomial outbreaks in NICU, particularly in neonates and infants receiving intravenous lipids solution. Additionally, *M. pachydermatis* has been associated with bloodstream infection in preterm with very low birth weight and the prolonged use of indwelling catheters and parenteral lipid formulations [18, 24].

3. Neonatal *Candida* infections

Candida species are correlated to invasive fungal infections among at-risk groups as neonatal patients admitted NICU in and have been ranked third to seventh as a cause of nosocomial bloodstream infection, defined as candidemia, depending on geographical patterns [25–28]. Studies on invasive candidiasis infections and candidemia are frequently focused on specific diagnoses and/or specific populations. In all published studies, ICU was the most frequent localization of the patients, even with different frequencies [29].

Candidemia is associated with high rates of illness and death and has an attributable mortality rate that varies widely in the literature, ranging from 29 to 76%, both in adult and pediatric patients [30, 31]. Furthermore, *Candida* species are common gastrointestinal flora that causes a wide range of severe manifestations when disseminated into the bloodstream. Thus, candidemia has been described as the most common manifestation of invasive candidiasis [32].

These yeasts are less frequent than those infections caused by Gram-positive or Gram-negative bacteria; nonetheless, they are higher rates of morbidity and mortality. Particularly, among newborn with extremely low weight, 10% may to develop candidemia that has until 30% mortality in this patient group. Among infants who survive these infections, several long-term neurological impairments such as cerebral palsy, blindness, hearing and cognitive deficits and periventricular leukomalacia may occur [9, 27].

Neonatal candidemia during the first week of life is less common and less well described than the later onset of this group of infections. According to Barton et al. [33], risk factors for candidemia among neonates had not been studied before their research, in early onset disease (EOD, ≤7 days) or compared to late onset disease (LOD, >7 days). After a 2-year study, the authors concluded that risk factors such as birthweight <750 g, gestation <25 weeks, chorioamnionitis and vaginal delivery were strongly associated with EOD. Infection with *Candida albicans*, disseminated disease, pneumonia and cardiovascular disease were significantly more common in EOD than in LOD. Also, neurodevelopmental impairment and mortality were also higher than controls.

Extremely low birth weight is considered a risk factor related to a poor prognosis in EOD. Also, the role of perinatal transmission is supported by its association with chorioamnionitis, vaginal delivery and pneumonia. Dissemination and cardiovascular involvement are common, and affected infants often die. Empiric treatment should be considered in these risk situations [33, 34].

Pereira et al. [34] developed a retrospective observational study to investigate the risks for sepsis in neonates, including *Candida* infections, and verified an association between healthcare-associated sepsis, antibiotic therapy in day 1, the duration of parenteral nutrition and the use of central vascular catheter. For each extra week on gestational age, the risks declined in 20%, and for each day of parenteral nutrition, the risk increased 22%.

Kung et al. [35] affirm that infants in NICU have a higher incidence of *Candida* infections than any other pediatric or adult population. The predisposing factors were evaluated in Taiwan using a retrospective matched case-control study conducted in the NICUs of a teaching hospital from July 2003 to June 2006. A total of 164 infants with culture-proven bloodstream infections were identified and the common etiologic pathogens included coagulase-negative staphylococci (28.7%), *Staphylococcus aureus* (16.5%), *Klebsiella pneumoniae* (14.6%) and *Candida* species accounting for 11 (6.7%) episodes. According to these authors, parenteral nutrition was a significant and independent risk of late-onset neonatal sepsis, including those caused by *Candida* species. This risk should be considered when implementing early parenteral nutrition in NICUs.

The collected potential risk factors consisted of: (1) prenatal and maternal history such as toxemia, multiple gestation, intra-uterine growth retardation and perinatal infections; (2) perinatal history such as premature rupture of membrane greater than 18 hours and delay in initial crying; (3) invasive procedures such as instrument insertion and its duration (e.g., placement of nasogastric tubes, endotracheal tubes, mechanical ventilation, peripherally inserted central catheters, chest tubes, blood transfusion or exchanged blood transfusion and lumbar puncture); (4) the concomitant use of medications such as parenteral nutrition and intravenous lipid, antibiotics and steroids and (5) comorbidities such as meconium aspiration syndrome (MAS), persistent pulmonary hypertension of the newborn (PPHN), intraventricular hemorrhage (IVH), necrotizing enterocolitis (NEC), respiratory distress syndrome (RDS), inborn error of metabolism and cardiac anomalies (except for patent ductus arteriosus and secundum type of atrial septal defect). However, transfusion, antimicrobial treatment, use of steroids and the presence of other comorbidities were not associated with *Candida* infections in neonates [35].

Invasive neonatal candidiasis presented an overall mortality rate of 35% during a study in Los Angeles (USA) in a neonatal intensive care unit. In general, every infant used a central venous catheter (CVC), required mechanical ventilation and previous administration of antibacterial agents. According to the authors, delayed institution of antifungal therapy was associated with increased mortality as well as length of hospitalization and the duration of prior antibacterial therapy [36].

Frequently, *C. albicans* is the most fungal clinical isolate; however, the incidence of bloodstream infections caused by *Candida* non-*albicans*, mainly *C. parapsilosis* complex and *C. glabrata*, has increased over the past 15 years. The current high rate of *Candida parapsilosis* infections may be attributed the capacity of this isolate to form biofilms and contaminate solutions, as those used in parenteral nutrition [8].

In recent Italian study, *C. albicans* was the most frequently identified strain, but nearly 20% of infections were due to *Candida* non-*albicans*, mainly *C. krusei* and *C. glabrata* [10]. Since both these strains can be resistant to fluconazole, that is the antifungal drug with the best urinary penetration [37], treatment of these patients could be challenging, despite a recent report that showed effective concentrations of micafungin in the urinary tract [38]. In these search, fungemia was the second most frequent diagnosis and was more frequent in children with malignancy/hematopoietic stem cell transplantation, those undergoing abdominal surgery and in low birth weight neonates, also in this case, confirming other recent pediatric data such as Ota et al. [39] and Steinbach et al. [40].

Invasive fungal infections in NICUs show high mortality. The better prognosis of the patient with invasive candidiasis/or candidemia admitted in NICU is associated with the early diagnosis and fast treatment. Evidence suggests an estimated mortality rate of 40% if therapy is not initiated early. Therefore, it is not a good practice to wait for cultures to become positive. This need for early therapy must be balanced against the need to use antifungal agents to avoid selection of resistant strains. Early empiric therapy guided by stratification systems for high-risk patients should help address these cases [41].

The score for exact risk measurement of invasive candidiasis has yet to be developed. The "Candida Score" presented by Spanish group in 2006 provides an easy-to-use tool to assist the health professionals with critically ill adults [42]. However, we believe that will should be adapted to pediatric patients, in the near future. In this stratification, the selected variables by logistic regression model with increasing weight are total parenteral nutrition, surgery, multifocal *Candida* species colonization and severe sepsis [42].

Recent Infectious Disease Society American guidelines suggest that "empirical antifungal therapy should be considered in critically ill patients with risk factors for invasive candidiasis and no other known cause of fever." Risk factors for invasive candidiasis are well identified. When analyzing clinical data, surveillance culture and levels of anti-*Candida* antibodies plus β-D-glucan in the serum, the same Spanish researchers showed a positive correlation among increasing values of the "*Candida* score" and the rate of invasive *Candida* infections. Such a score was calculated by variables such as total parenteral nutrition, surgery, multifocal *Candida* colonization and severe sepsis. Thus, *Candida* score ≥3 suggest patients at high risk for invasive candidiasis and enable to differentiate patients who would benefit from early antifungal treatment from those for whom invasive candidiasis is highly improbable [43].

4. Other neonatal fungal infections

Despite *C. albicans* is known to be primarily responsible for most neonatal fungal diseases, the prevalence of infections caused by other fungi in neonates and young infants is not significant, except for *Malassezia* species, which may occur in epidemic outbreaks [44–46].

Since 1980, this genus has been recognized in sepsis and systemic infections involving neonates receiving lipidic parenteral nutrition using a central venous catheter. It is believed that lipid supplementation facilitates the colonization of the catheter that used to infuse the nutrients. In newborns, colonization by *Malassezia* can progress to fungemia. The removal of the infected catheter is sufficient to limit infection in most cases [46, 47].

The vast majority of cases of fungemia occur in children less than 12 months old. In this population, this *Malassezia* infection rarely remains asymptomatic. Interstitial pneumonia and thrombocytopenia are common clinical manifestations in this group of patients, and the most frequent symptoms in systemic infections are fever and respiratory dysfunction with or without apnea [46, 48].

Other less common symptoms include lethargy, malnutrition, bradycardia and hepatosplenomegaly. However, no signs of erythema, swelling or purulence appear at the catheter entry site. Signs of skin rash are also not evident in children with systemic infections. Interstitial bronchopneumonia can be found in 40% of children [44–46].

The diagnosis of fungal infection by *Malassezia* is made by isolating the microorganism from blood collected through the catheter or by culturing the catheter tip after its removal. In suspected sepsis by *Malassezia*, the tip of the catheter should be cultured in broth enriched with lipids [45, 46].

The standard therapeutic management for systemic infections by *Malassezia* is still not well defined, since the fungemia by this microorganism is relatively unusual. However, some authors recommend the use of amphotericin B to treat these infections [45, 46, 49]. Morrison and Weisdorf [50] found that all patients enrolled in their study were cured without the administration of systemic antifungal therapy.

Studies have indicated that the most important factor for therapeutic success against systemic infection is the removal of the infected catheter and the interruption of lipid infusion, with or without antifungals [18, 45, 46].

5. Treatment of neonatal fungal infections

The appropriate use of antifungals agents is of particular importance in the prevention and treatment of invasive fungal infection in neonates; however, guidelines to facilitate the optimal therapy choice do not exist. The current therapeutic options that are available to treat fungemia among newborns and children are based on clinical trials in adults, since there are few comparative studies of antifungal agents in infants. The optimal treatment of fungal infection in this special population requires detailed studies on pharmacokinetics, safety and efficacy of antifungal therapies [51–54].

Similar to neonatal invasive infections by species of *Candida*, the management of *Malassezia* sp. fungemia requires the removal of any catheter as soon as the first positive blood culture occurs and the temporary discontinuation of parenteral nutrition in combination with an intravenous antifungal therapy. The most commonly used agents for the treatment of invasive fungal infections in NICU are classified into four different classes: polyene, azoles, analogs of pyrimidines and echinocandins. Among many years, the drugs of choice in this group of patients were amphotericin B alone or in combination with fluocitosin, liposomal formulation of amphotericin B or fluconazole. However, the development of a new generation of azoles and echinocandins, such as micafungin, has increased the therapeutic options for the treatment [45, 54].

Amphotericin B deoxycholate and lipid preparations are traditional choices for invasive fungal infections being active against a majority of clinical important *Candida* species and with reported use for *Malassezia* [45, 55]. Amphotericin B deoxycholate is well tolerated by neonates who do not exhibit many of the toxicities seen in older children and adults. However, liposomal amphotericin B has been found to be safe and efficacious in newborns with renal impairment. Another polyene agent, nystatin suspension, is administered orally to infants with gestational age ≤ 27 weeks or birth weight less than 750 g until removal of central venous catheters; this is shown to reduce colonization of the gastrointestinal tract and the rate of invasive candidiasis [55].

Among the azoles, fluconazole is more frequently used in NICUs for the treatment of oropharyngeal and systemic candidiasis, but has no inherent activity against the genus *Aspergillus*, which is rare pathogen in neonates. This antifungal agent is commonly recommended as prophylactic therapy in NICU with a high incidence in fungal infections. Fluconazole prophylaxis is effective in reducing the rate of colonization and progression to systemic infection in nursery; on the other hand, some studies have revealed that prophylactic or empiric therapy with antifungal agents may be associated with changes in *Candida* ecology and antifungal agent susceptibility. Actually, the fluconazole dose recommended for neonates is 6 mg/kg/day, and maintenance doses currently used in NICUs in Europe is often higher, between 6 and 12 mg/kg [53, 56–58].

New azoles such as voriconazole, posaconazole and ravuconazole have limited utility in the nursery and are rarely used to treat neonatal infections. Voriconazole is a second-generation triazole that has excellent activity against *Candida* and *Aspergillus* spp.; however, data on its use in neonates are limited. Posaconazole and ravuconazole are the newest agents of the triazole family with added action against zygomycetes, however there are scarces of survey involving these antifungal agents in infants and the use of ravuconazole is not already approved by the Food and Drug Administration (FDA) [59, 60].

The echinocandins (micafungin, caspofungin and anidulafungin) are increasingly used for treatment of *Candida* sp. infections. Their role in the nursery is not so clear, although accruing evidence suggests they may be safe and effective, especially for the treatment of invasive infections caused by *Candida* spp. Some point have to be taken under consideration before the use of echinocandins in NICUs: first, limited clinical data also suggest that these agents may be effective for the treatment of central nervous system infections. Second, a high incidence of *C. parapsilosis* in NICUs is usually reported and this species is related to higher minimum inhibitory concentration (MIC) front of echinocandins [56, 57].

Among the three representatives of the group, micafungin is the most recommended and its use is approved for adults, children and newborns, being considered the one with better description for neonatal population. The use of caspofungin is approved by the FDA, but only for adults and children over 3 months of age. There were no relevant clinical trials that support the administration of anidulafungin among neonates and children [56, 57].

Invasive fungal infections are devastating pathologies that still result in death or serious long-term morbidity in neonates; however, the management of this mycosis has progressed greatly, with the azole agents playing a significant role. Effective prophylactic strategies have recently become available; therefore, the choice and use of appropriate antifungal drugs need careful assessment of neonatal characteristics, the epidemiology and drug pharmacokinetics [53].

Author details

Rejane P. Neves[1]*, Ana Maria R. de Carvalho Parahym[2], Carolina M. da Silva[1], Danielle P.C. Macêdo[2], André F.G. Leal[1], Henrique J. Neves[1] and Reginaldo G. Lima-Neto[3]

*Address all correspondence to: rejadel@yahoo.com.br

1 Department of Mycology, Centre of Biosciences, Federal University of Pernambuco (UFPE), Recife, Brazil

2 Department of Pharmaceutical Sciences, Center for Health Sciences, UFPE, Recife, Brazil

3 Department of Tropical Medicine, Center for Health Sciences, UFPE, Recife, Brazil

References

[1] Montagna M, Lovero G, De Giglio O, Iatta R, Caggiano G, Montagna O, Laforgia N. Invasive fungal infections in Neonatal Intensive Care Units of Southern Italy: A multi-centre regional active surveillance (AURORA Project). Journal of Preventive Medicine and Hygiene. 2010;**51**:125-130

[2] Smith ER, Bergelson I, Constantian S, Valsangkar B, Chan GJ. Barriers and enablers of health system adoption of kangaroo mother care: A systematic review of caregiver perspectives. BMC Pediatrics. 2017;25;**17**(1):35. DOI: 10.1186/s12887-016-0769-5

[3] Chitnis AS, Magill SS, Edwards JR, Chiller TM, Fridkin SK, Lessa FC. Trends in *Candida* central line-associated bloodstream infections among NICUs, 1999-2009. Pediatrics. 2012;**130**(1):46-52. DOI: 10.1542/peds.2011-3620

[4] Kaufman DA. "Getting to Zero": preventing invasive *Candida* infections and eliminating infection-related mortality and morbidity in extremely preterm infants. Early Human Development. 2012;**88**:45-49. DOI: 10.1016/S0378-3782(12)70014-2

[5] Harriott MM, Noverr MC. Importance of *Candida*-bacterial polymicrobial biofilms in disease. Trends in Microbiology. 2011;**19**(11): 557-563. DOI: 10.1016/j.tim.2011.07.004

[6] Brissaud O, Guichoux J, Harambat J, Tandonnet O, Zaoutis T. Invasive fungal disease in PICU: Epidemiology and risk factors. Annals of Intensive Care. 2012;**22**(1):6. DOI: 10.1186/2110-5820-2-6

[7] Wu Y, Wang J, Li W, Jia H, Che J, Lu J, Liu L, Cheng Y. *Pichia fabianii* blood infection in a premature infant in China: Case report. BMC Research Notes. 2013;**6**:77

[8] Goel S, Mittal S, Chaudhary U. Role of non-albicans *Candida* spp. and biofilm in neonatal ICU. Infectious Disorders Drug Targets. 2016;**16**(3):192-198

[9] Vivas R, Beltran C, Munera MI, Trujillo M, Restrepo A, Garcés C. Fungemia due to *Kodamaea ohmeri* in a young infant and review of the literature. Medical Mycology Case Reports. 2016, 20;**13**:5-8. DOI: 10.1016/j.mmcr.2016.06.001

[10] Mesini A, Bandettini R, Caviglia I, Fioredda F, Amoroso L, Faraci M, Mattioli G, Piaggio G, Risso FM, Moscatelli A, Loy A, Castagnola E. *Candida* infections in paediatrics: Results from a prospective single-centre study in a tertiary care children's hospital. Mycoses. 2017;**60**:118-123

[11] Silva CM, Carvalho-Parahym AM, Macêdo DP, Lima-Neto RG, Francisco EC, Melo AS, da Conceição MSM, Jucá MB, Mello LR, Amorim RM, Neves RP. Neonatal candidemia caused by *Candida haemulonii*: Case report and review of literature. Mycopathologia. 2015;**180**(1-2):69-73. DOI: 10.1007/s11046-015-9872-7

[12] Arriaga Redondo M, Sanz López E, Rodríguez Sánchez de la Blanca A, Marsinyach Ros I, Collados Gómez L, Díaz Redondo A, Sánchez Luna M. Improving patient safety: Usefulness of safety checklists in a neonatal unit. Anales Pediatr (Barc). 2017;S1695-4033(16)30309-5. DOI: 10.1016/j.anpedi.2016.11.005. [Epub ahead of print]

[13] Simonsen KA, Anderson-Berry AL, Delair SF, Davies HD. Early-onset neonatal sepsis. Clinical Microbiology Reviews. 2014;**27**(1):21-47. DOI: 10.1128/CMR.00031-13

[14] Benjamin D, Stoll B, Gants M, Walsh M, Sánchez P, Das A, Walsh T. Neonatal candidiasis: Epidemiology, risk factors, and clinical judgment. Pediatrics. 2010;**126**(4):e865-e873

[15] Shane AL, Stoll BJ. Neonatal sepsis: Progress towards improved outcomes. The Journal of Infection. 2014;**68**(Suppl. 1):S24e32

[16] Bougnoux M, Kac G, Aegerter P. et al. Candidemia and candiduria in critically ill patients admitted to intensive care units in France: Incidence, molecular diversity, management and outcome. Intensive Care Medicine. 2008;**34**:292-299

[17] Brady MT. Healthcare-associated infections in the neonatal intensive care unit. American Journal of Infection Control. 2005;**33**(5):268-275

[18] Devlin R. Invasive fungal infections caused by *Candida* and *Malassezia* species in the neonatal intensive care unit. Advances in Neonatal Care. 2006;**6**(2):68-77

[19] Aliaga S, Clark RH, Laugh M. et al. Changes in the incidence of candidiasis in neonatal intensive care units. Pediatrics. 2014;**133**(2):236-242

[20] Huang Y, Lin R, Chou Y, Kuo C, Yang P, Hsieh W. Candidaemia in special care nurseries: Comparison of *albicans* and *parapsilosis* infection. The Journal of Infection. 2000;**40**:171

[21] Lupetti A, Tavanti A, Davini P, Ghelardi E, Corsini V, Merusi I, Boldrini A, Campa M, Senesi S. Horizontal transmission of *Candida parapsilosis* candidemia in a neonatal intensive care unit. Journal of Clinical Microbiology. 2002;**40**(7):2363-2369

[22] Fridkin S, Kaufman D, Edwards JR. et al. Changing incidence of *Candida* bloodstream infections among NICU patients in the United States: 1995-2004. Pediatrics. 2006;**117**(5):1680-1687

[23] Finkelstein R, Reinhertz G, Hashman N, Merzbach D. Outbreak of *Candida tropicalis* fungemia in a neonatal intensive care unit. Infection Control and Hospital Epidemiology. 1993;**14**:587-590

[24] Chryssanthou E, Broberger U, Petrini B. *Malassezia pachydermatis* fungaemia in a neonatal intensive care unit. Acta Paediatrica. 2001;**90**(3):323-327

[25] Magill SS, Edwards JR, Bamberg W, Beldavs ZG, Dumyati G, Kainer MA, et al. Emerging infections program healthcare-associated infections and antimicrobial use prevalence survey team. Multistate point-prevalence survey of healthcare-associated infections. The New England Journal of Medicine. 2014;**370**:1198-1208

[26] Yapar N. Epidemiology and risk factors for invasive candidiasis. Therapeutics and Clinical Risk Management. 2014;**10**:95-105

[27] Lovero G, De Giglio O, Montagna O, Diella G, Divenuto F, Lopuzzo M, Rutigliano S, Laforgia N, Caggiano G, Montagna MT. Epidemiology of candidemia in neonatal intensive care units: A persistent public health problem. Annali di Igiene. 2016;**28**:282-287

[28] Doi AM, Pignatari AC, Edmond MB, Marra AR, Camargo LF, Siqueira RA, et al. Epidemiology and microbiologic characterization of nosocomial candidemia from a Brazilian national surveillance program. PLoS One. 2016;**11**:e0146909

[29] Sobel JD, Fisher JF, Kauffman CA, Newman CA. *Candida* urinary tract infections epidemiology. Clinical Infectious Diseases. 2011;**52**(Suppl 6):S433-S436

[30] Wisplinghoff H, Ebbers J, Geurtz L, Stefanik D, Major Y, Edmond MB, et al. Nosocomial bloodstream infections due to *Candida* spp. in the USA: Species distribution, clinical features and antifungal susceptibilities. International Journal of Antimicrobial Agents. 2014;**43**:78-81

[31] Diekema D, Arbefeville S, Boyken L, Kroeger J, Pfaller M. The changing epidemiology of healthcare-associated candidemia over three decades. Diagnostic Microbiology and Infectious Disease. 2012;**73**:45-48

[32] Pfaller MA, Andes DR, Diekema DJ, Horn DL, Reboli AC, Rotstein C, et al. Epidemiology and outcomes of invasive candidiasis due to non-*albicans* species of *Candida* in 2496 patients: Data from the Prospective Antifungal Therapy (PATH) registry 2004-2008. PLoS One. 2014;**9**:e101510

[33] Barton M, et al. Early onset invasive candidiasis in extremely low birth weight infants: Perinatal acquisition predicts poor outcome. Clinical Infectious Diseases. 2017;**64**:cix001

[34] Pereira H, et al. Risk factors for healthcare associated sepsis in very low birth weight infants. Acta Médica Portuguesa. 2016;**29**(4):261-267

[35] Kung YH, et al. Risk factors of late-onset neonatal sepsis in Taiwan: A matched case-control study. Journal of Microbiology, Immunology and Infection. 2016;**49**:430-435

[36] Cahan H, Deville JG. Outcomes of neonatal candidiasis: The impact of delayed initiation of antifungal therapy. International Journal of Pediatrics. 2011;**2011**:Article ID 813871

[37] Felton T, Troke PF, Hope WW. Tissue penetration of antifungal agents. Clinical Microbiology Reviews. 2014;**27**:68-88

[38] Grau S, Luque S, Echeverría-Esnal D, et al. Urinary micafungin levels are sufficient to treat urinary tract infections caused by *Candida* spp. International Journal of Antimicrobial Agents. 2016;**48**:212-214

[39] Ota KV, McGowan KL. Declining incidence of candidemia in a tertiary inpatient pediatric population. Journal of Clinical Microbiology. 2012;**50**:1048-1050

[40] Steinbach WJ, Roilides E, Berman D, et al. Results from a prospective, international, epidemiologic study of invasive candidiasis in children and neonates. The Pediatric Infectious Disease Journal. 2012;**31**:1252-1257

[41] Leroy G, Lambiotte F, Thévenin D, Lemaire C, Parmentier E, Devos P and Leroy O. Evaluation of "*Candida* score" in critically ill patients: A prospective, multicenter, observational, cohort study. Annals of Intensive Care. 2011;**1**:50

[42] León C, Ruiz-Santana S, Saavedra P, et al. A bedside scoring system ("Candida score") for early antifungal treatment in nonneutropenic critically ill patients with *Candida* colonization. Critical Care Medicine. Mar 2006;**34**(3):730-737

[43] León C, Ruiz-Santana S, Saavedra P, Galván B, Blanco A, Castro C, Balasini C, Utande-Vázquez A, González de Molina FJ, Blasco-Navalproto MA, López MJ, Charles PE, Martín E, Hernández-Viera MA, Cava Study Group. Usefulness of the "*Candida* score" for discriminating between *Candida* colonization and invasive candidiasis in non-neutropenic critically ill patients: A prospective multicenter study. Critical Care Medicine. 2009;**37**:1624-1633

[44] Kaufman D, Fairchild KD. Clinical microbiology of bacterial and fungal sepsis in very-low-birth-weight infants. Clinical Microbiology Reviews. 2004;**17**(3):638-680

[45] Latta R, Cafarchia C, Cuna T, Montagna O, Laforgia N, Gentile O, Rizzo A, Boekhout T, Otranto D, Montagna MT. Bloodstream infections by *Malassezia* and *Candida* species in critical care patients. Medical Mycology. 2014;**52**:264-269

[46] Maraschin MM, Spader T, Mario DAN, Rossato L, Lopes PGM. Infections by *Malassezia*: New approaches. Saúde. 2008;**34**(1):4-8

[47] Marcon MJ, Powell DA. Human infection due to *Malassezia* spp. Clinical Microbiology Reviews. 1992;**5**(2):101-119

[48] Barder GR, Brown AE, Kiehn TE, Edwards FF, Armstrong D. Catheter-related *Malassezia furfur* fungemia in immunocompromised patients. The American Journal of Medicine. 1993;**95**(4):365-370

[49] Strippoli V, Piacentini A, D'Auria FD, Simonetti N. Antifungal activity of ketoconazole and azole against *Malassezia furfur in vitro* and *in vivo*. Infection 1997;**25**:303-306

[50] Morrison VA, Weisdorf DJ. The spectrum of *Malassezia* infections in the bone marrow transplant population. Bone Marrow Transplantation. 2000;**26**(6):645-648

[51] Blyth C, Chen S, Slavin M., Serena C, Nguyen Q, Marriott D, Ellis D, Meyer W, Sorrel T. Australian Candidemia Study. Not just little adults: Candidemia epidemiology, molecular characterization, and antifungal susceptibility in neonatal and pediatric patients. Pediatrics. 2009;**123**:1360-1368

[52] Ericson J, Manzoni P, Benjamin D. Old and new: Appropriate dosing for neonatal antifungal drugs in the nursery. Early Human Development. 2013;**89**:S25-S27

[53] Hassan M, Yasmeen B, Begum N. Fungal sepsis and Indications of antifungal prophylaxis and treatment in neonatal intensive care units: A review. Northern International Medical College Journal. 2015;**6**:6-8

[54] Pana Z, Kougia V, Roilides E. Therapeutic strategies for invasive fungal infections in neonatal and pediatric patients: An update. Expert Opinion on Pharmacotherapy. 2015;**16**:693-710

[55] Lsetner J, et al. Systemic antifungal prescribing in neonates and children: Outcomes from the antibiotic resistance and prescribing in European children (ARPEC) study. Antimicrobial Agents and Chemotherapy. 2015;**59**:782-789

[56] Hope W, et al. ESCMID* guideline for the diagnosis and management of *Candida* diseases 2012: Prevention and management of invasive infections in neonates and children caused by Candida spp. Clinical Microbiology and Infection. 2012;**18**:38-52

[57] Leroux S, et al. Randomized Pharmacokinetic Study of fluconazole and micafungin in preterm neonates with suspected or proven fungal infection. American Journal of Perinatology. 2016;**33**, n. S 01, p A006

[58] Manzoni P, Mostert M, Castagnola E. Update on the management of *Candida* infections in preterm neonates. Archives of Disease in Childhood-Fetal and Neonatal Edition 2015;**100**:F454-F459

[59] Shane A, Stoll B. Recent developments and current issues in the epidemiology, diagnosis, and management of bacterial and fungal neonatal sepsis. American Journal of Perinatology. 2013;**30**:131-142

[60] Watt K, et al. Triazole use in the nursery: Fluconazole, voriconazole, posaconazole, and ravuconazole. Current Drug Metabolismo. 2013;**14**(2):193-202

8

Hemodynamic Monitoring in Neonates

Petja Fister and Štefan Grosek

Abstract

Sick neonates are often hemodynamically unstable, hence their organs are inadequately supplied with oxygen. In order to maintain blood flow to vital organs, a number of compensatory mechanisms divert the blood flow away from the non-vital organs. If hemodynamic changes are detected early, the cardiovascular compromise can be recognized in compensated phase and thereby the escalation to decompensated phase of low cardiac output syndrome might be prevented. In the treatment of hemodynamically unstable neonate venous filling, contractility of the heart muscle, blood pressure in the aorta, systemic blood flow, and regional distribution of blood flow should be evaluated. There are many evaluation and measurement methods based on different physical basis, each of them having their advantages and disadvantages. For most of them, it has not been demonstrated that they improve outcomes of sick neonates. Using these methods, useful hemodynamic data for the treatment of sick neonates can be obtained. Using new techniques will clarify the pathophysiology of cardiovascular failure in sick neonates, assess the effects of drugs on blood pressure and perfusion of the heart and other organs.

Keywords: neonate, hemodynamics, oxygenation, perfusion, arterial blood pressure, cardiac output, peripheral vascular resistance

1. Introduction

In neonatal intensive care unit (NICU), hemodynamic instability is an important cause for admission and treatment after respiratory distress syndrome (RDS) and most common problems of prematurity [1]. Therefore, hemodynamic monitoring is important especially in transitional period to extrauterine life and during the next following days. Hemodynamic monitoring is also crucial in neonates with congenital heart defects (CHDs) and other complex surgical anomalies of neonates. During early transitional period, cardiac output (CO) is not dependent solely on the performance of the neonate's left ventricle but also on pulsating blood flow through the umbilical vein. This pulsating blood flow is extremely important especially if newborn is under fetal distress, and it is usually prudent to postpone ligation of umbilicus for a short period of time to add additional pulsatile and volume support to neonate's CO [2, 3]. Even later in the life, neonate with RDS requires hemodynamic monitoring due to disturbances related to RDS or other common problems of prematurity or immaturity. Besides prematurity, immaturity of cardiovascular system in the first days and weeks of life and altered physiology of systemic and pulmonary circulation in neonates with CHD may need frequent hemodynamic monitoring, whether invasively or noninvasively.

2. Methods

We conducted electronic searches of articles on hemodynamic management and care of neonates, using key terms: neonate, hemodynamics, oxygenation, perfusion, arterial blood pressure, cardiac output, and peripheral vascular resistance in the PubMed data base from the years 2000 to 2017 and reported the most relevant ones. The article lists the methods for the evaluation of the venous filling, cardiac output, blood pressure, regional blood flow, and microcirculation, from the clinical methods to the noninvasive and invasive ones. Some methods for monitoring the cardiovascular status of neonates are mainly used for research purposes. This chapter includes the impact of optimal arterial blood pressure, tissue perfusion, and persistent ductus arteriosus on the hemodynamic management in neonates. Also, the short- and long-term outcomes in respect of hemodynamic management of neonates in the intensive care unit are addressed.

3. Physiology of hemodynamics

Hemodynamics describes the dynamics of blood flow in the body. Blood flows in the circulatory system, which is composed of the central pump—the heart—and the blood vessels, and is controlled by homeostatic mechanisms. The pulsatile rate of blood flow out of the heart is called the cardiac output. The main role of the cardio-circulatory system is to match the oxygen and nutrient needs of the organs and tissues and elimination of the metabolic wastes. The cardio-circulatory system should provide an appropriate blood flow to the organs and by that an appropriate tissue perfusion. In the physiologic conditions, the tissue oxygen and nutrient needs are matched by their supply. In cardiovascular compromise, the compensatory mechanisms allow the redistribution of blood flow to the vital organs—the brain, heart, and suprarenal gland in the neonate—at the expense of decreased blood flow to the non-vital organs.

3.1. Hemodynamic monitoring

Hemodynamic monitoring encompasses the observation and measurement of hemodynamic parameters over time. The ultimate goals of hemodynamic monitoring is to alert the health-care team of impending cardiovascular crisis, to obtain information specific to the disease processes, which may facilitate diagnosis and treatment and allow one to monitor the response to therapy, and also to derive estimates of performances and physiological reserve that may in turn direct treatment [4]. The purpose of hemodynamic monitoring is to attain the optimal goals of cardiovascular therapy. Three functional-based questions should be addressed: (1) Will blood flow to the body increase (or decrease) if the neonates' intravascular volume is increased (or decreased), and if so, by how much? (2) Is the decrease in arterial blood pressure due to loss of vascular tone or merely due to inadequate blood flow? (3) Is the heart capable of maintaining an effective blood flow with an acceptable perfusion pressure without going into failure?

Physiologically, hemodynamic parameters can be divided into central or macro-hemodynamic parameters, which assess blood flow and pressure in the heart, vena cava, pulmonary artery, and the aorta, and the peripheral or micro-hemodynamic parameters, which assess the regional microvascular blood flow and tissue oxygenation (**Table 1**). The majority of existing hemodynamic monitoring assesses the central part of the cardio-circulatory system.

In the past, hemodynamic monitoring data were attained in neonates with CHD after heart surgery when the invasive and frequently inaccurate pulmonary artery catheters have been inserted [5]. Recently, efforts have been made to monitor the newborns as noninvasively

Hemodynamic parameter	Physiologic parameter	Clinical assessment	Noninvasive measurement	Invasive measurement
Central or macro	Preload—venous filling	Estimating jugular venous pressure, hand pressure on the liver, elevation of the legs	Inferior vena cava diameter and its collapsibility, lung ultrasonography	Central venous catheters*
	Cardiac output	Palpating peripheral pulses, heart rate*, capillary refill time, peripheral-core temperature difference	Echocardiography, cardiac magnetic resonance, electrical cardiometry*, arterial pulse waveform analysis*, electrocardiogram	Arterial catheters*
	Afterload—arterial blood pressure	Palpating peripheral pulses	Cuff oscillometry, Doppler ultrasound	Arterial catheters*
Peripheral or micro	Regional blood flow	Skin color, lactate	Perfusion index*, near-infrared spectroscopy*	
	Microcirculation		Laser-Doppler method, video microscopy, xenon clearance techniques	

*Continuous method, all others are intermittent.

Table 1. Physiologic hemodynamic parameters in neonates, assessed clinically, noninvasively, and invasively.

as possible and many new techniques have been applied in this vulnerable population to measure the central (arterial blood pressure and systemic blood flow) and peripheral hemodynamic parameters (peripheral vascular resistance). Arterial blood pressure is measured either noninvasively by sphygmomanometer or invasively through arterial catheters. Systemic blood flow is noninvasively assessed by echocardiography, cardiac magnetic resonance, electrical cardiometry, and arterial pulse waveform analysis. Invasive methods for measuring the systemic blood flow are applied through centrally inserted vascular catheters. It is not known whether laser-Doppler and spectroscopy in the near-infrared spectrum (near-infrared spectroscopy, NIRS) can reliably monitor peripheral vascular resistance (**Figure 1**) [6].

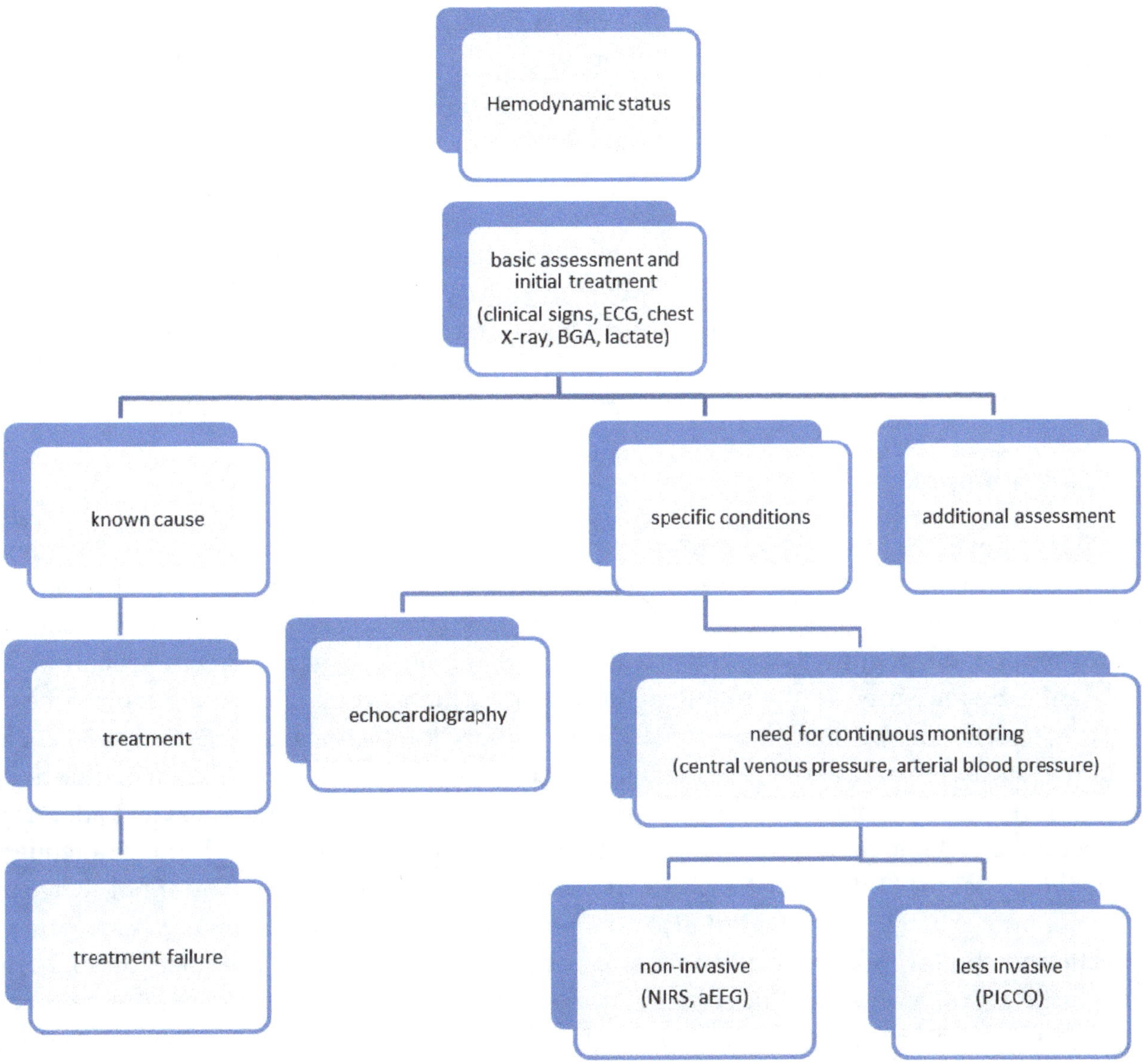

Figure 1. Assessment of hemodynamic status in neonatal intensive care unit. Adapted from Ref. [64]. aEEG, amplitude-integrated electroencephalogram; BGA, blood gas analysis; ECG, electrocardiogram; NIRS, near-infrared spectroscopy; PICCO, pulse-induced contour cardiac output.

4. The central hemodynamic monitoring

The central hemodynamic monitoring assesses the blood flow and the blood pressure in the heart and major vessels. The heart function and by that the stroke volume (SV) are determined by the preload—the venous filling, contractility of the heart muscle, and the afterload—which can be estimated only partially with the pressure in the aorta. The CO is the product of the SV and the heart rate (HR). Neonates increase their CO mainly by increasing the HR as they cannot sufficiently increase the SV. The HR is influenced by the body temperature, catecholamine secretion, and the autonomic nervous system.

4.1. The preload assessment

Clinically, the preload can be assessed visually assessing the jugular venous pressure, which is rarely possible in neonates with short neck. Using the hand pressure on the liver or elevation of the legs increases preload and is a simple method of assessing preload but less used in the NICU. The venous filling in neonates can be measured by inferior vena cava (IVC) diameter, and its collapsibility during respiration indicates volume responsiveness [7, 8]. IVC assessment is not an accurate marker of volume status and fluid responsiveness in cases of (1) increased right atrial pressure, (2) tricuspid or pulmonary valve regurgitation, (3) pulmonary hypertension, or (4) right ventricular dysfunction. Another method for assessing volume status of a neonate is lung ultrasonography (US) [9, 10]. Sonographic visualization of B-lines and measurement of extravascular lung water may aid diagnosing early volume overload in neonate. In a neonate with RDS after receiving surfactant, the B-lines are still visible [11].

4.2. Cardiac output

The measurement of CO is the most important parameter of the central hemodynamic monitoring, assessing the perfusion of organs. It is vital for the etiopathogenic diagnosis of low cardiac output syndrome, being due to either hypovolemia, myocardial dysfunction, vasodilatation, tamponade, pneumothorax, obstructive shock, pulmonary hypertension, or acute RDS. CO should be measured in the following clinical conditions: congenital and acquired heart diseases, shock, multiple organ failure, cardiopulmonary interactions during mechanical ventilation, clinical research, and assessment of new therapies [12]. The following three questions guide us in the interpretation of the adequacy of CO: (1) Is the delivery of oxygen adequate to meet the metabolic need of the patient? (2) Is oxygen delivery occurring with an adequate perfusion pressure? (3) Is the patient able to utilize the oxygen delivered, and if not, why so? [13]. Not only the measurement but also adequacy of CO and oxygen delivery is important, reflecting in clinical (capillary refill and core-peripheral temperature difference) and laboratory (lactic acid) parameters. But caveat is needed; normal values do not mean that regional perfusion is adequate, as well as abnormal values do not provide us with etiologic clue.

Clinically, CO with the systemic blood flow and perfusion can indirectly noninvasively be assessed by palpating the peripheral pulses and heart rate, capillary refill time, and measuring the peripheral-core temperature difference [14]. None of clinical methods for the evaluation of CO is definitely reliable [15]. The HR in neonate is affected by many factors and so it is not necessarily a good indicator of hemodynamic status. In hypovolemic state, the immature heart muscle and the autonomic nervous system impact the cardiovascular response differently in neonates in comparison to adults. The capillary refill time is affected by the pressure technique, variability among investigators, ambient temperature, drugs, and maturity of neonatal skin. The capillary refill time of >3 s has 55% sensitivity and 81% specificity for the prediction of the low systemic blood flow [16].

Noninvasive methods that are used in clinical practice to assess neonatal CO are echocardiography, cardiac magnetic resonance, electrical cardiometry, and arterial pulse waveform analysis. Functional echocardiography (fECHO) enables visualization of the shape and size of the chambers of the heart, the heart valves, contractility, and relaxation of the heart muscle. Various forms of Doppler echocardiography, such as color, continuous and pulsed Doppler echocardiography, enable the determination of both the blood flow direction and velocity. By assessing the velocity of blood flow, two more parameters can be calculated: the difference in pressure above and below the narrowing with the modified Bernoulli's equation and the blood flow through the blood vessel diameter and a mean flow velocity of the blood [17].

fECHO is daily used in the neonatal intensive medicine and constitutes an important part of an integrated bedside hemodynamic monitoring of a neonate. An appropriate training and experience is necessary for performing fECHO; so the obtained measurements are accurate and reliable. It should be noted that fECHO is not a substitute for formal echocardiographic assessment of the neonate by a pediatric cardiologist, especially if the newborn is suspected to have CHD or the latter has already been diagnosed [18, 19]. fECHO enables discontinuous hemodynamic assessment of neonate in real time. With fECHO, we can estimate the central venous pressure, and thus the volume of blood, and the contractility and filling of the right and left cavities, pulmonary arterial pressure, and the SV of the both ventricles, thereby CO. With neonatal fECHO, we can assess the presence, direction, and measure the blood flow velocity through the shunts, such as persistent ductus arteriosus (PDA) and open foramen ovale, the pressure in the pulmonary artery and the superior vena cava (SVC) and thereby assess heart function. The drawback is the limited accuracy of the measurements (10% with a single investigator and 20% among various investigators). Acquired measurements also depend on the blood flow: from the transitional to neonatal, shunts through connections between the pulmonary and systemic blood flow and immaturity or lability of the lung vasculature, and thus the pressure in the pulmonary artery [20].

fECHO is helpful in the treatment of neonates with cardiovascular instability, PDA, persistent pulmonary hypertension, preterm premature rupture of membranes, perinatal asphyxia, sepsis, and general management in intensive care for a sick neonate. In the case of hemodynamically significant PDA, fECHO has significant limitations in measuring CO. Significant left-right shunting through PDA apparently increases SV of the left ventricle, which is a measure of pulmonary blood flow; outflow from the right ventricle is a measure of the systemic blood flow. Similarly, the measurement of flow from the right ventricle is affected by the presence of left-right atrial shunting which apparently increases SV and the outflow from the right ventricle. For this reason, the assessment of the systemic blood flow is made through the measurement of the venous return to the heart through the SVC. The flow in the SVC is normally between 30 and 50% of the total systemic blood flow. Similarly, to assess the pulmonary blood flow, the blood flow velocity in the left pulmonary artery is measured [21].

Measuring the ejection fraction (EF) and fractional shortening (FS) in hemodynamic monitoring of the newborn is not very useful measurement, except in the case of severe myocardial dysfunction, when measurements are not really necessary, since the poor contractility of the heart muscle is obvious. We calculate them on the basis of measurement differences in dimensions of left ventricle in the long axis between diastole and systole. The problem of measurement in neonates is that the anterior wall of the ventricle is relatively stiff in comparison to the posterior and lateral wall of the left ventricle. To avoid this, they proposed measuring the dimensions of the left ventricle in short axis [22]. Two new US methods for assessing cardiac function are the measurement of diastolic function and tissue Doppler US. Diminished diastolic relaxation effects systolic function of the heart muscle, and thus the SV and CO. We may assess the diastolic function from the shape of Doppler wave of the inflow of blood into the ventricle. The filling of the ventricle has two phases: early ventricular filling during relaxation (E wave) and late active ventricular filling due to atrial systole (A wave). In a healthy neonate, 80% of the blood fills the left ventricle early in diastole, so the predominance of A wave indicates impaired diastolic function [23]. But when assessing impaired diastolic function, we have to be aware that diastolic function in premature and mature infants is already impaired because of immature contractile system of cardiac muscles [22]. The method of tissue Doppler echocardiography detects low frequency of high energy resulting from the movement of the ventricular wall which cannot be assessed by the standard Doppler investigation. In the four-chamber view of the heart in the longitudinal axis, we observe three different variables of ventricular wall motion: velocity, acceleration, and displacement [24]. Even if the method is advantageously used in adult patients, their clinical utility in the treatment of sick newborns is not yet fully understood [25].

Cardiovascular magnetic resonance (CMR) imaging is a method of nuclear magnetic resonance based on the spinning of hydrogen nuclei in a magnetic field, which are most numerous in the human body. CMR is the gold standard for the assessment of CO. Special expensive equipment, trained personnel, sedation, and transportation of a neonate are needed to perform CMR. In adults, CMR is used to assess the function of the ventricles, in complex congenital heart disease and cardiomyopathy. Compared with adults, it is necessary to increase the image resolution in neonates, both spatially (because of the size of the heart), as well as the time (due to the relatively high heart rate of newborn). The essential advantages of this method are detailed assessment of CO, cardiovascular anatomy, and good repeatability. CMR cannot measure the oxygen need and consumption [26]. Images obtained by CMR in real time have lower quality. Kino CMR enables improved anatomy imaging and the ventricular wall motion, by which the heart is imaged at specific phases of the cardiac cycle, depending on the electrocardiographic (ECG) recording. This creates a series of images that can be played as a movie (kino). End-diastolic and end-systolic endocardial and epicardial borders are followed and we reconstruct three-dimensional models of ventricles: end-systolic and end-diastolic volume, ejection fraction, and SV. CMR with a phase contrast allows the measurement of blood flow to the heart throughout the cardiac cycle [27]. This method quantifies the flow in IVC and descendent aorta, which indicates the systemic perfusion in the premature neonate. Similarly, we can measure the flow in the internal carotid and basilar arteries and thus the blood flow in the brain [28].

Electrical impedance cardiometry is the only available method that enables continuous noninvasive monitoring of SV and CO in a neonate [29, 30]. The method is based on a model of the electrical velocimetry, using four-surface ECG electrodes attached to the left side of the neck (two electrodes), and to the chest (two electrodes). Alternating electric current (AC) of constant amplitude flows through the pair of external electrodes toward the direction of the aorta. The ratio of the current and measured voltage is equal to the conductivity (or bioimpedance). Each tissue in the chest has its bioimpedance: that of the blood is very low, whole bone and lungs, filled with air, have high bioimpedance. Moreover, bioimpedance of bone is static, and bioimpedance of the lungs, which are filled and emptied of air, and of the heart and large blood vessels, which are filled with blood, is dynamic, in accordance with the respiratory or cardiac cycle. In case of sudden acceleration of blood flow into the aorta in systole, the conductivity dramatically increases. Electrical bioimpedance of the chest is strongly increased with every heartbeat. The neonate's movement causes artifacts in measuring the electrical impedance [31, 32].

Arterial pulse waveform analysis is a relatively good method for monitoring the dynamics of arterial blood pressure and assessment of CO. It is based on the analysis of the curve of arterial pulse waveform derived from arterial catheter and on the fact that the pulse pressure is proportional to SV [33]. The arterial pulse waveform changes in the case of arrhythmia, shock, or hypothermia, when it comes to peripheral vasoconstriction. Typically, the devices for calculating the SV and CO are based on the analysis of arterial pulse waveform, and require periodic, and in advance calibrations. An additional limitation of the method is that it assumes a constant rate of systemic vascular resistance [34]. So far, the methods of arterial pulse wave analysis have not been studied in neonates.

Invasive methods for assessing the CO have been developed in adults, and then applied in sick neonates, where their use is limited. Limitations of these methods are the invasiveness, complexity, and relatively long process (need for central vascular approach and taking sequential blood samples for laboratory analysis), for which reason they are seldom used in practice. Invasive methods for estimating average CO over time are based on a few physical principles. Fick's law is the law of mass/mass flow conservation. The amount of oxygen in the pulmonary artery and the amount of oxygen in the capillaries, flowing from the alveoli, is equal to the concentration of oxygen in the pulmonary vein [35].

Clinically, the O_2 consumption can be measured by measuring the concentration of oxygen in the inhaled and exhaled air and pulmonary ventilation. Consumption is estimated as the difference between the amount of oxygen in the inhaled and exhaled air. The concentration of oxygen in the peripheral arteries is the same as in the pulmonary veins. Pulmonary arteries have mixed venous blood. Samples for the analysis of O_2 are obtained from the pulmonary artery or the right ventricle through the cardiac catheter. Thus, we can calculate the CO (CO = O_2 consumption/AVΔO_2). Neonates compensate the reduced release of oxygen from fetal hemoglobin in tissues with higher hemoglobin concentrations, a larger volume of blood per unit of body weight, and increased CO. Instead of measuring O_2 consumption, we can measure the formation of CO_2 using capnography and assume that it is equal to the exchange of CO_2 in the lungs [36]. In neonates with a healthy alveolar-capillary membrane, the partial pressure of CO_2 in arterial blood is equal to the partial concentration of CO_2 in the exhaled air [37].

Stewart principle is a method of dilution of the indicator and provides calculation of the CO on the basis of change in the concentration of the dye (lithium-based dilution devices) or a change in the temperature of the solution (thermodilution-based devices). We inject a known amount/temperature of a substance proximally and measure its concentration/temperature distally. We calculate the total flow rate ($Q = m/\int cdt$) from the time profile (integral) curve and a known quantity of the injected substance [38]. Clinically, a known amount of dye or isotope is injected rapidly into a large central vein, or the right side of the heart. We measure the concentration of dye or isotope in arterial blood: the larger the CO the greater the dilution. The most common indicator is a small volume of cold saline; we calculate flow from the temperature change. The average blood flow through an organ can also be calculated from the change in the volume of the hollow body in time: dV/dt (volume of a cavity is imaged within a specified time sequence: by ultrasound, magnetic resonance, X-ray).

4.3. Arterial blood pressure

Arterial blood pressure in the newborn can be measured noninvasively using appropriate cuffs or through the invasive arterial catheters. In principle, the matching of both methods is good [39]. We currently do not know what the normal arterial blood pressure is for a given gestational and postnatal age. Also, we do not know what the value of blood pressure is when the blood flow to vital organs is diminished and the auto-regulatory mechanisms in the brain fail. Thus, neonatal hypotension is not precisely defined. In addition, there is currently no evidence that the treatment of hypotension has significant impact on the clinical outcome in neonates [40–42].

Global perfusion pressure is measured via invasive arterial blood pressure monitoring. However, "adequate" blood pressure does not signify an "adequate" CO; therefore, an increase in blood pressure does not necessary mean an increment of CO. However, without measuring CO we can only assume that adequate mean blood pressure means also adequate CO, which is not always true. Second, the increase in blood pressure does not always mean the elevation of CO (failing myocardium poorly responds to a high vascular resistance). In neonates, the threshold heart rates and perfusion pressure are different depending on gestational and postmenstrual age of premature neonates [42, 43].

5. The peripheral hemodynamic monitoring

Hemodynamic failure results in low cardiac output syndrome with inadequacy of oxygen and nutrients delivered to peripheral tissues and cells. Clinically, peripheral perfusion of organs can be assessed by observing the skin color of a neonate. The method is vastly subjective. A laboratory method of defining the peripheral perfusion is the measurement of the concentration of lactic acid in the peripheral blood. In case of lowered peripheral perfusion tissue hypoxia occurs, which leads to anaerobic metabolism and lactic acid formation. Lactic acid is present in the less perfused tissues and therefore it is primarily not present centrally in systemic circulation; therefore, lactic acidosis (>2.5 mmol/L) is a late sign of low cardiac output syndrome. Consequently, the concentration of lactic acid in the systemic blood rises after the reanimation. Moreover, the production of lactic acid is increased in the case of adrenaline treatment, which increases glycogenolysis and glycolysis in the liver [44]. The plasma concentration of the lactic acid is associated with the stage of the disease and a higher mortality in neonates [45].

Noninvasively, the peripheral perfusion may be assessed by the perfusion index [46]. It is based on an analysis of the pulse oximetry signal. The perfusion index is the ratio between pulsatile and non-pulsatile pulse oximetry signal (AC/DC × 100). It reflects the difference between the amount of blood in the tissue between systole and diastole. The perfusion index correlates well with the capillary refill time, the surface-core body temperature difference [47], and also the severity of the disease in neonates [48].

Assessing the function of peripheral organs is another way of assessing the peripheral hemodynamics. Using amplitude-integrated electroencephalogram (aEEG), we assess the brain function. Observing respiratory rate and pattern indicates the lung function and myocardial contractility indicates the heart function. By measuring the urine output and cleared substances, we assess the renal function. Measurement of diuresis in the neonate for hemodynamic monitoring has many caveats, especially in premature neonates, since immature renal tubules are not able to concentrate the urine. Moreover, the accurate monitoring of diuresis is an invasive method. Laboratory measurements of liver enzymes, clotting factors, and ammonia concentration assess liver function, and measurements of muscle enzyme assess the muscle function [49].

The peripheral monitors enable measuring the micro-vascular blood flow to the peripheral organs by perfusion index and laser-Doppler method and regional tissue oxygenation by NIRS.

5.1. The regional blood flow monitoring in the peripheral organs in the neonate

Regional blood flow is a complex and dynamic variable that changes depending on the functional activity of the body. In pathological conditions, like, for example, a sudden change in blood pressure or hypoxia, blood flow through the body can change very quickly. Like CO also the regional blood flow is measured in mL/min and expressed either normalized by body weight either by 100 g of tissue, or as a percentage of the CO. Assessing and measuring the blood flow is not a part of the permanent clinical practice in neonatal intensive care units, because the methods are generally complicated, inaccurate, invasive, and expensive, and currently their use is not showing clinical welfare for sick newborns.

With the help of the abovementioned physical principles and listed methods for CO monitoring, it is also possible to estimate the regional blood flow in peripheral organs. Using Fick's law, we can calculate blood flow through the peripheral organ, knowing its oxygen consumption. By applying this principle, several methods for the evaluation of blood flow in the brain—through the inhalation of 15% nitrous oxide [50] and the clearance of a radioactive isotope of xenon [51]—have been developed. Regional blood flow to peripheral organs can be measured using Doppler ultrasound [52]. The method is based on measuring the blood flow velocity through the blood vessel. The product of the flow rate and maximum vessel diameter allows us to evaluate blood flow in the vessel, and if the vessel supplies the oxygen and nutrients to the organ we can estimate the blood flow to the organ. Blood flow to the brain can also be measured using magnetic resonance imaging (MRI) techniques. Blood flow to the brain is supplied by four arteries in the neck; hence, it can be evaluated using a scan through the arteries: the cross section of the vessels is multiplied by the blood flow velocity. The blood flow velocity is measured by the loss of magnetization caused by the fresh blood flowing into the plane of imaging (imaging with phase contrast) [28]. For quantitative measurement of the flow, a contrast agent containing gadolinium can be used [53]. The blood flow in each blood vessel can be measured with an electromagnetic flowmeter: the moving particles-ions are deflected to right angles to the direction of movement in an electric field and by that deflection the electric current is measured. Blood flow can also be measured by thermodilution method: the faster the blood flow, the cooler the tip of the heated sensor. Using the plethysmography, the displaced blood volume from the vessels is measured [38].

Frequently used noninvasive and continuous method for the indirect assessment of blood flow in various organs is the spectroscopy in the near-infrared spectrum [54–56]. The method is based on the principle of different absorption patterns of oxyhemoglobin and deoxyhemoglobin. It measures the index of tissue oxygenation and enables the calculation of the extraction of oxygen of the tissues in the target organ. If we assume that changes in the regional tissue oxygenation are not accompanied by changes in the arterial blood oxygen saturation (SaO_2), oxygen consumption, the amount of blood in the arteries and veins, and hemoglobin concentration, then the measured tissue oxygenation can be used to assess organ perfusion. NIRS optodes can be placed practically anywhere on the surface of the body, they measure tissue oxygenation approximately 4 cm below the surface (in the brain, kidneys, intestines, liver, and muscle) [57].

5.2. Microcirculation monitoring in the neonate

Microcirculation encompasses arterioles, capillaries, arteriolar-venous connections, venules, and lymphatic vessels. It supplies the target organs with oxygen and nutrients. Capillary filling or opening depends on the tone of arterioles and precapillary sphincters, whose diameter changes in parallel to the contractions/relaxations of smooth muscle in the vessel wall. The humoral factors, endothelial vasodilators (NO, CO, and H_2S), vasoconstrictors (epinephrine, norepinephrine, and endothelin-1), myogenic mechanism, local metabolites, and the parasympathetic nervous system affect the tone of smooth muscles. Blood flow in the microcirculation reflects the function of the central elements of the blood flow and is thus the ultimate indicator of cardiovascular efficiency. Microcirculation in individual organs also operates globally and represents one of the largest virtual organs in the body. In adults, it is estimated that 5% of the total blood volume is located in the capillaries, which may increase its capacity to fourfold [58].

Microcirculation in the newborn can be assessed using a variety of methods, the most commonly used is the evaluation of flow by laser-Doppler method, video microscopy (dynamic capillaroscopy), and xenon clearance techniques [59]. Flow measurement by laser-Doppler method is based on the fact that the frequency of the light beam, which passes through the tissue, changes as a result of reflection from the moving parts—red blood cells (the Doppler effect). The flow is proportional to the concentration and speed of moving red blood cells in the microcirculation. Since the flow in microcirculation is highly variable, we usually assess microcirculatory response to some of the challenge tests and monitor the dynamics of change. The most commonly used provocation methods are the postocclusive reactive hyperemia (hyperemia after a transitional cuffing of the proximal artery), thermal methods (local heating or cooling), and iontophoresis of vasoactive substances [60, 61]. In the first days after birth, the blood flow is very fragile and the peripheral blood flow in the microcirculation is unstable. The myogenic and nervous controls of skin blood flow enable thermoregulation. The blood flow to the skin in the first days after birth is reduced. The blood flow is related to gestational and postnatal age and the incidence of morbidity and cardiovascular function [62]. The deterioration of peripheral blood flow regulation in microcirculation causes vasodilation and decreased peripheral vascular resistance and contributes to the vulnerability of blood flow. The peripheral blood flow in the first days after birth differs in boys and girls; boys have stronger vasodilation; the mechanism is possibly associated with an increased incidence of hypotension in newborn males [63].

6. Limitations

The described methods for hemodynamic monitoring of neonates have many limitations. The clinical ones are vastly subjective and do not correlate well with the laboratory methods. The continuous bedside noninvasive methods are less accurate and sometimes demand complex deducement to what is happening. There are no trials on resuscitation using the noninvasive methods. The more sophisticated noninvasive methods require expensive equipment and are time consuming, measuring the parameters in the moment of measurement and not continuously.

7. Conclusion

Hemodynamic monitoring, which was for a long time not available in neonates and prematures, is becoming an indispensable tool for understanding how cardiovascular system adapts to extrauterine life. This is especially important when treating the smallest premature with peculiar and very vulnerable hemodynamics. This article adds some of the latest information on hemodynamic monitoring in neonates with specific emphasis on the methods which are available, cost-effective, noninvasive, and easy to manage and understand.

Author details

Petja Fister[1]* and Štefan Grosek[2,3]

*Address all correspondence to: petja_fister@yahoo.com

1 Department of Neonatology, University Children's Hospital, University Medical Center Ljubljana, Ljubljana, Slovenia

2 Department of Pediatric Surgery and Intensive Therapy, Surgical Service, University Medical Center Ljubljana, Ljubljana, Slovenia

3 Department of Pediatrics, Medical Faculty, University of Ljubljana, Ljubljana, Slovenia

References

[1] Ziegler KA, Paul DA, Hoffman M, Locke R. Variation in NICU admission rates without identifiable cause. Hospital Pediatrics. 2016;**6**(5):255-260

[2] Popat H, Robledo KP, Sebastian L, Evans N, Gill A, Kluckow M, et al. Effect of delayed cord clamping on systemic blood flow: A randomized controlled trial. Journal of Pediatrics. 2016;**178**:81-6.e2

[3] Kluckow M, Hooper SB. Using physiology to guide time to cord clamping. Seminars in Fetal and Neonatal Medicine. 2015;**20**(4):225-231

[4] Pinsky MR, Payen D. Functional hemodynamic monitoring. Critical Care. 2005;**9**(6): 566-572

[5] Muralidhar K, Dixit MD, Shetty DP. A safe technique to monitor pulmonary artery pressure during and after paediatric cardiac surgery. Anaesthesia and Intensive Care. 1997;**25**(6):634-636

[6] Soleymani S, Borzage M, Seri I. Hemodynamic monitoring in neonates: Advances and challenges. Journal of Perinatology. 2010;**30**(Suppl):S38-S45

[7] Kluckow M, Evans N. Superior vena cava flow in newborn infants: A novel marker of systemic blood flow. Archives of Diseases in Childhood—Fetal and Neonatal Edition. 2000;**82**(3):F182–F187

[8] Evans N, Kluckow M, Simmons M, Osborn D. Which to measure, systemic or organ blood flow? Middle cerebral artery and superior vena cava flow in very preterm infants. Archives of Diseases in Childhood—Fetal and Neonatal Edition. 2002;**87**(3):F181-F184

[9] Copetti R, Cattarossi L, Macagno F, Violino M, Furlan R. Lung ultrasound in respiratory distress syndrome: A useful tool for early diagnosis. Neonatology. 2008;**94**(1):52-59

[10] Vergine M, Copetti R, Brusa G, Cattarossi L. Lung ultrasound accuracy in respiratory distress syndrome and transient tachypnea of the newborn. Neonatology. 2014;**106**(2):87-93

[11] Cattarossi L, Copetti R, Poskurica B, Miserocchi G. Surfactant administration for neonatal respiratory distress does not improve lung interstitial fluid clearance: Echographic and experimental evidence. Journal of Perinatal Medicine. 2010;**38**(5):557-563

[12] Thompson AE. Pulmonary artery catheterization in children. New Horizon. 1997;**5**(3): 244-250

[13] Tibby SM, Murdoch IA. Monitoring cardiac function in intensive care. Archives of Disease in Childhood. 2003;**88**(1):46-52

[14] Tibby SM, Hatherill M, Murdoch IA. Capillary refill and core-peripheral temperature gap as indicators of haemodynamic status in paediatric intensive care patients. Archives of Disease in Childhood. 1999;**80**(2):163-166

[15] Tibby SM, Hatherill M, Marsh MJ, Murdoch IA. Clinicians' abilities to estimate cardiac index in ventilated children and infants. Archives of Disease in Childhood. 1997;**77**(6):516-518

[16] Osborn DA, Evans N, Kluckow M. Clinical detection of low upper body blood flow in very premature infants using blood pressure, capillary refill time, and central-peripheral temperature difference. Archives of Diseases in Childhood—Fetal and Neonatal Edition. 2004;**89**(2):F168-F173

[17] El-Khuffash AF, McNamara PJ. Neonatologist-performed functional echocardiography in the neonatal intensive care unit. Seminars in Fetal and Neonatal Medicine. 2011;**16**(1):50-60

[18] Singh Y, Gupta S, Groves AM, Gandhi A, Thomson J, Qureshi S, et al. Expert consensus statement 'Neonatologist-performed Echocardiography (NoPE)'-training and accreditation in UK. European Journal of Pediatrics. 2016;**175**(2):281-287

[19] Kluckow M, Seri I, Evans N. Echocardiography and the neonatologist. Pediatric Cardiology. 2008;**29**(6):1043-1047

[20] de Waal K, Kluckow M. Functional echocardiography; from physiology to treatment. Early Human Development. 2010;**86**(3):149-154

[21] Kluckow M. Use of ultrasound in the haemodynamic assessment of the sick neonate. Archives of Diseases in Childhood—Fetal and Neonatal Edition. 2014;**99**(4):F332–F337

[22] Osborn DA, Evans N, Kluckow M. Left ventricular contractility in extremely premature infants in the first day and response to inotropes. Pediatric Research. 2007;**61**(3):335-340

[23] Schmitz L, Stiller B, Pees C, Koch H, Xanthopoulos A, Lange P. Doppler-derived parameters of diastolic left ventricular function in preterm infants with a birth weight <1500 g: Reference values and differences to term infants. Early Human Development. 2004;**76**(2): 101-114

[24] Nestaas E, Støylen A, Brunvand L, Fugelseth D. Tissue Doppler derived longitudinal strain and strain rate during the first 3 days of life in healthy term neonates. Pediatric Research. 2009;**65**(3):357-362

[25] Isaaz K. Tissue Doppler imaging for the assessment of left ventricular systolic and diastolic functions. Current Opinion in Cardiology. 2002;**17**(5):431-442

[26] Groves AM, Chiesa G, Durighel G, Goldring ST, Fitzpatrick JA, Uribe S, et al. Functional cardiac MRI in preterm and term newborns. Archives of Diseases in Childhood—Fetal and Neonatal Edition. 2011;**96**(2):F86–F91

[27] Fogel MA. Assessment of cardiac function by magnetic resonance imaging. Pediatric Cardiology. 2000;**21**(1):59-69

[28] Benders MJ, Hendrikse J, De Vries LS, Van Bel F, Groenendaal F. Phase-contrast magnetic resonance angiography measurements of global cerebral blood flow in the neonate. Pediatric Research. 2011;**69**(6):544-547

[29] Song R, Rich W, Kim JH, Finer NN, Katheria AC. The use of electrical cardiometry for continuous cardiac output monitoring in preterm neonates: A validation study. American Journal of Perinatology. 2014;**31**(12):1105-1110

[30] Coté CJ, Sui J, Anderson TA, Bhattacharya ST, Shank ES, Tuason PM, et al. Continuous noninvasive cardiac output in children: Is this the next generation of operating room monitors? Initial experience in 402 pediatric patients. Paediatric Anaesthesia. 2015;**25**(2): 150-159

[31] Noori S, Drabu B, Soleymani S, Seri I. Continuous non-invasive cardiac output measurements in the neonate by electrical velocimetry: A comparison with echocardiography. Archives of Diseases in Childhood—Fetal and Neonatal Edition. 2012;**97**(5):F340–F343

[32] Lien R, Hsu KH, Chu JJ, Chang YS. Hemodynamic alterations recorded by electrical cardiometry during ligation of ductus arteriosus in preterm infants. European Journal of Pediatrics. 2015;**174**(4):543-550

[33] Hofer CK, Ganter MT, Zollinger A. What technique should I use to measure cardiac output? Current Opinion in Critical Care. 2007;**13**(3):308-317

[34] Gödje O, Höke K, Goetz AE, Felbinger TW, Reuter DA, Reichart B, et al. Reliability of a new algorithm for continuous cardiac output determination by pulse-contour analysis during hemodynamic instability. Critical Care Medicine. 2002;**30**(1):52-58

[35] Osypka M, Soleymani S, Seri I, Noori S. Assessment of cardiac output in neonates: Techniques using the Fick principle, pulse wave form analysis and, electrical impedance. In: Kleinman CS, Seri I, editors. Neonatology Questions and Controversies: Hemodynamics and Cardiology. 2nd ed. Philadelphia: Saunders/Elsevier; 2012. pp. 125-149

[36] Coates BM, Chaize R, Goodman DM, Rozenfeld RA. Performance of capnometry in non-intubated infants in the pediatric intensive care unit. BMC Pediatrics. 2014;**14**:163

[37] Singh BS, Gilbert U, Singh S, Govindaswami B. Sidestream microstream end tidal carbon dioxide measurements and blood gas correlations in neonatal intensive care unit. Pediatric Pulmonology. 2013;**48**(3):250-256

[38] Greisen G. Methods to assess systemic and organ blood flow in the neonate. In: Kleinman CS, Seri I, editors. Neonatology Questions and Controversies: Hemodynamics and Cardiology. Philadelphia: Saunders/Elsevier; 2012. pp. 81-94

[39] Dannevig I, Dale HC, Liestøl K, Lindemann R. Blood pressure in the neonate: Three noninvasive oscillometric pressure monitors compared with invasively measured blood pressure. Acta Paediatrics. 2005;**94**(2):191-196

[40] Batton B, Li L, Newman NS, Das A, Watterberg KL, Yoder BA, et al. Early blood pressure, antihypotensive therapy and outcomes at 18-22 months' corrected age in extremely preterm infants. Archives of Diseases in Childhood—Fetal and Neonatal Edition. 2016; **101**(3):F201–F206

[41] Batton B, Li L, Newman NS, Das A, Watterberg KL, Yoder BA, et al. Use of antihypotensive therapies in extremely preterm infants. Pediatrics. 2013;**131**(6):e1865–e1873

[42] Dempsey EM, Barrington KJ. Treating hypotension in the preterm infant: When and with what: A critical and systematic review. Journal of Perinatology. 2007;**27**(8):469-478

[43] Munro MJ, Walker AM, Barfield CP. Hypotensive extremely low birth weight infants have reduced cerebral blood flow. Pediatrics. 2004;**114**(6):1591-1596

[44] Valverde E, Pellicer A, Madero R, Elorza D, Quero J, Cabañas F. Dopamine versus epinephrine for cardiovascular support in low birth weight infants: Analysis of systemic effects and neonatal clinical outcomes. Pediatrics. 2006;**117**(6):e1213–e1222

[45] Deshpande SA, Platt MP. Association between blood lactate and acid-base status and mortality in ventilated babies. Archives of Diseases in Childhood—Fetal and Neonatal Edition. 1997;**76**(1):F15–F20

[46] Piasek CZ, Van Bel F, Sola A. Perfusion index in newborn infants: A noninvasive tool for neonatal monitoring. Acta Paediatrics. 2014;**103**(5):468-473

[47] Alderliesten T, Lemmers PM, Baerts W, Groenendaal F, van Bel F. Perfusion index in preterm infants during the first 3 days of life: Reference values and relation with clinical variables. Neonatology. 2015;**107**(4):258-265

[48] De Felice C, Latini G, Vacca P, Kopotic RJ. The pulse oximeter perfusion index as a predictor for high illness severity in neonates. European Journal of Pediatrics. 2002; **161**(10):561-562

[49] Azhibekov T, Noori S, Soleymani S, Seri I. Transitional cardiovascular physiology and comprehensive hemodynamic monitoring in the neonate: Relevance to research and clinical care. Seminars in Fetal and Neonatal Medicine. 2014;**19**(1):45-53

[50] Top AP, Ince C, Schouwenberg PH, Tibboel D. Inhaled nitric oxide improves systemic microcirculation in infants with hypoxemic respiratory failure. Pediatric Critical Care Medicine. 2011;**12**(6):e271–e274

[51] Greisen G, Pryds O. Intravenous 133Xe clearance in preterm neonates with respiratory distress. Internal validation of CBF infinity as a measure of global cerebral blood flow. Scandinavian Journal of Clinical and Laboratory Investigation. 1988;**48**(7):673-678

[52] Bada HS, Hajjar W, Chua C, Sumner DS. Noninvasive diagnosis of neonatal asphyxia and intraventricular hemorrhage by Doppler ultrasound. Journal of Pediatrics. 1979;**95** (5 Pt 1):775-779

[53] Tanner SF, Cornette L, Ramenghi LA, Miall LS, Ridgway JP, Smith MA, et al. Cerebral perfusion in infants and neonates: Preliminary results obtained using dynamic susceptibility contrast enhanced magnetic resonance imaging. Archives of Diseases in Childhood—Fetal and Neonatal Edition. 2003;**88**(6):F525–F530

[54] Hou X, Ding H, Teng Y, Zhou C, Zhang D. NIRS study of cerebral oxygenation and hemodynamics in neonate at birth. Conference Proceedings of IEEE Engineering in Medicine and Biology Society. 2011;**2011**:1229-1232

[55] Mittnacht AJ. Near infrared spectroscopy in children at high risk of low perfusion. Current Opinion in Anaesthesiology. 2010;**23**(3):342-347

[56] Goff DA, Buckley EM, Durduran T, Wang J, Licht DJ. Noninvasive cerebral perfusion imaging in high-risk neonates. Seminars in Perinatology. 2010;**34**(1):46-56

[57] Noori S, McCoy M, Anderson MP, Ramji F, Seri I. Changes in cardiac function and cerebral blood flow in relation to peri/intraventricular hemorrhage in extremely preterm infants. Journal of Pediatrics. 2014;**164**(2):264-270.e1-3

[58] Wright IM, Stark MJ, Clifton VL. Assessment of the microcirculation in the neonate. In: Kleinman CS, Seri I, editors. Neonatology Questions and Controversies: Hemodynamics and Cardiology. Philadelphia: Saunders/Elsevier; 2012. pp. 215-234

[59] Weindling M, Paize F. Peripheral haemodynamics in newborns: Best practice guidelines. Early Human Development. 2010;**86**(3):159-165

[60] Turner J, Belch JJ, Khan F. Current concepts in assessment of microvascular endothelial function using laser Doppler imaging and iontophoresis. Trends in Cardiovascular Medicine. 2008;**18**(4):109-116

[61] Agarwal SC, Allen J, Murray A, Purcell IF. Comparative reproducibility of dermal microvascular blood flow changes in response to acetylcholine iontophoresis, hyperthermia and reactive hyperaemia. Physiological Measurement. 2010;**31**(1):1-11

[62] Stark MJ, Clifton VL, Wright IM. Microvascular flow, clinical illness severity and cardiovascular function in the preterm infant. Archives of Diseases in Childhood—Fetal and Neonatal Edition. 2008;**93**(4):F271–F274

[63] Stark MJ, Clifton VL, Wright IM. Sex-specific differences in peripheral microvascular blood flow in preterm infants. Pediatrics Research. 2008;**63**(4):415-419

[64] Voga G. Assessment of cardiac function and circulatory status in critically ill patients. Zdravstveni Vestnik. 2007;**76**:I-19-27

9

Neonatal Gene Therapy for Inherited Disorders

Koichi Miyake, Noriko Miyake and Takashi Shimada

Abstract

In spite of developments of neonatal intensive care medicine, it is still difficult or impossible to treat several inherited genetic disorders using conventional pharmacological methods. Gene therapy is a promising alternate approach for treating a variety of genetic disorders. By the time the patient reaches adulthood, however, it is often too late for effective treatment. But in several of these cases, neonatal gene therapy appears potentially useful against inherited disorders that are not obviously treatable through any other methods. This chapter describes the strategy for neonatal gene therapy for inherited disorders and presents preclinical neonatal gene therapy data for two inherited disorders, metachromatic leukodystrophy and hypophosphatasia. We also discuss the utility, advantages, problems and potential of neonatal gene therapy for inherited disorders.

Keywords: neonatal gene therapy, AAV vectors, metachromatic leukodystrophy, hypophosphatasia

1. Introduction

Although there have been significant advances in neonatal intensive care medicine, several neonatal disorders remain major causes of mortality and morbidity. Consequently, there is an urgent need for development of new safe and effective therapies to improve the outcomes of these intractable and devastating neonatal disorders. Gene therapy is an exciting and promising approach to treat many diseases for which there are still no effective therapies. To date, more than 2400 clinical trials of gene therapy protocols have been attempted in effort to treat various genetic diseases as well as many types of cancers and infectious diseases (http://www.abedia.com/wiley/continents.php). The results of preclinical studies suggest that neonatal gene therapies represent potentially effective treatments for currently intractable neonatal disorders [1–6]. However, although neonatal gene therapies have several advantages over similar therapies used in adult patients, there is as yet no clinical protocol for use of gene therapy in newborn infants. This chapter describes a strategy for the use of neonatal gene therapy in the treatment of inherited disorders and presents preclinical neonatal gene therapy data for two inherited disorders, metachromatic leukodystrophy (MLD) and hypophosphatasia (HPP). We also discuss the utility, advantages, problems and the potential of neonatal gene therapeutic approaches for the treatment of inherited disorders.

2. Adeno-associated virus-mediated gene transfer to neonate

Among the numerous viral and nonviral vectors that have been developed to deliver genes of interest into target cells, adeno-associated virus (AAV) vector has emerged as a particularly promising tool for gene delivery, thanks to its safety (AAV is not pathogenic) and its ability to transduce nondividing cells [7–9]. We are now using several AAV vector serotypes (mainly 1–12), depending on the target [10–13]. **Figure 1** shows the results after intravenous injection into neonatal

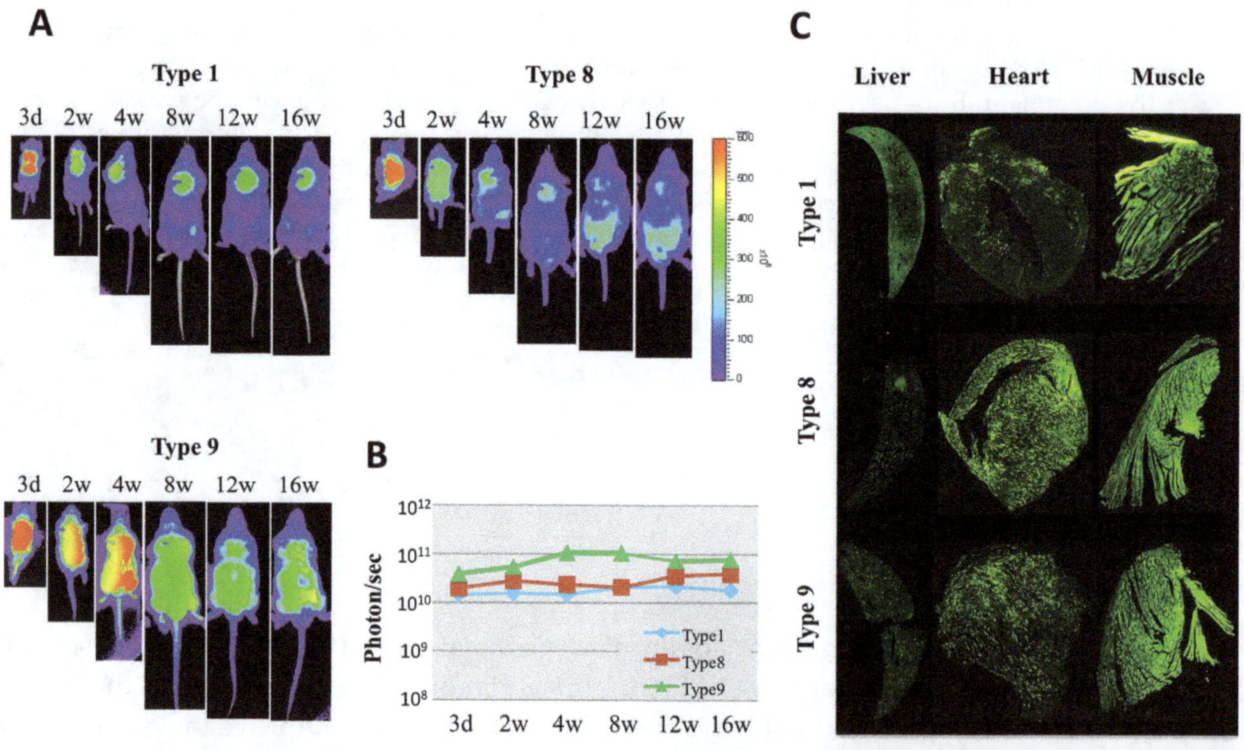

Figure 1. Systemic intravenous injection of AAV vectors into neonatal mice. (A) Approximately 5.0×10^{11} vector genomes (vg) of recombinant AAV vectors encoding the luciferase gene (AAV/Luc) (serotype 1, 8, 9) were injected into the external jugular vein of neonatal mice using a syringe with a 29-G needle. Bioluminescent images of mice were obtained using a Xenogen IVIS imaging system 3 days and 2, 4, 8, 12 and 16 weeks after administration. Color scale bar indicates radiant efficiency (photons s^{-1} cm^{-2} $steradian^{-1}$ per μW cm^{-2}). (B) Radiant efficiency of serotype 1 (blue), 8 (red), and 9 (green) AAV vectors injected mice was quantified. (C) Approximately 5.0×10^{11} vg of AAV vectors encoding green fluorescent protein (serotype 1, 8, 9) were injected into the external jugular vein of neonatal mice. Sixteen weeks after injection, liver, heart and muscle were stained with anti-GFP antibody.

mice of AAV vector serotypes 1, 8 and 9, harboring the luciferase gene. Expression of luciferase was detected within 3 days and continued for more than 16 weeks with no decrease in expression. Serotype 9 mediated the highest expression during the observation period (**Figure 1A, B**). In addition, using an AAV vector encoding green fluorescent protein (GFP), we determined that the organs most efficiently transduced are the liver, heart and muscle (**Figure 1C**). Moreover, although transduction efficiency was not as high, the central nervous system (CNS) was also transduced after intravenous injection of AAV vector, which apparently passes through the blood-brain barrier (BBB) [14] in neonatal mice [15]. Thus, a systemically administered AAV vector was able to transduce several important target organs in neonatal mice, including the CNS, and mediate expression of a gene of interest for a prolonged period of time.

3. Advantages of neonatal gene therapy

Systemic gene transfer to neonates has several advantages over treatment of the adults (**Table 1**). First, as mentioned above, neonatal gene therapy has the potential to overcome the limitation imposed by the BBB on treating genetic disorders of the CNS. Because the BBB is developmentally immature during the perinatal period, AAV-mediated neonatal gene therapy is a highly promising strategy for treating genetic neurological diseases. Second, because the immune system is immature, neonates are immunologically tolerant of the transgene and/or viral vector [16–18]. Immune rejection of the transgene product by neutralizing antibodies is a severe problem for gene therapy in adults. Third, treatment administered soon after birth may enable prevention of early-onset genetic disease. Finally, neonates can be effectively treated with a smaller amount of viral vector than adults. Using smaller amounts of viral vector is superior with respect to both safety and cost. Taken together, these advantages make systemic neonatal gene therapy a promising method for treating systemic genetic diseases.

- Penetrates the blood-brain barrier
- Induces immune tolerance
- Prevents early-onset genetic diseases
- Enables the use of smaller amounts of vector

Table 1. Advantages of neonatal gene therapy.

4. Application of neonatal gene therapy

4.1. Neonatal gene therapy for metachromatic leukodystrophy

Metachromatic leukodystrophy is an inherited, autosomal recessive lysosomal storage disease (LSD) caused by a deficiency in the lysosomal enzyme arylsulfatase A (ASA), which catalyzes the degradation of galactosyl-3-sulfate ceramide (sulfatide (Sulf)), a major myelin sphingolipid [19]. This disease is characterized by myelin degeneration, mainly in the CNS, and clinically by progressive motor and mental deterioration that is ultimately lethal. Therefore, the major target organ for treatment of this disease is the CNS, and the aim is to arrest or reverse the progression of the neurological symptoms. A major obstacle, however, is the BBB, which limits delivery of systemically administered therapeutic molecules to the brain [14]. It is therefore hoped that systemic administration of an AAV vector harboring ASA during the neonatal period would be useful for treating the CNS. We previously showed that a single systemic injection of AAV vector encoding human ASA (AAV/hASA) into neonatal ASA knockout (MLD) mice results in the wide distribution of ASA in the brain and correction of the biochemical and neurological phenotypes [20]. **Figure 2A** shows that a single systemic injection of AAV/hASA enables transduction of the CNS in neonates but not

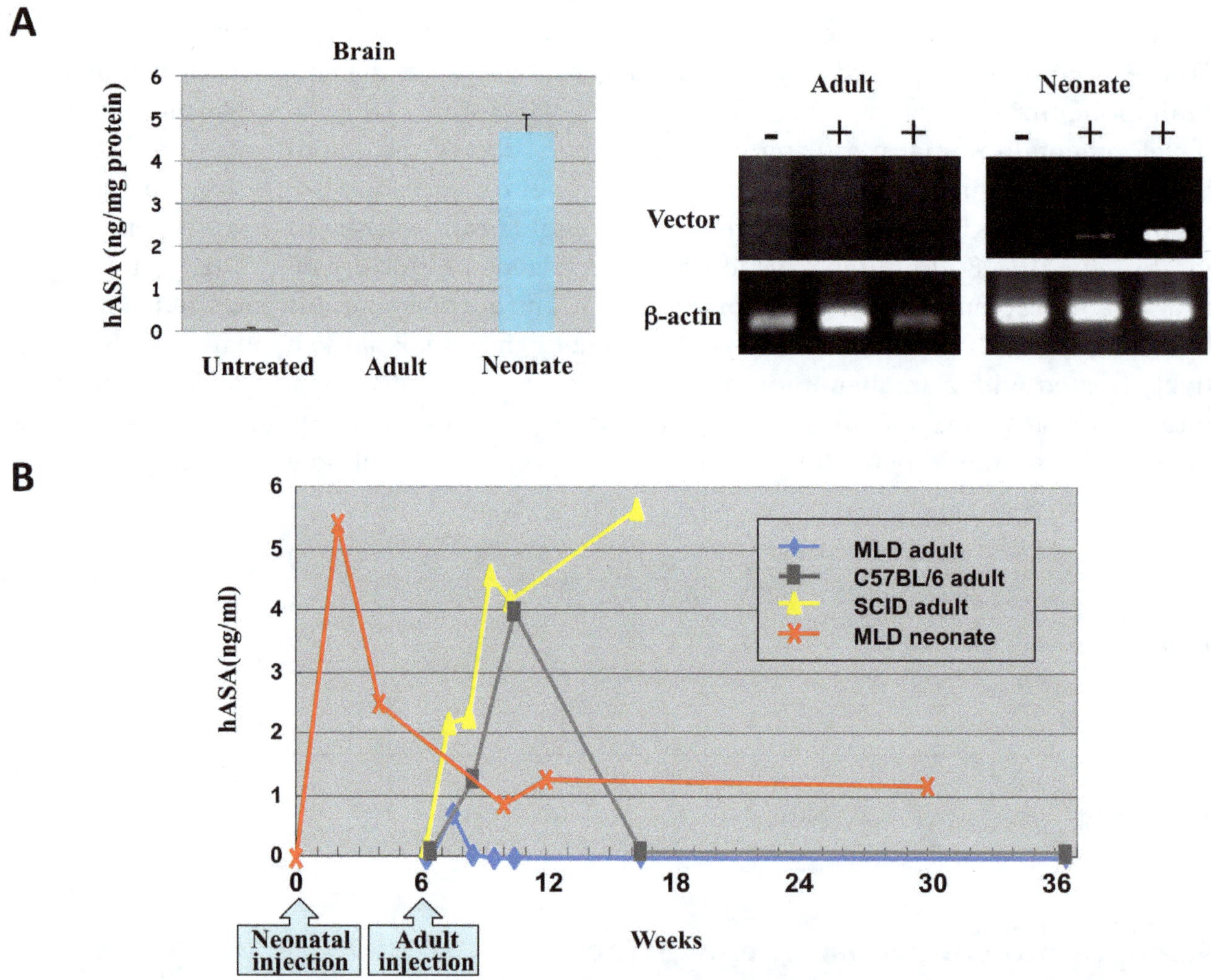

Figure 2. hASA expression of MLD mice following neonatal systemic administration of AAV/hASA vectors. (A) Fifty-two weeks after AAV/hASA injection, hASA concentration in the brain was determined by an indirect sandwich enzyme-linked immunosorbent assay (ELISA) (left panel). DNA from the brain was extracted and analyzed using PCR with hASA-specific primers (right panel). (B) hASA expression in plasma of AAV/hASA-injected mice. hASA concentration in plasma was determined by ELISA. Sustained expression was observed after neonatal injection of AAV/hASA.

in adults. Efficient hASA expression was detected in the brain of AAV/hASA treated at the neonatal period of MLD mice. PCR analysis confirmed that AAV vector genome was observed only in neonatal-treated MLD mice. Moreover, sustained expression of hASA in plasma was detected for at least 30 weeks after intravenous injection into neonatal MLD mice, while only transient increase in plasma hASA was obtained when injected into either adult MLD mice or wild-type C57Bl/6 mice (**Figure 2B**). Vector injection into adult NOD-SCID mice led to sustained secretion of hASA into the circulation, suggesting that immune responses to hASA are a major hurdle for successful gene therapy in immunocompetent adult MLD mice. It thus appears that the systemic injection of AAV vector during the neonatal period is a potentially useful means of treating neurological disorders.

4.2. Neonatal gene therapy for hypophosphatasia

Hypophosphatasia is an inherited disease caused by a deficiency of tissue-nonspecific alkaline phosphatase (TNALP) [21, 22]. The major symptom of human HPP is hypomineralization,

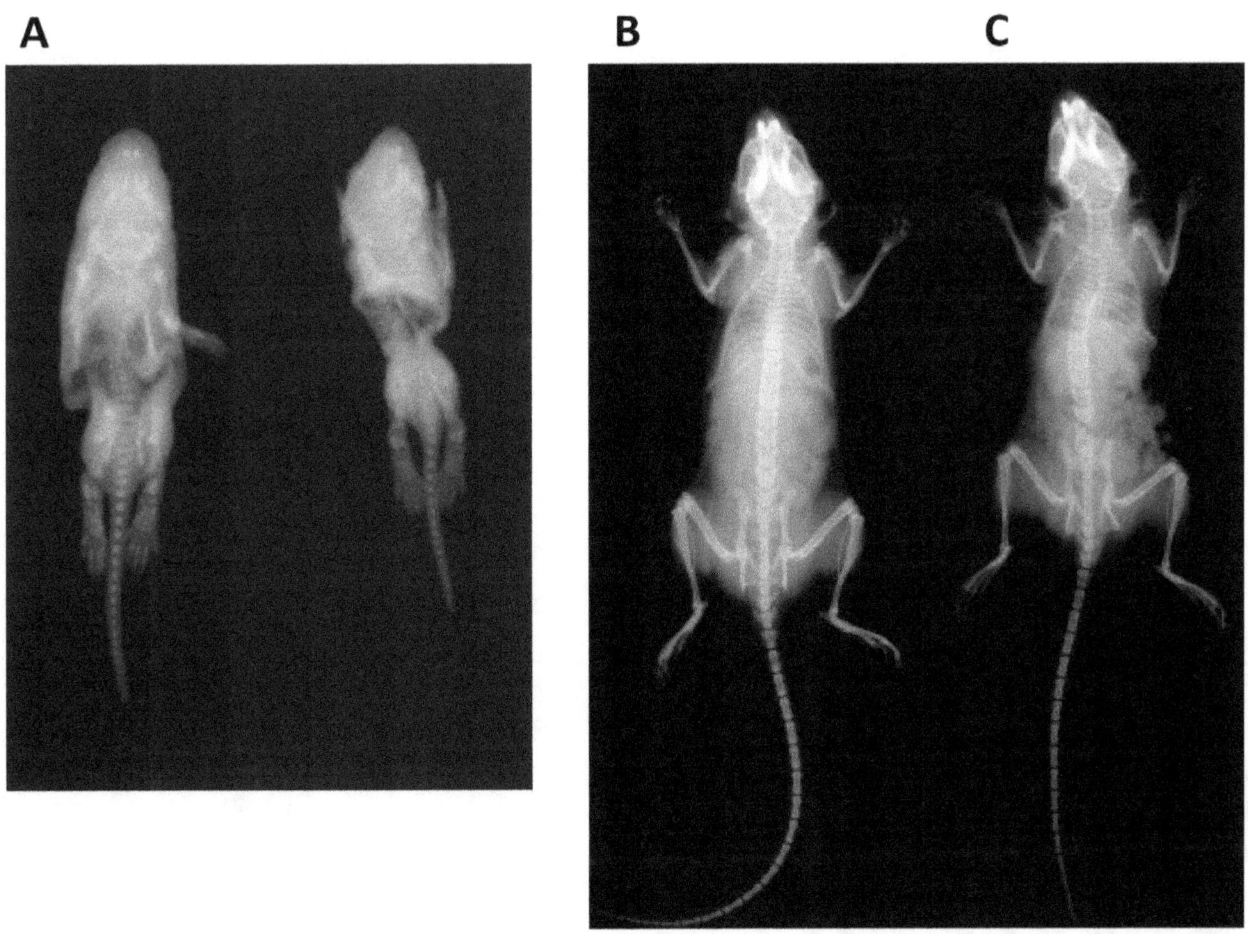

Figure 3. X-ray images of the whole bodies of TNALP knockout mice. Radiographic images were obtained on IFX1000 film (Fujifilm Corp., Tokyo, Japan) using a setup for analysis of small animals. The energy level was 25 kV, and the exposure time was 90 s for 10-day-old untreated TNALP knockout (A), normal wild-type (B) and AAV/TNALP-D10-treated TNALP knockout mice (C).

rickets or osteomalacia, although the clinical severity is highly variable. Patients with infantile HPP may appear normal at birth but gradually develop rickets before reaching 6 months of age. Neonatal gene therapy is a promising strategy for treating infantile HPP by preventing early onset. We have shown that the phenotype of TNALP knockout mice [23–25], which mimics the severe infantile form of HPP, can be prevented by a single neonatal injection of AAV vector encoding bone-targeted TNALP in which a deca-aspartate tail is linked to the C-terminus of soluble TNALP (AAV/TNALP-D10). Sustained expression of TNALP and phenotypic correction of TNALP knockout mice were observed following the neonatal gene therapy [26]. X-ray analysis showed that treated TNALP knockout mice grow as well as normal wild-type mice (**Figure 3**).

5. Problems of neonatal gene therapy

There are several problems that must be overcome before neonatal gene therapies can be used in humans. First, safety concern must be addressed, as there is the possibility of tumor development and of germ-line transmission. It was reported that liver and lung cancers appeared in some mice treated using AAV-mediated neonatal gene therapy [27, 28]. In addition, differences in developmental stages of organs in mice and humans may be another problem. The immune system in mice is less mature at birth than that in larger animals, and the human BBB is functionally mature before birth. It is therefore not clear whether the same beneficial effect of neonatal gene therapy seen in mice would be achieved in human infants. These problems must be overcome before there can be clinical trials of neonatal gene therapy.

6. Summary and future developments

We have shown that AAV-mediated gene transfer in neonatal mice has characteristics that could potentially overcome the problems encountered with current gene therapy protocols. However, before applying neonatal gene transfer to humans, several important issues must be addressed. In particular, the safety of neonatal gene transfer must be carefully evaluated using large animal models, including nonhuman primates. Nonetheless, because of its advantages over gene therapies used to treat genetic disorders in adults, safe and effective neonatal gene therapy has the potential to be an invaluable method for treating genetic diseases.

Acknowledgements

We thank Dr. James Wilson (University of Pennsylvania), Dr. R. Jude Samulski (University of North Carolina), Dr. Robert M. Kotin (National Institutes of Health) and Dr. David W. Russell (University of Washington) for kindly providing AAV packaging or vector plasmids and Dr. Volkmar Gieselmann (Rheinische Friedrich-Wilhelms-University) and Dr. Jose Luis Millán (Stanford Children's Health Research Center) for kindly providing MLD and HPP model mice. We also thank Dr. Tae Matsumoto and Dr. Yukihiko Hirai for joint research and helpful discussions. This chapter was supported in part by grants from the Ministry of Health and Welfare of Japan and the Ministry of Education, Science and Culture of Japan.

Author details

Koichi Miyake*, Noriko Miyake and Takashi Shimada

*Address all correspondence to: kmiyake@nms.ac.jp

Department of Biochemistry and Molecular Biology, Division of Gene Therapy Research Center for Advanced Medical Technology, Nippon Medical School, Japan

References

[1] Cantero G, Liu XB, Mervis RF, Lazaro MT, Cederbaum SD, Golshani P, Lipshutz GS. Rescue of the functional alterations of motor cortical circuits in arginase deficiency by neonatal gene therapy. The Journal of Neuroscience. 2016;**36**(25):6680-6690

[2] Heldermon CD, Qin EY, Ohlemiller KK, Herzog ED, Brown JR, Vogler C, Hou W, Orrock JL, Crawford BE, Sands MS. Disease correction by combined neonatal intracranial AAV and systemic lentiviral gene therapy in Sanfilippo syndrome type B mice. Gene Therapy. 2013; **20**(9):913-921

[3] Iijima O, Miyake K, Watanabe A, Miyake N, Igarashi T, Kanokoda C, Nakamura-Takahashi A, Kinoshita H, Noguchi T, Abe S, Narisawa S, Millan JL, Okada T, Shimada T. Prevention of lethal murine hypophosphatasia by neonatal ex vivo gene therapy using lentivirally transduced bone marrow cells. Human Gene Therapy. 2015;**26**(12):801-812

[4] Lattanzi A, Salvagno C, Maderna C, Benedicenti F, Morena F, Kulik W, Naldini L, Montini E, Martino S, Gritti A. Therapeutic benefit of lentiviral-mediated neonatal intracerebral gene therapy in a mouse model of globoid cell leukodystrophy. Human Molecular Genetics. 2014;**23**(12):3250-3268

[5] Mearini G, Stimpel D, Geertz B, Weinberger F, Kramer E, Schlossarek S, Mourot-Filiatre J, Stoehr A, Dutsch A, Wijnker PJ, Braren I, Katus HA, Muller OJ, Voit T, Eschenhagen T, Carrier L. Mybpc3 gene therapy for neonatal cardiomyopathy enables long-term disease prevention in mice. Nature Communications. 2014;**5**:5515

[6] Xing EM, Wu S, Ponder KP. The effect of Tlr4 and/or C3 deficiency and of neonatal gene therapy on skeletal disease in mucopolysaccharidosis VII mice. Molecular Genetics and Metabolism. 2015;**114**(2):209-216

[7] Grieger JC, Samulski RJ. Adeno-associated virus vectorology, manufacturing, and clinical applications. Methods in Enzymology. 2012;**507**:229-254

[8] Skubis-Zegadlo J, Stachurska A, Malecki M. Vectrology of adeno-associated viruses (AAV). Medycyna Wieku Rozwojowego. 2013;**17**(3):202-206

[9] Wright JF, Qu G, Tang C, Sommer JM. Recombinant adeno-associated virus: Formulation challenges and strategies for a gene therapy vector. Current Opinion in Drug Discovery and Development. 2003;**6**(2):174-178

[10] Gao G, Vandenberghe LH, Wilson JM. New recombinant serotypes of AAV vectors. Current Gene Therapy. 2005;**5**(3):285-297

[11] Gao GP, Alvira MR, Wang L, Calcedo R, Johnston J, Wilson JM. Novel adeno-associated viruses from rhesus monkeys as vectors for human gene therapy. Proceedings of the National Academy of Sciences of the United States of America. 2002;**99**(18):11854-11859

[12] Miyake K, Miyake N, Yamazaki Y, Shimada T, Hirai Y. Serotype-independent method of recombinant adeno-associated virus (AAV) vector production and purification. Journal of Nippon Medical School. 2012;**79**(6):394-402

[13] Summerford C, Samulski RJ. AAVR: A multi-serotype receptor for AAV. Molecular Therapy. 2016;**24**(4):663-666

[14] Tajes M, Ramos-Fernandez E, Weng-Jiang X, Bosch-Morato M, Guivernau B, Eraso-Pichot A, Salvador B, Fernandez-Busquets X, Roquer J, Munoz FJ. The blood-brain barrier: Structure, function and therapeutic approaches to cross it. Molecular Membrane Biology. 2014;**31**(5):152-167

[15] Miyake N, Miyake K, Yamamoto M, Hirai Y, Shimada T. Global gene transfer into the CNS across the BBB after neonatal systemic delivery of single-stranded AAV vectors. Brain Research. 2011;**1389**:19-26

[16] Hinderer C, Bell P, Louboutin JP, Katz N, Zhu Y, Lin G, Choa R, Bagel J, O'Donnell P, Fitzgerald CA, Langan T, Wang P, Casal ML, Haskins ME, Wilson JM. Neonatal tolerance induction enables accurate evaluation of gene therapy for MPS I in a canine model. Molecular Genetics and Metabolism. 2016;**119**(1-2):124-130

[17] Hinderer C, Bell P, Louboutin JP, Zhu Y, Yu H, Lin G, Choa R, Gurda BL, Bagel J, O'Donnell P, Sikora T, Ruane T, Wang P, Tarantal AF, Casal ML, Haskins ME, Wilson JM. Neonatal systemic AAV induces tolerance to CNS gene therapy in MPS I dogs and nonhuman primates. Molecular Therapy. 2015;**23**(8):1298-1307

[18] Hu C, Lipshutz GS. AAV-based neonatal gene therapy for hemophilia A: Long-term correction and avoidance of immune responses in mice. Gene Therapy. 2012;**19**(12):1166-1176

[19] von Figura K, Gieselmann V, Jaeken J. Metachromatic leukodystrophy. The Metabolic and Molecular Bases of Inherited Disease. New York: McGraw-Hill; 2001

[20] Miyake N, Miyake K, Asakawa N, Yamamoto M, Shimada T. Long-term correction of biochemical and neurological abnormalities in MLD mice model by neonatal systemic injection of an AAV serotype 9 vector. Gene Therapy. 2014;**21**(4):427-433

[21] Mornet E. Hypophosphatasia. Orphanet Journal of Rare Diseases. 2007;**2**:40

[22] Whyte MP. Physiological role of alkaline phosphatase explored in hypophosphatasia. Annals of the New York Academy of Sciences. 2010;**1192**:190-200

[23] Narisawa S, Fröhlander N, Millán JL. Inactivation of two mouse alkaline phosphatase genes and establishment of a model of infantile hypophosphatasia. Developmental Dynamics: An Official Publication of the American Association of Anatomists. 1997;**208**(3):432-446

[24] Narisawa S, Yadav MC, Millán JL. In vivo overexpression of tissue-nonspecific alkaline phosphatase increases skeletal mineralization and affects the phosphorylation status of osteopontin. Journal of Bone and Mineral Research : The Official Journal of the American Society for Bone and Mineral Research. 2013;**28**(7):1587-1598

[25] Yadav MC, Simão AM, Narisawa S, Huesa C, McKee MD, Farquharson C, Millán JL. Loss of skeletal mineralization by the simultaneous ablation of PHOSPHO1 and alkaline phosphatase function: a unified model of the mechanisms of initiation of skeletal calcification. Journal of Bone and Mineral Research : The Official Journal of the American Society for Bone and Mineral Research. 2011;**26**(2):286-297

[26] Matsumoto T, Miyake K, Yamamoto S, Orimo H, Miyake N, Odagaki Y, Adachi K, Iijima O, Narisawa S, Millán JL, Fukunaga Y, Shimada T. Rescue of severe infantile hypophosphatasia mice by AAV-mediated sustained expression of soluble alkaline phosphatase. Human Gene Therapy. 2011;**22**(11):1355-1364

[27] Chandler RJ, LaFave MC, Varshney GK, Burgess SM, Venditti CP. Genotoxicity in mice following AAV gene delivery: A safety concern for human gene therapy? Molecular Therapy. 2016;**24**(2):198-201

[28] Walia JS, Altaleb N, Bello A, Kruck C, LaFave MC, Varshney GK, Burgess SM, Chowdhury B, Hurlbut D, Hemming R, Kobinger GP, Triggs-Raine B. Long-term correction of Sandhoff disease following intravenous delivery of rAAV9 to mouse neonates. Molecular Therapy. 2015;**23**(3):414-422

10

Neonatal Care for Anesthesiologists

Esra Caliskan

Abstract

In recent years, developments in obstetrics and neonatology have significantly improved the survival and quality life time of neonates. Therefore, anesthesiologists are more confronted with these patients due to surgical and non-surgical procedures. For a safe anesthetic approach and safe care, anesthesiologist must have necessary knowledge and equipment on the physiology of the newborn and should be better understand how immature organs respond to surgery and anesthetic. The purpose of this section is to present spot information that will allow clinicians and anesthesiologists to better understand the problems of neonatal patients and to perform safe care for these patients in the light of the physiologic characteristics of neonates. General principles of anesthetic management of neonatal patients are also reviewed and discussed.

Keywords: neonatal physiology, anesthetic management, perioperative evaluation, postoperative care, neonatal surgery

1. Introduction

Differently from the adult patients, pediatric, especially neonatal age group is a patient population that is difficult to assess. It should not be forgotten that children are not miniaturized adults. Therefore, the preoperative evaluation of the neonate is admittedly the most important part of anesthetic evaluation. The developments in the field of neonatal medicine over the past two decades have increased our probability of encountering a healthy and unhealthy neonatal population [1]. Surgical procedures especially emergency surgical conditions can be represent a significant anesthetic challenge and life threatening in neonatal period [2, 3].

Therefore, the anesthetist needs to take into account the immature function of many vital organ systems, the normal course of development, the effects of the underlying pathologic disease processes, which can frequently lead to serious physiological instability [4, 5].

In this chapter will be discussed issues that related to the anesthetic approach and postoperative care to neonatal patients.

2. Physiological feature in neonatal period

2.1. Organ and system differences in neonate

The neonatal period shows anatomical and physiological differences when compared to adult period. In this section, will be mentioned to physiological characteristics of neonates, also anatomical differences of neonates will be discussed in the part of anesthetic management.

It is important to know the anatomical airway differences between adults and children and newborns for a complete anesthesia assessment [6]. These differences can be listed as follows:

- Proportionately larger head and tongue,
- Narrower nasal passages,
- An anterior and cephalad larynx,
- A longer epiglottis,
- Shorter trachea and neck.

Because of these anatomical features, nasal breathing is dominant in neonates and infants until about 5 months of age [6].

In the newborn period, many vital organ and system functions are immature [7]. In respiratory system, high pulmonary vascular resistance (PVR) which is characteristics in fetal circulation decreases by approximately 10% after labor, but the apparent decrease occurs with the first breath [8, 9]. When the transition period to the adult circulation is examined, pulmonary blood flow, increased alveolar and arterial PO_2 appear to be important factors.

The characteristics of the neonatal respiratory system can be listed as follows: [1, 6].

- Immature hypoxic response, lower functional residual capacity (limits oxygen reserves during period of apnea, rapid desaturation in prolonged intubation attempt),
- Central control of ventilation is not fully develop,
- Peripheral feedback mechanisms are not sufficiently mature,
- Neonatal oxygen consumption 6 cc kg^{-1} per minute is twice that of resting adult (this value increases 10 cc kg^{-1} in the first week of life).

Cardiovascular system changes are also observed during neonatal period. The circulation of a newborn infant is a dynamic state which may revert to a transitional characteristic at any time. This means that the adult series circulation accompanies fetal parallel circulation [10].

The onset of spontaneous breathing is the main factor that reduces high PVR which is characteristic of fetal circulation. This decrease in pulmonary pressure is followed by an increase in systemic vascular resistance and left atrial pressure. Some clinical situations such as hypoxia and acidosis may lead to reduction of pulmonary blood flow which causes a return the fetal circulation features that is called persistent fetal circulation (PFC) [11].

Cardiac function is heart rate dependent in healthy neonates because the immature myocardium has limited compliance [2, 12].

The parasympathetic system is predominant in neonates [10], so that vagal stimulus by laryngoscopy and hypoxia may cause bradycardia. Therefore, it should be avoided bradycardia and treated aggressively when it is observed.

Liver and kidney function are also closely related to the anesthetic management of neonates. In the neonatal period, both organs have not yet completed maturation. The liver serves a critical role in carbohydrate, protein, lipid metabolism, coagulation. And is the primary site for biotransformation of drugs [13]. Hepatic oxidation, reduction and hydrolysis maturation process is rapid and these functions reaches adult rates around 6 month of ages [14]. Because of this, newborns may metabolize drugs (include anesthetic drugs) and toxins less efficiently than adults in the early months of their lives, as the pathway of degradation is immature [1]. Also, one of the changes in early infancy is the lower concentration of total serum protein, albumin and α1-acid glycoprotein. These proteins reach the adult level at about 1 year old [14].

One of the main routes of clearance of drugs and metabolites are the kidneys too. Glomerular filtration rate (GFR), active secretion and passive reabsorption are functions that determine renal excretion of drugs [15].

The kidneys also play an important role in the maintaining of acid base homeostasis and fluid electrolyte balance. GFR and reabsorption are increase age dependent manner. A neonate's kidney takes approximately 6–12 months to achieve adult performance.

In the perioperative period, fluid electrolyte balance is affected and the metabolism of commonly used anesthetic drug altered [10]. Drug metabolism and protein binding are also reduced due to immature organ (hepatic and renal) function [16].

Maturational physiologic changes are most prominent in neonatal period and infancy. The distribution of total body fluid component in neonates is different from adults. Body fluid constitute a greater proportion of body weight in the neonate (approximately 70–75%) and higher than adults. In neonate, the intracellular and extracellular fluid compartments are approximately 45 and 33% of body weight, respectively [17]. These body component changes affect volumes of distribution of drugs.

2.2. Thermoregulation

The newborn baby has a greater surface area relative to weight and a thin layer subcutaneous fat tissue [3]. These properties cause more heat loss to the environment in neonates than older children and adult. Nonshivering thermogenesis is regulated by brown fat is the primary mechanism in heat generation in the neonates [1]. Brown fat tissue is located in the posterior neck along the interscapular and vertebral regions and it is responsible for heat generation in newborns.

There are four different mechanisms of heat loss [18]:

- Evaporation,
- Convection,
- Conduction,
- Radiation,

Cold intravenous fluids, exposure to cold sterilization solutions, drying of anesthetic gases and the direct effect of anesthetic agents on temperature regulation are the factors that increase this loss.

For this reason mentioned above, caution should be exercised in serious temperature changes in the perioperative period. Hypothermia may cause undesirable effects such as acidosis, myocardial depression, and delay recovery from anesthesia [19, 20].

Maximum precautions should be taken to prevent hypothermia in the perioperative period. These precautions are mentioned in the intraoperative management section.

Characteristics of neonates and infants that differentiate them adult patients are summarized in **Table 1**.

Anatomical differences	Physiological differences	Pharmacological differences
Head and neck • Relatively larger head and tongue • Narrower nasal passage • Anterior and cephalad larynx • Relatively longer epiglottis and shorter trachea Circulation • Left ventricle –noncompliant • Transitional circulation Respiratory • Weak intercostal and diaphragmatic muscles • Increased resistance to airflow	Increasing parameters • Heart rate (dependent cardiac output) • Respiratory rate • Metabolic rate • Total body water content • Chest wall compliance • Ratio of body surface area to body weight Decreasing parameters • Blood pressure • Functional residual capacity • Lung compliance	Hepatic function • Immature biotransformation • Decreased protein, decreased binding for drug Respiratory changes • More rapid rise in *FA/FI • more rapid induction and recovery from inhaled anesthetics • Increased minimum alveolar concentration Body fluid changes • Relatively larger volume distribution for water- soluble drugs • Immature neuromuscular junction

*FA/FI: Fractional alveolar concentration/fractional inspired concentration.
Table has modified by Lange Clinical Anesthesia 2015.

Table 1. Characteristics of neonates and infants that differentiate them adult patient.

3. General principles of anesthesia in neonate

Neonatal period, which is the most vulnerable time period in terms of anesthetic risk and perioperative mortality, is a challenging period for pediatric anesthetists.

Drug interactions, physiological and anatomical differences, and knowledge of risk factors are also important to reduce these risks.

What are the risks associated with neonatal anesthesia? In addition to the neonatal differences, prematurity, congenital anomalies, asphyxia at birth, and emergency situations that required surgery are risk factors. At the same time, there is a very narrow margin of error, including airway management, vascular access and drug administration. Some of these risk factors are summarized in **Table 2**.

Therefore, a safe aesthetic approach depends on a good understanding of the variables and physiological and anatomical changes taking place in the transition from fatal to neonatal life.

Anatomical differences

Airway anomalies
- Difficult airway: Micrognathia, macroglossia, cleft palate-lift

Prematurity, Immature organ and system function
- Respiratory
- Apnea (especially premature neonates)
- Respiratory failure, mechanical ventilatory support, supplemental oxygen
- Oxygenation: avoid high FiO_2 (high FiO_2 risk of retinopathy, NEC)

Cardiac
- Transitional circulation
- Persistent pulmonary hypertension
- Immature myocardium
- Parasympathetic dominance

Neurological problems
- Intraventricular/periventricular hemorrhage (IVH, PVH)

Congenital syndromes and disorders (especially associated with risk of difficult airway, comorbidities of cardiac defect)

- Pierre-Robin syndrome
- Treacher-Collins syndrome (mandibulofacial dysostosis)
- Goldenhar syndrome
- Klippel-Feil syndrome
- Down syndrome

Pharmacological differences
- Anesthetic drugs – dilutional changes, prolonged effect

Fluid management
- Glucose: avoid hypoglycemia
- Intolerance for rapid fluid infusion
- Problems of vascular access

Temperature management
- Prevent hypothermia

Emergency surgery

Table 2. Risk factors in neonatal anesthesia.

3.1. Effects of anesthetic drugs and inhalation anesthetics on neonates

Effective and safe drug administration in neonates should be based on detailed knowledge on the physiological characteristics of the neonates and pharmacokinetics and pharmacodynamics of given drug. Clinical pharmacology in neonates is recognized with extensive variability. The effect of anesthetic agents varies with organ maturation, body water content and metabolic differences and, coexisting disease in neonatal patient population.

Inhalation anesthesia is a commonly used anesthetic technique in neonatal population. However, intravenous and regional anesthesia methods also can be applied as anesthetic technique in this patient population. The minimum alveolar concentration (MAC) of an inhaled anesthetic is the alveolar concentration that prevents movement in 50% of patients in response to a standardized stimulus (e.g., surgical incision) and changes with age [1, 6, 21]. MAC for inhalational agents is less in neonates than in infants (up to 6 months of age [12, 21]. In newborns, cardiac and respiratory functions and blood pressure are very sensitive to volatile anesthesia. Immature myocardium and less developed compensatory mechanisms are responsible for this result. Therefore, these anesthetics can cause dose dependent cardiac and respiratory depressant effect and can be seen bradycardia, hypotension and postoperative apnea. These effects are more pronounced during the induction period [12, 22].

Intravenous anesthetic agents may be used for induction of anesthesia when inhalational anesthetics are not preferred and/or not practices.

Factors affecting the administration of intravenous anesthesia can be listed as follows:

- Larger intravascular and extracellular fluid compartments,
- Immaturity of hepatic biotransformation pathways,
- Decreased protein binding,
- Increased organ blood flow,
- Higher metabolic rate.

These factors mentioned above affect the properties of the intravenous anesthetics such as duration of effect (onset and termination), doses and toxicity limits of drugs.

An opioid agent causes fewer hemodynamic changes but it should be noted that increase the risk of postoperative apnea and late-onset re-sedation in recovery in preterm and term neonates [2, 4].

Thus, it is crucial that intravenous lines are flushed and cleared of any medication (e.g. opioid, neuromuscular blocker).

Muscle relaxant may be required for some surgical procedures (especially abdominal surgical procedures such as necrotizing enterocolitis, abdominal wall defect). The response of neonates to nondepolarizing muscle relaxant is quite variable. Neuromuscular junction is immature in preterms and this increases the susceptibility to muscle relaxants. However, the large extracellular distribution volume will dilute the drug concentration, while those metabolized in the liver will prolong the duration.

4. Anesthesia preparation in neonates before surgical procedure

4.1. Preoperative evaluation

Anesthetic management in neonatal patients can be challenging but careful preoperative assessment means that a safe and smooth preparation process for the neonates and anesthetic team. This evaluation is also an approach that encourages confidence for their parents.

A careful preoperative examination allows the anesthetist to determine the risk of anesthesia based on the general state of health of newborn. It is aimed to establish an appropriate plan for anesthesia, postoperative care and analgesia in the light of acquired information.

Preoperative assessment in neonates should include a comprehensive examination of the neonate's perinatal history (such as prematurity, apnea-hypoxic episode history, duration of oxygen dependency, neurological damage etc.), congenital anomalies, previous anesthesia applications, and general state of health (acute, chronic lung disease, cardiac pathologies, etc.) [23].

Premature, ex-premature and term neonates are highly heterogeneous group within newborn period and needs various surgical interventions. Most of them come directly from the neonatal intensive care unit (NICU) and require urgent intervention. Many unusual congenital syndromes occur in childhood. These congenital anomalies in newborn period may accompany emergency surgical procedures [24]. Congenital anomalies that may cause difficult intubation should be noted and the anesthesia plan should be made accordingly.

In addition, a more detailed examination should be performed to reveal early postnatal problems that may be seen (such as hypoglycemia, infection and sepsis, etc.).

Risk factors which are important in neonatal anesthesia are summarized in **Table 2**.

A systematic approach to preoperative evaluation will prevent important problems from being overlooked. Many healthy neonates undergoing elective simple surgery and procedures are fit and do not require compressive physical examination. However, evaluation of the head and neck (such micrognathia, limited neck mobility, macroglossia, etc.) and cardiorespiratory examination (cardiac congenital anomalies, breathing sounds, respiratory pathologies associated with increased secretion and inflammation etc.) should be performed before surgical procedures. Also in cardiac examination, previously undiagnosed murmur with pathological qualities (e.g. loud, continuous, diastolic and or/associated with a trill) may be noticeable.

Evaluation of the airway is critical to the delivery of safe anesthesia. In neonates with a syndrome associated with airway anomalies, the potential presence of a difficult airway (**Table 2**) (*e.g. Pierre-Robin, Goldenhar, Treacher-Collins Syndrome, cleft palate and lip, maxilla mandibular synechia, etc.*) can be identified preoperatively.

It is also important to identify any concomitant (such as necrotizing enterocolitis, hyaline membrane syndrome, cardiac pathologies, sepsis, etc.) disease which might increase the risk of anesthesia and surgery. Familial, genetic, and neuromuscular diseases are important for anesthetic management. The presence of these diseases should be questioned.

Body weight, height, head circumference size must be recorded in order to evaluate newborn's physical status. For example, microcephaly is associated with some genetic disorders and may cause neurological sequel, which may pose a risk for anesthesia.

In laboratory evaluation, a baseline hemoglobin measurement should be obtained for minor surgical procedures [24]. If there is no indication for emergency surgery, anemia should be treated before surgical procedure. Because, even if it is a minor surgery, anemia may precipitate postoperative apnea and bradycardia in neonate. In addition to hemoglobin, in infants with fluid and electrolyte deficit, initial electrolyte values are also important. In major surgeries (e.g. oesophageal atresia, necrotizing enterocolitis, congenital cardiac surgery, neurosurgery) full blood count, blood electrolyte values, renal function and clotting test are recommended [25].

Fasting time before elective surgery should be pointed out. Clear liquid, breast milk and formula milk intake should be prohibited at according to the recommended fasting times (2 hours for clear liquids, 4 hours for breast milk, 6 hours for formula/non-human milk) before elective surgery [12, 14, 25]. Since prolonged period of fasting time pose a risk for hypoglycemia and dehydration, dextrose containing intravenous maintenance fluids should be instituted early period.

A systematic approach the preoperative assessment is summarized in **Table 3**.

Gathering of patient information
History of neonate
Perinatal
Medical conditions (co-morbidities, congenital syndromes, genetic disease)
Medications
Previous anesthesia and surgical experience
Examination
Body weight, height
Physical observation
Airway (especially pathologies that can cause difficult intubation, micrognathia)
Respiratory System
Prematurity
Bronchopulmonary dysplasia
Laryngeal pathologies, stridor
Breathing sounds
Cardiovascular system
Auscultation of heart
Neurological (intracranial hemorrhage history-treatment, seizure activation)
Previous resuscitation history
Previous anesthesia experience
Optimize medical condition
Determination of anesthesia risk
Determination of anesthetic plan

Table 3. Systematic approach to preoperative assessment.

4.2. Preparation of the operating theater

Anesthesia preparation should be based on the information obtained from the preoperative visit. But, anesthesia preparation does not include preparation of anesthetic equipment, drugs and anesthesia station only. It also includes preparations for the operating theater, such as proper heating of the surgery room, preparations for aspiration materials and arrangements for the patient's position.

The newborn baby has a high ratio surface area to body weight and a thin layer subcutaneous fat tissue. Therefore, neonates lose heat rapidly more than older children and adult [1]. The operating room temperature must be set to maintained neonate's thermoneutral temperature in order to minimize heat loss. In addition, the following applications can be used to reduce heat loss:

- Humidify and warm inspired anesthetic gases
- Many devices such as warmed blanket, overhead radiant heater, a forced air warmer mattress, clear plastic drapes
- Using heating solution for cleansing the skin
- Warm blood and intravenous solutions
- Transport the neonate in a heated incubator

Gas resources and suction materials must be checked.

The patient position is one of the issues to be considered. Different materials such as soft foam padding, rolls and tapes can be used safely for the position.

4.3. Assessment of patient and anesthetic equipment

Proper anesthesia preparation is very important for safe anesthetic management. This is one of the goals of the preoperative visit.

4.3.1. Airway

No matter what anesthetic method is used (sedation or general anesthesia), the airway must be guaranteed in every situation. Difficult, immature airway and respiratory system can lead to airway obstruction during sedation or mask ventilation. Therefore, appropriately size face mask, oropharyngeal airway, laryngoscope blades, endotracheal tube and suction catheters must be available. The use of transparent face masks are recommended for early recognition of cyanosis, vomiting and secretions.

Endotracheal Intubation Study Group [26] demonstrated that the use of Microcuffed tracheal tubes is effective and safe in neonates and young children. But, most anesthetist prefer to use according to the clinical condition of the patient rather than routine.

The laryngeal mask airway (LMA) can be used as an alternative to endotracheal intubation in the presence of difficult airway and for some short surgical procedures. Against possibility of difficult pediatric airway, advanced airway devices (such as Glidescope, Airtraq) which allow indirect visualization of the larynx should be available [27].

4.3.2. Anesthesia devices

The anesthesia device must be pre-checked before surgical procedure and anesthesia practice. It is essential that the anesthesia ventilator has the ability to provide neonatal compliance, small tidal volume (usually in pressure controlled ventilator mode) and positive end-expiratory pressure [24]. In recent years, new generation anesthesia machines have been developed which is able to small tidal volumes [28] and to provide the ability to ventilate using pressure support ventilation (PSV) [29].

4.3.3. Monitoring

Heart rate-electrocardiography, non-invasive blood pressure, pulse oximetry, and temperature monitorizations are sufficient for basic monitorizations in a healthy newborn.

In neonates whom more risky for surgical procedures, in major surgical procedures and a special circumstances (such as congenital cardiac surgery, oesophageal atresia, congenital diaphragmatic hernia, expected ventilation-perfusion anomalies, hemodynamic changes, and acid-base imbalance), invasive arterial blood pressure and central venous pressure should be monitored.

Two oxygen saturation probes (the right arm probe – pre ductal, the leg probe - post ductal) must be plugged. This approach may provide the diagnosis as, with reverting to transitional circulation and is important to evaluate possible PDA mediated shunt development.

In last three decades, continuous monitoring of respiratory gases (inspiratory oxygen and expiratory end-tidal carbon dioxide and monitoring of gas flows) and continuous use of ventilator disconnection devices are observed routinely in most anesthesia clinic [27].

The precordial oesophageal stethoscope is a traditional and still valid method of monitoring the newborn. With this method, changes in heart rate and respiratory parameters can be identified in early phase.

5. Intraoperative management of anesthesia

5.1. Induction of anesthesia

The anesthesia station is the working area of the anesthetist. Before the surgical procedure, all drugs and equipments required for anesthetic administration should be checked. The neonate should be properly monitored and placed on a forced-air warming mattress before the induction of anesthesia. A safe intravenous access should be established for drug use and fluid therapy. The use of a topical anesthetic such as EMLA cream facilitates awake placement of intravenous cannula [30].

In addition to routine monitoring, direct observation of the neonate is also an important monitoring method. This observation allows the anesthetist to recognize early signs of certain clinic situations (such as cyanosis and pallor).

Inhalation agents or intravenous anesthetics may be used for induction of anesthesia. Although depending on the choice of anesthetist, induction with inhalation anesthetics is a more preferred method. One of the characteristics of the newborns that are different from older children and adults is that they have relatively high alveolar ventilation but low functional residual capacity [6, 14, 24]. This higher minute ventilation to FRC ratio with relatively higher blood flow to vessel rich organs contributes to a rapid increase in alveolar anesthetic concentration. These features enable rapid induction and rapid recovery in general anesthesia [6].

Inhalational induction has the advantage of protection of spontaneous ventilation (especially, important in neonates with potentially difficult airway).

With the advantages we have mentioned above, volatile anesthetics cause dose dependent cardiac and respiratory depressant effect in neonates. These effects can result bradycardia, hypotension and postoperative apnea. This hypotensive effect is also more pronounced in neonates and preterms with cardiovascular instability than older children.

Also, immature airway and respiratory system may cause airway obstruction in mask ventilation during induction phase. Laryngospasm is a frequent occurrence in neonatal anesthesia in this period [31] and if it is intervened early is usually easy to manage. However, laryngospasm, hypoventilation, hypoxia are among the causes of apnea during induction (especially in cases of late notice) [32].

In short surgical procedures, mask ventilation or laryngeal mask airway may be suitable to support respiration. However, endotracheal intubation is frequently performed in patients with emergency surgical procedures, long and major surgical interventions, conditions that requiring muscle relaxation and aspiration risk.

In situation that where inhalation anesthetics are contraindicated or not preferred, intravenous anesthetics may be used to induce and maintain anesthesia.

As we have already mentioned, total body water and extracellular fluid are increased in neonates [16]. These different fluid component affect volumes of distribution of intravenous anesthetic drugs (this means increasing the volume of distribution, especially for water-soluble drugs).

In addition, due to the immaturity of hepatic functions, duration of action will be prolonged in neonates if the drug depends on hepatic metabolism [6].

Muscle relaxant may be required for some neonatal surgical procedures. However, due to immaturity of the neuromuscular junction, neonates have an increased sensitivity to the effects of nondepolarizing neuromuscular blocking drugs [33]. For this reason, prolonged effects may occur at additional doses.

5.2. Intraoperative period

Balanced general anesthesia management is usually achieved by inhalation anesthesia supplemented with different class and wide range of drugs and/or muscle relaxants and regional techniques or achieved by total intravenous anesthesia.

Barbiturates, opioids, propofol, ketamine listed among these intravenous drugs [14]. Long-acting agents such as morphine should be avoided especially in day-case surgery or procedures and postoperative apnea risk should be kept in mind.

In neonatal patients, reduced hepatic glycogen stores, inadequate muscle glycogen reserve and gluconeogenesis enzyme activity require close monitoring of blood glucose concentration [34].

Intravenous glucose infusion may be required to maintain normoglycemia (serum glucose concentration of 40–90 mg dL [1, 24].

All maintenance fluids and blood products used intraoperatively must be warmed before use. Intravenous fluids should be titrated with an infusion pump or a fluid-adjusted burette to avoid excessive fluid loading and to give a controlled fluid.

Following the first few days of baby's life, in all newborns of gestational age, adequate intake of sodium is essential for continued normal developmental activity [1]. In full term neonates, it is not usually necessary to add sodium in maintenance fluids in the first 24 hours of life. However, sodium is added to the maintenance fluids after the second day to replace the sodium losses from the renal and gastrointestinal tract [35]. Also, non-hypotonic, dextrose-containing fluids for sodium replacement may also be used. But, hypotonic fluids should be avoided. These fluids are most common cause of potentially lethal postoperative hyponatremia [35, 36].

Intraoperative fluid requirement should also be met, depending on pre-existing fluid deficits, quality and duration of operation, and the extent of blood loss.

It should not be allowed hypothermia during the intraoperative period. Hypothermia may cause stress in the newborn, leading to postoperative respiratory insufficiency and ventilatory support [10]. On the other hand, the only stressor factor that to avoid in newborns is not hypothermia. Many stress factors (such as hypotension episodes, hypoxia, hypercapnia, acidosis, anemia) can occur during intraoperative period. These factors leads increase PVR and can cause return of the transitional circulation [Ivanova-24]. Different therapeutic maneuvers such as hyperventilation, deepening anesthesia, increased inspired oxygen, and volume expansion may also help in treatment [10].

5.3. Postoperative period and pain practices in neonate

Many neonates undergoing day-case surgery can be anesthetized using mask ventilation and/or LMA by continuing spontaneous breathing without the use of muscle relaxants and intubation.

However, in some situations (such as in major surgical procedures, urgent surgery, full stomach, etc.) endotracheal intubation must be done to secure the airway.

In these patients, in these patients there are many factors that determine postoperative extubation (including surgical conditions).

In major surgeries, (such as NEC, oesophageal atresia, diaphragmatic hernia) endotracheal intubation safer for these neonatal patients. In these neonates usually require elective postoperative mechanical ventilator support in early postoperative period in NICU.

Estuation period is a critical as intubation. Likewise, it requires to be careful and attentive.

It should be take care with regard to residual neuromuscular block and the neuromuscular blocker drugs should be reversed. In extubation period, we may encounter with side effects such as bradycardia, hypoxia, bronchospasm, which can be seen in induction of anesthesia. Intubation equipments and drugs should be available in the anesthesia theater for immediate intervention.

Post-conceptional age (PCA) is important factor in ex-premature babies, for day case surgical procedures. Most ex-premature babies are suitable for day case surgical procedures at greater than 60 weeks post-conceptional age (PCA). Prior to 60 weeks PCA, especially in premature infants less than 44 weeks PCA, postoperative apnea risk increased. In these neonates is recommended postoperative saturation and apnea monitoring in postoperative 24 hours period.

Pain in neonatal patients has for many years been ignored. However, the theory that newborns do not feel pain has become a subject that has lost its validity nowadays.

Recent studies have shown that neuroanatomical and neuroendocrine systems of premature newborns are sufficient for the transmission and perception of pain [37].

Untreated pain causes restlessness, increased oxygen consumption, ventilation/perfusion deficiency, and reduced food intake in early period of neonatal life. Long-term effects are learning disability and developmental retardation. Surgical trauma causes pain and a hormonal stress response that is directly related to the severity and urgency of surgery. Opioids (such as fentanyl, ultra-short acting remifentanil or traditional longer acting morphine) reduce the stress response and catecholamine release in response to painful stimuli. In addition, opioids provide effective pain control so decrease the pulmonary vasoconstrictor responses to painful stimuli in NICU.

In recent years, intravenous paracetamol has begun to be used in the treatment protocol of pain in neonates [38].

6. General anesthesia and developing brain. A special highlight for neonatal anesthesia

One of the most interesting topics in the last 20 years is the general anesthetic effect on the developing brain and neurocognitive functions.

Animal studies show that exposure to general anesthetics (especially these acting through the NMDA and GABA receptors) during the critical period of neuronal development in the developing brain leads to an apoptotic cell death and neurocognitive impairment especially in immature brain [39, 40]. It is reported that this effect to be related to drug dosages and exposure time.

Long-term neurobehavioral effects of sedative and anesthetic agents should be supported by long-term human studies. In recent years, early results of international, multidisciplinary, prospective clinical trials such as GAS and PANDA have begun to be published [41, 42].

In these studies and in Wilder et al. study, it has been reported that multiple exposures to anesthesia, rather than single exposure to anesthesia, pose a risk factor for later development learning disability in children [41–43].

However, to withhold sedation and anesthesia when necessary, would result in ethical consequences, in addition will trigger many negative consequences of painful stimulation in neonatal patients.

7. Conclusion

Approximately 1.5 million neonates receive general anesthesia each year for a surgical procedure according to literature data on neonatal patients [44].

In recent years, it has seen significant improvements in pediatric and neonatal anesthesia practice such as patient safety, advanced monitoring methods and new anesthesia equipments. Nevertheless, the neonatal period is still challenging for the anesthesiologist.

Anesthetic approach in neonatal population has to take into consideration the many immature vital organ functions as well as the effects of the underlying disease processes, which can frequently lead to severe physiological derangements.

Therefore, reliable anesthesia management is possible with a good understanding of the anatomical, physiological and pharmacological differences of the neonatal period.

Also, basic understanding of risk factors in neonatal anesthesia is a starting point for the reduction of risk. A careful preoperative examination of the child and the child's medical record, careful and close perioperative monitoring and follow-up and effective pain treatment would reduce mortality and morbidity.

The basics of safe anesthetic management in neonatal patients are summarized in this chapter, based on feature of neonatal period. The approach in neonatal emergency surgical procedures has not been mentioned in this chapter, since it was described another chapter.

Author details

Esra Caliskan

Address all correspondence to: duru5654@gmail.com

Department of Anesthesiology and Reanimation, Baskent University Faculty of Medicine, Ankara, Turkey

References

[1] Gregory GA, Brett C. Neonatology for anesthesiologists. In: Davis PJ, Cladis FP, Motoyoma EK, editors. Smith's Anesthesia for Infants and Children. 8th. Chapter 17 ed. Philadelphia: Elsevier Mosby; 2011. pp. 512-553 ISBN: 978-0-323-06612-9.ch3

[2] Brusseau R, McCann ME. Anaesthesia for urgent and emergency surgery. Early Human Development. 2010;**86**:703-714. DOI: 10.1016/j.earlhumdev.2010.08.008

[3] Dierdorf SF, Krishna G. Anesthetic Management of Neonatal Surgical Emergencies. Anesthesia and Analgesia. 1981;**60**:204-214 ISSN: 0003-2999

[4] Thomas J. Reducing the risk in neonatal anesthesia. Pediatric Anesthesia. 2014;**24**:106-113. DOI: 10.1111/pan.12315

[5] Davidson AJ. Editorial: In search of the big question. Pediatric Anesthesia. 2012;**22**:613-615. DOI: 10.1111/j.1460-9592.2012.03808.x

[6] Buttterforth JF, Mackey DC, Washnick DC. Pediatric Anesthesia. Morgan & Mikhail's Lange Clinical Anesthesiology. 5th. Chapter 42 ed. United States of America: McGraw-Hill Medical Publishing; 2013. pp. 849-873

[7] Cote CJ. Neonatal anaesthesia. Southern African Journal of Anaesthesia and Analgesia. 2010;**16**:6-11. DOI: 10.1080/22201173.2010.10872624

[8] Finnemore A, Groves A. Physiology of the fetal and transitional circulation. Seminars in Fetal & Neonatal Medicine. 2015;**20**:210-216. DOI: 10.1016/j.siny.2015.04.003

[9] Motoyama EK, Finder JD. Respiratory physiology in infants and children. In: Davis PJ, Cladis FP, Motoyoma EK, editors. Smith's Anesthesia for Infants and Children. 8th. Chapter 3 ed. Philadelphia: Elsevier Mosby; 2011. pp. 23-79. ISBN: 978-0-323-06612-9.ch3

[10] McCann ME, Soriano SG. Progress in anesthesia and management of the newborn surgical patient. Seminars in Pediatric Surgery. 2014;**23**:244-248. DOI: 10.1053/j.sempedsurg.2014.09.003

[11] Jain A, McNamara PJ. Persistent pulmonary hypertension of the newborn: Advances in diagnosis and treatment. Seminars in Fetal & Neonatal Medicine. 2015;**20**:262-271. DOI: 10.1016/j.siny.2015.03.001

[12] Cote CJ. Pediatric Anetshesia. In: Miller RD, editor. Miller's Anesthesia. 7th ed. Philadelphia: El Churchill Livingstone; 2010. pp. 2559-2597. ISBN: 978-0-443-06959-8.ch

[13] de Wildt SN. Profound changes in drug metabolism enzymes and possible effects on drug therapy in neonates and children. Expert Opinion on Drug Metabolism & Toxicology. 2011;**7**:935-948. DOI: 10.1517/17425255.2011.577739

[14] Brett C, Davis PJ. Anesthesia for general surgery in the neonate. In: Davis PJ, Cladis FP,

Motoyoma EK, editors. Smith's Anesthesia for Infants and Children. 8th. Chapter 18 ed. Philadelphia: Elsevier Mosby; 2011. pp. 554-588. ISBN: 978-0-323-06612-9. ch3

[15] Allegaert K, Velde MV, Anker JV. Neonatal clinical pharmacology. Paediatric Anaesthesia. 2014;**24**:1-14. DOI: 10.1111/pan.12176

[16] Anderson BJ. Pharmacology in the very young: Anaesthetic implications. European Journal of Anaesthesiology. 2012;**29**:261-270. DOI: 10.1097/EJA.0b013e3283542329

[17] O'Brien F, Walker IA. Fluid homeostasis in the neonate. Paediatric Anaesthesia. 2014;**24**:49-59. DOI: 10.1111/pan.12326

[18] Tourneux P, Libert JP, Ghyselen L, et al. Heat exchanges and thermoregulation in the neonate. Archives de Pédiatrie. 2009;**16**:1057-1062. DOI: 10.1016/j.arcped.2009.03.014.

[19] Friedman M, Baumgart S. Thermal regulation. In: MacDonald MG, Seshia MMK, Mullett MD, editors. Avery's Neonatology: Pathophysiology and Management of the Newborn. 6th ed. Philadelphia: Lippincott Williams & Wilkins; 2005. pp. 445-455

[20] Pearce B, Christensen R, Voepel-Lewis T. Perioperative hypothermia in the pediatric population: Prevalence, risk factors and outcomes. Journal of Anesthesia and Clinical Research. 2010;**1**:102. DOI: 10.4172/2155-6148.1000102

[21] Lerman J. Pharmacology of inhalational anaesthetics in infants and children. Paediatric Anaesthesia. 1992;**2**:191-203. DOI: 10.1111/j.1460-9592.1992.tb00200.x

[22] LeDez KM, Lerman J. The minimum alveolar concentration (MAC) of isoflurane in preterm neonates. Anesthesiology. 1987;**67**:301-307

[23] Short JA, Gordon JK. Preoperative assessment and preparation for anaesthesia in children. Anaesthesia and Intensive Care Medicine. 2015;**16**:381-388. DOI: 10.1016/j.mpaic.2015.06.003

[24] Ivanova I, Pittaway A. Principles of anaesthesia for term neonates: An updated practical guide. Anaesthesia and Intensive Care Medicine. 2014;**15**:103-106. DOI: 10.1016/j.mpaic.2014.01.008

[25] Pittaway A. Principles of anaesthesia for the term neonate. Anaesthesia and Intensive Care. 2008;**12**:95-98. DOI: 10.1016/j.mpaic.2016.11.002

[26] Weiss M, Dullenkopf J, Fischer E, et al. Prospective randomised controlled multi-centre trial of cuffed or un-cuffed endotracheal tubes in small children. British Journal of Anaesthesia. 2009;**103**:867-873. DOI: 10.1093/bja/aep290

[27] Cambell S, Graham W, Engelhart T. Equipment and monitoring – What is in the future to improve safety? Pediatric Anesthesia. 2011;**21**:815-824. DOI: 10.1111/j.1460-9592.2011.03553.x

[28] Bachiller PR, McDonough JM, Feldman JM. Do new anesthesia ventilators deliver small tidal volumes accurately during volume-controlled ventilation? Anesthesia and Analgesia. 2008;**106**:1392-1400. DOI: 10.1213/ane.0b013e31816a68c6

[29] Garcia-Fernandez J, Tusman G, Suarez-Sipmann F, Llorens J, Soro M, Belda JF. Programming pressure support ventilation in pediatric patients in ambulatory surgery with a laryngeal mask airway. Anesthesia and Analgesia. 2007;**105**:1585-1591

[30] Intravenous Anesthetics. Morgan & Mikhail's Lange Clinical Anesthesiology. 5th. Chapter 9 ed. United States of America: McGraw-Hill Medical Publishing; 2013. pp. 175-189

[31] Paterson N, Waterhouse P. Risk in pediatric anesthesia. Pediatric Anesthesia. 2011;**21**:848-857. DOI: 10.1111/j.1460-9592.2010.03366.x.

[32] Sale SM. Neonatal apnoea. Best Practice & Research Clinical Anaesthesiology. 2010;**24**:323-336. DOI: 10.1016/j.bpa.2010.04.002

[33] Meretoja OA. Neuromuscular block and current treatment strategies for its reversal in children. Paediatric Anaesthesia. 2010;**20**:591-604. DOI: 10.1111/j.1460-9592.2010.03335.x

[34] Mitanchez D. Glucose regulation in preterm newborn infants. Hormone Research. 2007;**68**:265-271

[35] Sümpelmann R, Becke K, Crean P, et al. European consensus statement for intraoperative fluid therapy in children. European Journal of Anaesthesiology. 2011;**28**(9):637. DOI: 10.1097/EJA.0b013e3283446bb8

[36] Datta PK, Pawar DK, Baidya DK, Maitra S, Aravindan A. Dextrose-containing intraoperative fluid in neonates: In randomised controlled trial. Pediatric Anesthesia. 2016;**26**:599-607

[37] Lee SJ, Ralston HJ, Drey EA, Partridge JC, Rosen MA. Fetal pain: A systematic multidisciplinary review of the evidence. JAMA. 2005;**24**(294):947-954

[38] Härmä A, Aikio O, Hallman M, Saarela T. Intravenous Paracetamol decreases requirements of morphine in very preterm infants. The Journal of Pediatrics. 2016;**168**:36-40. DOI: 10.1016/j.jpeds.2015.08.003

[39] Sinner B, Becke K, Engelhard K. General anaesthetics and developing brain. An overview. Anaesthesia. 2014;**69**:1009-1022

[40] Sun L. Early childhood general anesthesia exposure and neurocognitive development. British Journal of Anaesthesia. 2010;**105**:i61-i68. DOI: 10.1093/bja/aeq302

[41] Davidson AJ, Disma N, Graaff JC, et al. Neurodevelopmental outcome at 2 years of age after general anaesthesia and awake-regional anaesthesia in infancy (GAS): An international multicentre randomised controlled trial. Lancet. 2016;**387**:239-250. DOI: 10.1016/S0140-6736(15)00608-X

[42] Miller TL, Park R, Sun LS. Report of the fourth PANDA symposium on "anesthesia and neurodevelopment in children". Journal of Neurosurgical Anesthesiology. 2014;**26**:344-348. DOI: 10.1097/ANA.0000000000000109

[43] Wilder RT, Flick RP, Sprung J, et al. Early exposure to anesthesia and learning disabilities in a population-based birth cohort. Anesthesiology. 2009;**110**:796-804. DOI: 10.1097/01.anes.0000344728.34332.5d

[44] Nasr VG, Davis JM. Anesthetic use in newborn infants: The urgent need for rigorous evaluation. Pediatric Research. 2015;**78**:2-6. DOI: 10.1038/pr.2015.58

11

Update on Neonatal Male Circumcision: A Public Health Perspective

Kriengkrai Srithanaviboonchai

Abstract

Male circumcision (MC) is an effective preventive health intervention. WHO and UNAIDS jointly recommend that the international community considers MC as a potential long-term HIV prevention measure. Neonatal male circumcision (NMC) is a type of MC performed within 1 month after birth. There are several advantages in favor of NMC over circumcision at a later age; it is simpler, safer, and cheaper. Maximum benefits of MC are achieved through NMC. NMC is also more convenient and risk compensation after the surgery is unnecessary. Concerns over NMC include child rights, pain during the surgery, possibility of reduced sexual pleasure, and a long timeframe before achieving HIV reduction benefits. The local HIV epidemic and medical guidelines, policies and strategies, public education and demand creation, finance, readiness of health system, staff training, monitoring and evaluation (M&E), and quality assurance should be considered before and during the implementation of NMC. This chapter uses Thailand as an example of how a country might benefit from introducing NMC as a public health measure. Parents should be informed about the benefits and risks of NMC where service is available to allow them to decide whether their children should be circumcised.

Keywords: circumcision, neonatal male circumcision, HIV prevention, STI prevention, Thailand

1. Introduction

Whether to promote neonatal male circumcision (NMC) as a preventive health measure has long been a contentious subject among health professionals and the general public. NMC has been performed as a modern health intervention in English-speaking countries for health and hygiene since the mid-nineteenth century [1]. Although NMC lessened in popularity in the United Kingdom before World War II [2] and later in the United States over the last few decades [3], recent findings in several randomized controlled trials (RCT) confirming that male circumcision reduces heterosexual HIV acquisition [4–6], have renewed interest in NMC and debates continue on whether it should be promoted as a public health measure.

NMC, similar to other clinical procedures, has associated medical benefits and risks. However, current academic debates seem riddled with subjective feelings on the issue rather than a dispassionate analysis of recent scientific findings. Internet searches reveal many scientific articles written from the point of view of certain mind-sets, either concurring with NMC or deprecating NMC. These biases are also true regarding dedicated websites discussing circumcision. These articles and websites fall prey to social acceptability biases, which are not surprising given the sensitive nature of MC due to religious beliefs, cultural or religious rites, and sexuality. This conflicting information creates a lot of confusion among physicians and parents of newborn males. Many parents decide not to circumcise their babies, while many NMCs are routinely performed without support of factual scientific knowledge.

Other factors must be considered besides the theoretical medical benefits and risks for each individual. These include the characteristics of targeted localities, for example, real-life clinical circumstances, readiness of health staff, the local HIV epidemic, finance and costs, and related laws and regulations. The unique situation of each area will determine whether NMC should be promoted as a public health measure. Ethical and legal issues such as child rights are also important to explore.

After circumcision was confirmed as an effective HIV prevention measure, the author led a series of studies to evaluate the possibility of using NMC as a public health measure in Thailand [7–10]. The results and conclusions of those studies have been included in this chapter. The lessons learnt from Thailand might be useful for other countries with similar contexts.

This chapter starts by elaborating on how NMC is different from other forms of circumcision and why it is worth be considered as a public health measure. Traditional circumcisions practiced under religious rituals are beyond the scope of this article. An objective summary of the pros and cons of NMC from up-to-date scientific evidence follows. This chapter touches upon important aspects of NMC as a public health measure. The author also discusses his views toward implementation of NMC impartially. Readers should consider this information with care and adapt it to suit their local context. The article ends with recommendations and conclusions. Finally, the author hopes that this article is valuable for those who hope to gain more insight on this very interesting health intervention.

2. Distinguish NMC from other forms of circumcision

2.1. Types of circumcision

Many varieties of circumcisions are currently performed. They can be classified according to their characteristics and purposes. Acknowledging the whole spectrum of circumcision will help distinguish NMC from other procedures. **Figure 1** shows how different types of the

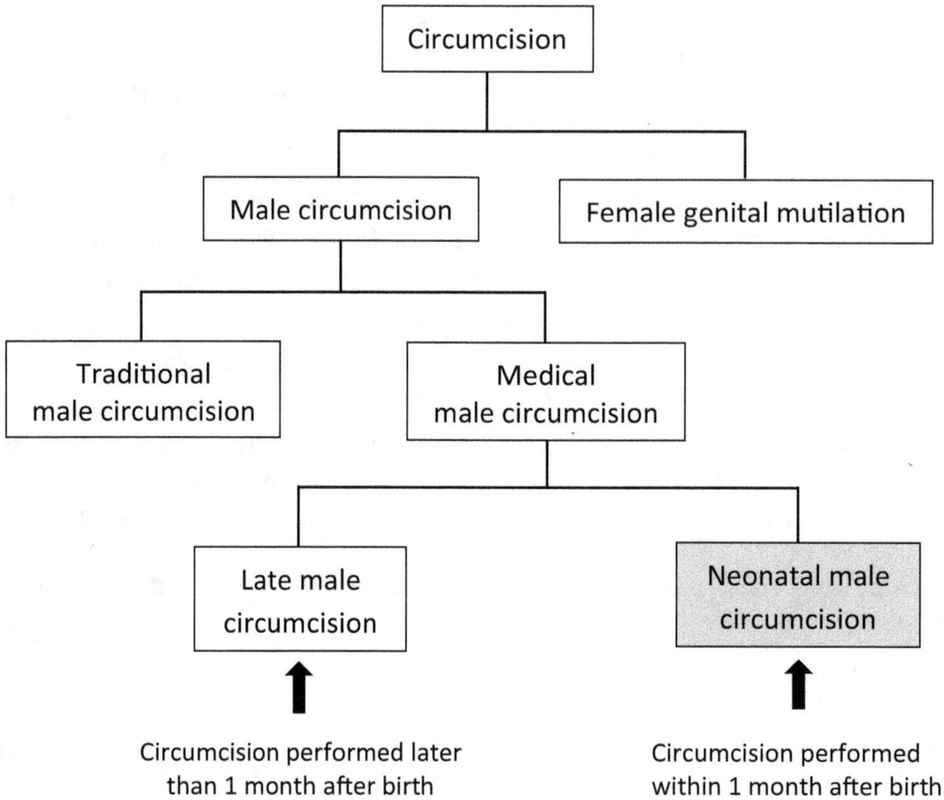

Figure 1. Schematic presentation of types of circumcision.

surgeries are categorized and pinpoints the whereabouts of NMC within the broad range of circumcision types. NMC is highlighted and discussed because of its favorable characteristics over other types of circumcision. It should be noted that other terms are used to refer to NMC such as "early infant male circumcision" and "newborn male circumcision."

2.1.1. Exclusion of female genital mutilations

First, the word "male" is intentionally added into the term to make sure that we are specifically talking about circumcision in males. All forms of female genital mutilations, described by some as female circumcision, procedures that intentionally alter or cause injury to the female genital organs for non-medical reasons [11] are excluded from this article. These procedures, which occur in some regions of the world, have no medical benefit and harm girls and women in many ways. The complications can be short and long term and include excessive bleeding, infection, urinary problems, keloid, sexual problems, and psychological trauma [12]. Female genital mutilations are a clear example of human rights violation. Collective efforts to prohibit and eliminate this practice are fully warranted.

2.1.2. Traditional MC

The prevalence of global male circumcision is estimated at 39% [13]. MC can be classified as traditional and medical. About half of the circumcisions are performed traditionally and are generally associated with certain religious or cultural beliefs [13]. In Muslim and Jewish cultures, MC is mandatory and conducted as part of a religious ceremony. Circumcision in Muslim male child varies from birth to puberty. For instance in Thailand, Muslim boys are usually circumcised between the ages of 6 and 15. The circumcision rate among men in the Philippines is very high. Circumcision is performed as a rite of passage to welcome boys to the next phase in life and is believed to be a remnant of pre-colonial Islamic influence. Jews traditionally conduct a circumcision ceremony on the eighth day of a male infant's life. Traditional MC normally takes place outside of established medical settings. Those performing the circumcision mostly are not trained health professionals, so there are concerns about possible complications such as excessive bleeding and infections. Efforts have been made to reduce the risk of adverse events associated with traditional circumcision. Traditional MCs are ruled out from this article since they are inevitable and not considered public health interventions.

2.1.3. Medical MC

Medical MC was introduced in English-speaking countries in the mid-nineteenth century. The primary purpose was to reduce masturbation which was considered an unhealthy behavior [14]. It was also performed to improve genital hygiene since the foreskin was believed to serve as a pouch that allows the accumulation of smegma. Medical MC is usually performed in established health facilities by trained medical practitioners. It is generally carried out a few days after birth. The surgery is performed only if the infant is healthy and may be postponed if the infant has a medical condition. Currently, medical MC is relatively prevalent in the United States, Canada, and Republic of Korea. Almost universal MC in the Republic of Korea is the result of the influence of the United States [15].

2.1.4. Focus on NMC

MC performed under 1 year of age is called infant MC. NMC is a specific type of infant MC which is administered within 1 month of birth. There are several advantages in favor of NMC over circumcision at a later age. In this chapter, we focus on NMC performed as a preventive medical measure in established health facilities.

2.2. Why NMC is worth being considered as a public health measure?

2.2.1. NMC carries potential health benefits of MC

Since NMC is performed early in life, it generally includes all the potential health benefits of MC. In this section, proven medical benefits of MC are presented and discussed.

2.2.1.1. Improved genital hygiene

Penile cleanliness is easier to maintain for a circumcised penis because there is no pocket underneath the prepuce that needs to be exposed before cleaning, which could be problematic in young boys. While most children eventually learn to retract the foreskin and cleanse the area as routine hygienic practice before puberty, some might find this difficult. There is a great variability in when the foreskin is fully retractable, with about 40% of boys having a fully retractable foreskin by age 10 [16]. Parents and boys are sometimes unclear whether they should try to force the foreskin open to clean the under area or leave it alone. This is not a dilemma for circumcised boys. The pouch under foreskin's inner surface is where smegma is compiled. Smegma is the accumulation of sebum combined with dead skin cells produced by the foreskin's inner surface. A build-up of smegma due to lack of routine cleaning may produce foul odors which are caused by the colonization of bacteria and chemical transformations.

2.2.1.2. Elimination of the chance to have phimosis and paraphimosis

Phimosis is defined as the inability to retract the foreskin over the glans penis in uncircumcised males. Male infants are born with congenital physiologic phimosis resulting from adhesions between the epithelial layers of the inner prepuce and glans. As mentioned earlier, this condition will go away in most boys with age after intermittent foreskin retraction and erections. Un-retractable foreskin that occurs after previously retractable or after puberty is considered a health problem and called pathologic phimosis when nonretractability is associated with local or urinary complaints caused by the phimotic prepuce [17]. Most pathologic phimosis in adults is the result of distal scarring of the foreskin due to poor hygiene, balanitis, balanoposthitis, and forceful retraction of the foreskin. It can also occur because of infections or inflammations. For the elderly, increased risk of phimosis is caused by the loss of skin elasticity and infrequent erections. Symptoms of phimosis are difficulty or pain during urination, collection of urine in prepuce, painful erection, and paraphimosis.

Paraphimosis is the condition where the foreskin is trapped behind the glans penis for a long time and can no longer be pulled forward over the tip of the penis. Paraphimosis is common among children who have forgotten to retract their foreskin after voiding or bathing [18]. Other causes of paraphimosis are infection, physical trauma, trying to retract the foreskin back too forcefully, and leaving the foreskin in a pulled back position for an extended period of time. Persons who have phimosis are at risk for developing paraphimosis. When paraphimosis occurs, the prepuce and the distal part of glans may be swollen and painful. Paraphimosis is considered a medical emergency as blood supply to the tip of the penis is diminished [18]. The condition requires immediate medical attention. If left unattended, paraphimosis may lead to serious complications such as severe infection and loss of the penis due to gangrene.

2.2.1.3. Reduction of balanitis and exclusion of balanoposthitis

Balanitis refers to inflammation of the glans penis and can occur at any age. Data from meta-analyses showed that circumcised males have a 68% lower prevalence of balanitis than uncircumcised males [19]. Symptoms may include tight and shiny skin on the glans, redness on the glans, itchiness, unpleasant smelling discharge, painful urination, and localized pain. There are many possible causes of balanitis including poor hygiene, irritation, physical trauma, skin conditions, phimosis, and various infections. Pathologic phimosis is a possible complication of balanitis. It can occur especially when balanitis is frequent since the preputial orifice may be scarred and reduced elasticity. Meatal stenosis is another possible complication of balanitis but is uncommon.

If the foreskin is also affected together with the glans penis, the condition is called balanoposthitis [20]. Therefore, balanoposthitis affects uncircumcised males only. Balanitis usually leads to balanoposthitis except in circumcised males. Signs and symptoms of balanoposthitis are similar to those of balanitis only if they also involve the foreskin, not just the glans. Diabetes is an important underlying cause of both balanitis and balanoposthitis especially in the patients with poorly controlled blood sugar [21]. Prophylaxis circumcision reduces the risk of balanitis and eliminates the chance of developing balanoposthitis. Circumcision is also an effective treatment for both conditions.

2.2.1.4. HIV reduction

Reduction of the risk of HIV acquisition during heterosexual sexual intercourse is perhaps the most significant and most discussed benefit of MC. Researchers have speculated about this benefit early on in the HIV epidemic as it was observed that the rates of circumcision inversely correlated with the rates of HIV infections [22, 23]. In Asia, for example, the prevalence of HIV was high where the rate of circumcision was low (e.g., Thailand and Cambodia) and the prevalence of HIV was low where the rate of circumcision was high (e.g., the Philippines and Korea).

Three randomized controlled trials conducted in South Africa [4], Kenya [5], and Uganda [6] later confirmed that MC reduces the risk of female-to-male HIV transmission by 51–60%. All three studies were stopped early by their respective data and safety monitoring boards due to the obvious differences in HIV incidence between the intervention and the control arms. The protective effect seemed to be sustainable as the effect was maintained at 58% for 72 months of follow-up compared to 60% at 24 months of follow-up among Kenyan trial participants [24]. MC is seen as surgical vaccination as it can be done once and does not rely on consistent health behaviors.

There is scientific evidence that explains why circumcised males would have lower risk of acquiring HIV infection through heterosexual intercourse. Unlike the glans penis, the inner surface of the prepuce is lined with mucosal epithelium with no protective keratin layer. Histologically, the lining of inner foreskin is similar to the lining of nasal mucosa and vagina which are the common entry points of infectious organisms. Thin mucosal epithelium and lack of a protective keratin layer also make the foreskin more susceptible to minor trauma during sexual intercourse [25]. Therefore, the existence of foreskin serves as an entry point for HIV. Langerhans dendritic cells are antigen-presenting immune cells. They are abundant close to the mucosal lining surface of the inner foreskin [26]. In general, their primary function is to take up and process microbial antigens to become fully functional antigen-presenting cells. Langerhans cells in the foreskin and other HIV target cells are the major targets for the HIV, since they have surface CD4 receptors and cofactors that HIV bind to when infecting cells. It is possible that HIV may stay alive longer in the preputial cavity between the non-retracted foreskin and the glans penis since the micro-environment is suitable for its survival [25]. Lower rates of other sexually transmitted infections (STIs) among circumcised men may indirectly reduce the risk of HIV infection [27]. Results from an RCT found a reduction of symptomatic genital ulcer disease and herpes simplex virus type 2 (HSV-2) infections due to circumcision accounted for an 11.2% and 8.6% reduction in the contraction of HIV infection, respectively [28].

2.2.1.5. *Reduction of other STIs*

Reduction of the risk of acquiring other STIs in circumcised men is less pronounced compared to HIV. Early observational studies revealed conflicting results. Respectable information came from a meta-analysis that concluded that circumcised men are at lower risk for chancroid and syphilis [29]. RCTs conducted in Uganda and South Africa found a 35% and 34% lower prevalence of high-risk HPV genotypes in circumcised men [30, 31]. The study in Uganda also found a 28% lower incidence of herpes simplex virus type-2 (HSV-2) [31]. The South African trial also found protection for *Trichomonas vaginalis* [32]. There is no concrete evidence supporting the preventive effect of MC on the risk of contracting gonorrhea or Chlamydia.

The female partners of circumcised men receive indirect health benefits from MC. Female partners had a lower prevalence of genital ulcers, *T. vaginalis* infection, and bacterial vaginosis compared to female partners of uncircumcised men [33].

2.2.1.6. *Cancer reduction*

Penile cancer is quite rare in developed countries but is more prevalent in developing countries [34]. Being uncircumcised is a strong risk factor for penile cancer. A systematic review found a 67% reduced risk of invasive penile cancer in circumcised men compared to uncircumcised men [35]. This preventive effect probably occurs through the elimination of phimosis, a strong risk factor for penile cancer [36]. Another explanation is that circumcised men are less likely to acquire HPV as mentioned earlier. High-risk HPV is suspected to be involved in the causation of penile cancer as it is found in a large proportion penile cancer cases [37]. The odds of detecting HPV are lower in circumcised men compared to uncircumcised men [38]. Chronic relapsing balanitis and balanoposthitis due to poor hygiene and circumcision may also increase the risk of invasive penile cancer.

It is well established that most cervical cancer cases are caused by high-risk HPV. Given that circumcised males are less likely to contract HPV, their female partners also are less likely to be infected with HPV. There is evidence showing that these associations help reduce the risk of cervical cancer. A meta-analysis of case-controlled studies found that monogamous women whose male partners had six or more sexual partners and were circumcised had a lower risk of cervical cancer than women whose partners were uncircumcised [38].

2.2.2. *Advantages of NMC over circumcision at later age*

There is unanimous consensus from the scientific community that MC, if implemented as a non-therapeutic preventive health measure, should be done as early as possible. The procedure is preferably performed within a few days after birth for healthy boys. Following are the list of advantages supporting the rational to perform MC early in life rather than waiting.

2.2.2.1. *Maximum benefits of circumcision are achieved*

Late circumcision reduces the risk of urinary tract infections (UTIs) which occur mostly during the first year of life by almost 10 times [39]. Thus, there is a loss of this preventive health benefits when circumcision happens late in life, from adolescent onward. Protection against UTIs and kidney damage in infancy is lost if it is not performed during the first year of life.

Avoiding childhood phimosis and balanoposthitis is also lost if circumcision is not performed early. Some benefits associated with STI prevention would be lost if circumcision is done after sexual debut. As penile cancer is associated with phimosis and HPV infection, late circumcision means increased risk of cancer.

From a public health perspective, a disease prevention measure has to be implemented on a scale large enough to have an impact at the population level. Circumcision could resemble a vaccination program against HIV. The indirect benefits of MC in women would not occur unless a sufficient number of men are circumcised to allow the effect of herd immunity [40]. Higher MC coverage can be achieved easier through NMC. All pregnant women and their husbands could be educated about NMC during antenatal care sessions and decide about the procedure prior to delivery. Circumcisions can be conducted within a few days of birth for healthy infants while the mother recovers from labor and delivery. This would allow mothers and infants to be discharged together.

2.2.2.2. *Simpler, safer, and cheaper*

Circumcision is much easier to perform during the neonatal period than at a later age. General anesthesia is not required which diminishes the possible adverse events associated with it. The procedure also takes less time, usually just a few minutes to complete. The tissues and blood vessels involved are so tiny that there is no need for stitches.

Bleeding and infection are the two main serious side effects of MC. When performed by trained health personnel at well-equipped health care facilities, NMC is safe and has a low rate of complications [41].

It is cost saving to conduct MC during the neonatal period than at an older age. A study in the US found that NMC was about 10 times cheaper than circumcision performed later [42]. This advantage is especially important in developing countries.

2.2.2.3. *More convenient*

Circumcising infants during their first few days of life is a lot more convenient than to circumcise older boys or adolescents. Neonates are ready for surgery and would not require the counseling required for older boys. There is no need to do HIV counseling and testing for newborns, since they are considered HIV negative, except for those born to HIV-infected mothers. Older boys need to be informed of the benefits and risks of the procedure and must give their informed consent. Confounding factors include fear of the surgery and psychological difficulties. If the procedure is done during school age, students will have to take time off school. Healing is also faster at around 1 week for NMC compared to at least 2–3 weeks for circumcision in adults [43]. Sexually active persons must abstain from sexual intercourse for 6 weeks to ensure proper healing. Having sex during this period would make patients prone to infections including HIV thus negating the main benefit to be gained from procedure.

Other benefits of NMC over circumcision at later age include no long-term memory of the surgery and a better cosmetic outcome.

2.2.2.4. No risk compensation

Risk compensation is a phenomenon by which people adjust their health behavior in response to the perceived level of risk. People become more careful where they sense greater risk and less careful if they feel more protected. Sexually active males who were circumcised as an adult may engage in greater sexual risks due to a perception they have less HIV risk following MC. This could occur among female partners of circumcised men as well if they perceive lower risk. There is little chance of risk compensation for NMC. Boys who are circumcised very early in life would not sense any change in risk as they have been circumcised their whole lives.

2.2.3. Concerns over MC

Besides the low probability of medical risks associated with the surgery such as bleeding, infection, and unsatisfactory cosmetic result, several concerns have been raised. Some of the issues raised are considered controversial, while others have no evidence to support them. In following section, each topic is discussed citing the ongoing conversation and debate as well as up-to-date scientific information.

2.2.3.1. Ethical issues

Since the surgery is performed on an infant who cannot provide consent, NMC has repeatedly raised ethical-related concerns [44]. The decision to circumcise children is usually taken by the parents who act in their child's best interests. People argue that the authority to perform interventions on a child should be limited to ones proven to be medically necessary. Scholars who do not view NMC as a necessary medical intervention suggest that it should be delayed until boys are mature enough to decide for themselves. Thus, this ethical issue boils down to whether people perceive NMC as a medical necessity based on the available scientific evidence. The guidelines and recommendations issued by relevant authorized bodies and medical committees might help determine its necessity.

There are a lot of discussions and debates in the literature whether NMC is a violation of child rights to bodily integrity [45–49]. The principle of bodily integrity refers to the right of each human being to autonomy and self-determination over their own body. Scholars and activists who favor an intact penis and oppose circumcision promote a concept of "Genital Integrity" which refers to the condition of having complete and unaltered genital organs. In their view, NMC is an unconsented physical intrusion and a human rights violation.

2.2.3.2. Pain during NMC

There is concern that NMC introduces unnecessary pain to the newborn. Children who have undergone NMC do experience pain as evidenced by increased heart rate, decreased oxygen saturation, and facial expressions indicative of pain during the procedure [50]. Pain experienced during the procedure has long-lasting effects on the circumcised child. Circumcised infants have been observed to have a stronger pain response to subsequent routine vaccination than uncircumcised infants [51]. Various interventions, in single and in combinations, have been used to minimize pain during NMC, e.g., sucrose syrup, oral acetaminophen, topical analgesic cream, and local nerve block. Sucrose alone has not been proven effective in reducing pain from circumcision [52], while topical analgesia may have some effect [53].

2.2.3.3. Reduced sexual pleasure

There are abundance of neurones which are sensitive to the touch in the foreskin. This leads many to believe that circumcised men might have less sexual pleasure than uncircumcised men [54]. This issue is not limited to NMC but is relevant to circumcision at any age. However, most studies testing this hypothesis have not found this to be true. Recent reviews concluded that loss of the foreskin by circumcision had no adverse effect on sexual pleasure during sexual acts [55, 56].

2.2.3.4. Effectiveness in preventing HIV in men who have sex with men (MSM)

MC reduces the risk of heterosexual HIV transmission in men, but its effect on male-to-male sexual transmission is uncertain. As the current HIV epidemic is concentrated in men who have sex with men (MSM) in many parts of the world, the lack of evidence to support that MC could reduce the risk of HIV acquisition among this population raises concerns over the implementation of this measure as a public health intervention. Observational studies on the protective effect of MC against HIV infection among MSM revealed conflicting results, with some studies showing positive results [57, 58] and others negative results [59–61]. A systematic review concluded that MC might offer HIV protection only among MSM who practice primarily insertive anal sex, but not for those who practice primarily receptive anal sex [62]. An RCT is needed to confirm this finding.

2.2.3.5. Long timeframe to see the HIV reduction benefits

Another concern on the implementation of NMC is a long waiting period to see the HIV prevention effect. Since NMC is conducted among newborns, it may take at least 15 years before they are sexually active and for the NMC to yield HIV prevention benefits. However, if this public health intervention is to be done, sooner is better than later. The only intervention that could have yield similar effect on the HIV epidemic is a preventive vaccine. According to the current status regarding HIV vaccine development, it is probable that NMC will yield an effect before an HIV vaccine is available.

3. NMC as a public health measure

A lot of factors come into play in deciding whether to promote NMC as a public health measure in a country or at a specific locality. Following are the issues that need to be considered before implementation of this health intervention.

3.1. Local HIV epidemic

Promoting NMC as a public health measure depends largely on the characteristics of the local HIV epidemic. Generally, the main reason to step up NMC service in health care facilities is to reduce the risk of HIV infection in the population. It may be not worth promoting NMC, if HIV is not a major public health problem in the country or of the target locality. As MC is proven to reduce only the risk of HIV acquisition through heterosexual transmission, it will not be appropriate to promote NMC where new HIV infections occur mainly through other routes of transmission, namely through same sex intercourse in males or intravenous drug use. An economic study using information on the local HIV epidemic as part of the analysis would help determine if NMC is justifiable for the country in the event that the country has to bear the majority of the costs of the intervention.

3.2. Medical guidelines on NMC

Soon after MC was proven to reduce the risk of HIV contraction among heterosexual males, global health authorities such as the World Health Organization and the Joint United Nations Programme on HIV/AIDS recommended that MC, including NMC, be adopted as part of comprehensive national HIV prevention strategies in countries with high prevalence of heterosexually transmitted HIV infection and low rates of male circumcision. The American Academy of Pediatrics determined that the preventive benefits of neonatal circumcision outweigh the risks of the procedure and should be offered to the families who have boy infants [63]. This statement has also been endorsed by the American College of Obstetricians and Gynecologists [64] and the American Urologic Association [65].

While these international recommendations influence some local practitioners, most health care personnel need national guidelines on NMC before they can start providing the service. Hence, local medical professional organizations should be included as important stakeholders while planning for the intervention. Their statements in favor of NMC would assist program implementation in a big way.

3.3. Policies and strategies

Clear policies and strategies will guide the respective details regarding NMC service. The magnitude and characteristics of the program will depend on the policies from a high-level authorized body, usually the Ministry of Health. The NMC implementation strategy can range from promotion of routine NMC to offering NMC only on a case-by-case basis or per request. The overall strategic plan should translate into action plans for each time interval including target numbers of NMC. The policies will also clearly specify the financial aspect of the program mainly on the payment scheme for the service.

3.4. Public education and demand creation

The general public needs to be educated about NMC before the service is promoted. Public education can be rolled out in a variety of ways. Educational materials should be straightforward, comprehensive, and attractive. The main contents of the media should include benefits and risks of NMC as well as other supporting information such as availability and cost. The design of the education campaign should follow dedicated steps starting with a formative research targeting different audiences such as the general population and pregnant mothers. The formative research and subsequent baseline survey will define the content of the message and explore its suitability along with other relevant issues such as the dissemination channels.

Clear and scientifically accurate information about NMC can prevent misconceptions and rumors about the procedure in the community. Perceived benefits of NMC at the societal level together with high level of satisfaction among early adopters will help increase the demand for the services.

3.5. Finance

NMC represents an added expenditure for the health care system even though the unit cost of NMC is lower than for circumcision at a later age. How the expenses are covered will depend on the nature of the program. However, the parents of the newborns should not have to pay for the total cost if NMC is promoted as a public health intervention. In developing countries, where resources are limited and a high number of recruitments are targeted in a short period of time, local governments usually do not have to pay, as the programs are supported by international agencies. In some other circumstances, the health insurance system may pay for the service. Partial payment by the parents is another possible option.

3.6. Readiness of health system and staff training

A baseline assessment of the readiness and capability of the health system should be conducted. For health facilities, the issues to be assessed should include the antenatal and child delivery service and availability of necessary medical equipment and supplies. Knowledge and attitudes toward NMC should be explored among health care personnel. The information gained from the surveys will help identify the basic elements needed for the service that are still lacking and the aspects that should be emphasized while training health care personnel.

Safety is the first priority when implementing NMC as a public health measure. The surgery should be performed by trained health staff. The health staff who performs the surgery should be educated comprehensively on all aspects related to delivery of NMC, and not just the operation. A training package on NMC developed by the WHO and its partners is available online [66].

3.7. Monitoring and evaluation (M&E) and quality assurance

A system to routinely monitor the performance of the NMC program should be established. The indicators should cover both medical and public health aspects of the intervention. Newly trained staff should conduct first NMC cases under the supervision of more experienced persons. The results of the monitoring system will indicate whether the program is being implemented as intended and should be used to adjust the program to meet the goals in a timely manner. On an interval basis, the outcomes of the program should be comprehensively evaluated. The evaluators could be from internal and/or external entities as appropriate. The information from the M&E system should be analyzed and used to improve the service and guarantee the quality of the service.

4. Thailand and NMC

Soon after it was confirmed that MC was effective in reducing the heterosexual transmission of HIV among men, the author formed a research team at Chiang Mai University, in Northern Thailand, to investigate the possibility of adopting NMC as a public health intervention in Thailand. A critical review compiling related information and the author's thoughts was the first publication [7]. A series of surveys have been conducted to gain insight on related issues in the country including knowledge and opinions of health staff on the intervention [10], the experiences of health staff on the procedure and capability of the Thai health care system to implement NMC [8], and acceptability as well as concerns of NMC among postpartum mothers [9].

Following are the findings of the abovementioned studies. This case study can serve as an example for other countries that share a similar context to Thailand and are considering adopting NMC as a public health measure.

4.1. Background on Thailand

Thailand is an upper middle income country [67] and located in Southeast Asia. The country was categorized as a "high" human development country according to the most recent Human Development Index (HDI) report [68]. Thailand has a well-established health care system. The infant mortality rate is considered low at 11:1000 live births [69]. The coverage of antenatal care among pregnant women and rate of delivery at the health facilities are high. The country has three major health insurance systems that cover almost all of its citizens namely the Universal Health Coverage Scheme, the Civil Servant Medical Benefit Scheme, and Social Security Scheme. People who can afford or have private health insurance could go to private hospitals for convenience.

Thailand was one of the Asian countries hardest-hit by the HIV epidemic during the early 1990s. The AIDS Epidemic Model (AEM) estimates that more than 1 million Thais were infected by the HIV virus. High quality and good coverage of antiretroviral treatment has saved a lot of lives. It is estimated that there are currently more than 400,000 people living with HIV in the country [70]. Thailand's MC rate in general is quite low [13]. It is prevalent only in Muslim communities especially in the southern most provinces.

4.2. Why should Thailand consider promoting NMC?

Thailand is a good candidate country for promoting NMC as a public health measure for many reasons. Most HIV infections in Thailand occur through heterosexual transmission, of which the risk is substantially reduced by MC. Theoretically, the effect of MC on HIV risk reduction should be of significant magnitude in countries where the baseline MC rate is low and achievement of high coverage of MC is possible. Thailand has a relatively strong health care infrastructure as evidenced by the relatively low infant mortality rate [69]. An NMC program could possibly be built on this existing capability. The country has high coverage of maternal and child healthcare services including family planning, antenatal care, and deliveries that almost universally occur in the hospitals [71]. Thailand was the first developing country to eliminate mother-to-child HIV infection [72]. Health care personnel can educate pregnant mothers and their families about the benefits of having their children circumcised. Offering NMC could occur during the antenatal period if the fetus is identified as a boy intrapartum. Mothers can also be advised on how to care for their child after NMC and can be discharged from the hospital with the infant. Lastly, most Thais are Buddhists. Buddhism does not have any prohibition or negative beliefs toward circumcision. Further details on this issue were published in a critical review [7].

4.3. Readiness of the Thai health care system to implement NMC

A nation-wide survey was conducted in 2011 to gather baseline information on the capability of hospitals in Thailand to provide NMC [8]. Two questionnaires were sent to all hospitals in Thailand providing obstetric services and considered potentially able to perform NMC. The first questionnaire requested information about the facility's characteristics and its provision of NMC in 2010. The second questionnaire, directed to doctors or nurses who are familiar with delivery and postpartum care, contained opinion questions about NMC, and whether the procedure should be offered in the respondents' hospital. Of the hospitals that had deliveries in 2010, only 8.2% provided at least one NMC. Thirty-eight percent of private hospitals and 2.3% of government hospitals provided the service during 2010. The primary reason for performing NMC was parental request. Only a minority of the respondents thought that NMC was easy to perform (31.3%), was safe (39.1%), and should be offered in their health care facilities (29%). Ninety-two percent stated that physicians should perform the procedure instead of nurses. When asked about who should decide whether or not to conduct NMC, 55% indicated the choice should be left to parents. Forty-three percent believed that the service should be free of charge, while the same proportion felt that the parents should pay for some or all of the cost.

In another study conducted during 2011–2012, Thai health care providers' knowledge and attitudes toward NMC were assessed using face-to-face interviews [10]. The participants were physician administrators, practicing physicians, and nurses whose jobs involved NMC clinical procedures or oversight. The subjects were drawn to represent various hospital sizes and regions of the country using a multi-stage sampling technique. The participants were initially asked whether they agreed that MC had an effect on HIV prevention. Subsequently, printed educational materials on the benefits of NMC were presented to the participants for review. The participants were then asked whether NMC should be implemented at their facilities. Of the 133 health staffs who participated in the study, only 38% initially agreed that NMC reduced the risk of sexual HIV transmission. After reviewing the written information about the benefits of NMC, 59% of the participants thought that NMC should be offered in their hospitals. HIV aside, 96% recognized the benefits of MC on hygiene, 74% knew about the effect of MC on cancer prevention, and 65% recognized that NMC could prevent STIs. Major concerns about NMC raised were safety and child rights. Physicians and nurses who had previous experience in performing circumcision on patients of all ages were more reluctant to have NMC performed in their hospitals.

4.4. Thai postpartum mothers' acceptability of NMC

In 2011–2012, a survey was conducted among 593 postpartum Thai mothers to determine their perceptions, concerns, and acceptability of NMC [9]. The study found that 70% of postpartum mothers knew or had heard of MC. Their biggest concerns were safety and pain of the procedure. After receiving information about the benefits and risks of NMC, one-third of the participants would choose to have their infants circumcised, one-third would not allow their sons to undergo NMC, and the last third were undecided. Mothers were the most influential person in deciding about NMC followed by fathers. Having a higher level of formal education, a circumcised husband, and knowing of at least one circumcised child were independent predictors of acceptability of NMC among postpartum mothers.

4.5. NMC in Thailand, the way forward

The study showed that NMC was rarely performed in government hospitals where the intervention meant to take place. The health care staffs were unaware of the health benefits of NMC. Most health staffs were concerned about the difficulty and safety of the procedure. However, the fact that a large proportion of health staff agreed that NMC should be offered in their health facility after being educated about the benefits of NMC revealed an opportunity for the program to be adopted by the health staff. The majority of postpartum mothers did not know about the benefits of NMC and were concerned about safety issues. The results suggest that NMC may be culturally neutral with evidence that even modest educational efforts can impact mothers' decisions in favor of NMC.

An education campaign on NMC for health professionals and general public is needed before NMC is promoted as a public health practice in Thailand. An economic study demonstrating the cost-effectiveness of NMC in Thailand is also needed in order to effectively advocate for policies to introduce NMC as an established, offered in health facilities.

Though Thailand might gain considerable benefits from the implementation of NMC as a public health measure, its actual occurrence seems to be impassable according to our research findings. Knowledge and technologies on HIV prevention have evolved rapidly and there are a lot of other options to choose from. For Thailand, other interventions are regarded as more attractive strategies, e.g., routine HIV testing among key populations at higher risk of HIV infection, treatment as prevention, and pre-exposure prophylaxis. Another reason why NMC is overshadowed by other interventions is the lack of proof of an HIV prevention effect on MSM who are the current target population. Unless all necessary things have been done, NMC will not be administered as a public health intervention in Thailand and will only be performed by request and on a case-by-case basis.

5. Conclusion

NMC is as an effective preventive health measure. The medical benefits of NMC outweigh the risks, especially after the effect on HIV prevention has been added. Nevertheless, NMC has not been used to its full potential due to controversies and concerns over the subject. Many issues need to be addressed, if NMC is to be implemented as a public health measure. Implementation of NMC shall vary according to the local context. Parents should be informed about the benefits and risks of NMC where the service is available so that they can decide whether their children should be circumcised. NMC is and will be a health intervention under debate in the years to come.

Author details

Kriengkrai Srithanaviboonchai[1,2]*

*Address all correspondence to: kriengkrai@rihes.org

1 Faculty of Medicine, Chiang Mai University, Chiang Mai, Thailand

2 Research Institute for Health Sciences, Chiang Mai University, Chiang Mai, Thailand

References

[1] Wallerstein E. Circumcision. The uniquely American medical enigma. The Urologic Clinics of North America. 1985;**12**(1):123-132

[2] Rickwood AM, Kenny SE, Donnell SC. Towards evidence based circumcision of English boys: Survey of trends in practice. BMJ (Clinical Research Edition). 2000;**321**(7264):792-793

[3] Maria Owings SU, Williams S. Trends in circumcision for male newborns in U.S. hospitals: 1979-2010. US Center for Disease Control and Prevention. https://www.cdc.gov/nchs/data/hestat/circumcision_2013/circumcision_2013.pdf [Accessed:2017-09-11]

[4] Auvert B, Taljaard D, Lagarde E, Sobngwi-Tambekou J, Sitta R, Puren A. Randomized, controlled intervention trial of male circumcision for reduction of HIV infection risk: The ANRS 1265 Trial. PLoS Medicine. 2005;**2**(11):e298

[5] Bailey RC, Moses S, Parker CB, Agot K, Maclean I, Krieger JN, et al. Male circumcision for HIV prevention in young men in Kisumu, Kenya: A randomised controlled trial. Lancet (London, England). 2007;**369**(9562):643-656

[6] Gray RH, Kigozi G, Serwadda D, Makumbi F, Watya S, Nalugoda F, et al. Male circumcision for HIV prevention in men in Rakai, Uganda: A randomised trial. Lancet (London, England). 2007;**369**(9562):657-666

[7] Srithanaviboonchai K, Grimes RM. Why Thailand should consider promoting neonatal circumcision? The Southeast Asian Journal of Tropical Medicine and Public Health. 2012;**43**(5):1218-1226

[8] Srithanaviboonchai K, Grimes RM, Suwanteerankul J, Thaikla K, Korana J, Pruenglampoo B. Capability of Thailand to implement newborn male circumcision: A nation-wide survey. AIDS Care. 2014;**26**(1):20-25

[9] Pruenglampoo BSK, Grimes RM, Grimes DE, Suwanteerangkul J, et al. Perception, concern and acceptability of neonatal male circumcision among postpartum mothers in Thailand. Journal of AIDS & Clinical Research. 2015;**6**(487)

[10] Srithanaviboonchai K, Pruenglampoo B, Thaikla K, Srirak N, Suwanteerangkul J, Khorana J, et al. Thai health care provider knowledge of neonatal male circumcision in reducing transmission of HIV and other STIs. BMC Health Services Research. 2015;**15**:520

[11] Little CM. Female genital circumcision: Medical and cultural considerations. Journal of Cultural Diversity. 2003;**10**(1):30-34

[12] World Health Organization. Female Genital Mutilation [Internet]. 2017. Available from: http://www.who.int/mediacentre/factsheets/fs241/en/ [Accessed:2017-09-11]

[13] Morris BJ, Wamai RG, Henebeng EB, Tobian AA, Klausner JD, Banerjee J, et al. Estimation of country-specific and global prevalence of male circumcision. Population Health Metrics. 2016;**14**:4

[14] Darby R. The masturbation taboo and the rise of routine male circumcision: A review of the historiography. Journal of Social History. 2003;**36**(3):737-757

[15] Pang MG, Kim DS. Extraordinarily high rates of male circumcision in South Korea: History and underlying causes. BJU International. 2002;**89**(1):48-54

[16] Circumcision Information and Resorce Pages. Normal development of the prepuce: Birth through age 18 [Internet]. 2008. Available from: http://www.cirp.org/library/normal/ [Accessed:2017-09-11]

[17] Shahid SK. Phimosis in children. ISRN Urology. 2012;**2012**:707329

[18] McGregor TB, Pike JG, Leonard MP. Pathologic and physiologic phimosis: Approach to the phimotic foreskin. Canadian Family Physician Medecin de Famille Canadien. 2007;**53**(3):445-448

[19] Morris BJ, Krieger JN. Penile inflammatory skin disorders and the preventive role of circumcision. International Journal of Preventive Medicine. 2017;**8**:32

[20] Edwards S. Balanitis and balanoposthitis: A review. Genitourinary Medicine. 1996;**72**(3):155-159

[21] Kalra S, Chawla A. Diabetes and balanoposthitis. JPMA—The Journal of the Pakistan Medical Association. 2016;**66**(8):1039-1041

[22] Kelly R, Kiwanuka N, Wawer MJ, Serwadda D, Sewankambo NK, Wabwire-Mangen F, et al. Age of male circumcision and risk of prevalent HIV infection in rural Uganda. AIDS (London, England). 1999;**13**(3):399-405

[23] Gray RH, Kiwanuka N, Quinn TC, Sewankambo NK, Serwadda D, Mangen FW, et al. Male circumcision and HIV acquisition and transmission: Cohort studies in Rakai, Uganda. Rakai Project Team. AIDS (London, England). 2000;**14**(15):2371-2381

[24] Mehta SD, Moses S, Agot K, Odoyo-June E, Li H, Maclean I, et al. The long-term efficacy of medical male circumcision against HIV acquisition. AIDS (London, England). 2013;**27**(18):2899-2907

[25] Alanis MC, Lucidi RS. Neonatal circumcision: A review of the world's oldest and most controversial operation. Obstetrical & Gynecological Survey. 2004;**59**(5):379-395

[26] Patterson BK, Landay A, Siegel JN, Flener Z, Pessis D, Chaviano A, et al. Susceptibility to human immunodeficiency virus-1 infection of human foreskin and cervical tissue grown in explant culture. The American Journal of Pathology. 2002;**161**(3):867-873

[27] Boily MC, Desai K, Masse B, Gumel A. Incremental role of male circumcision on a generalised HIV epidemic through its protective effect against other sexually transmitted infections: From efficacy to effectiveness to population-level impact. Sexually Transmitted Infections. 2008;**84**(Suppl 2):ii28-ii34

[28] Gray RH, Serwadda D, Tobian AA, Chen MZ, Makumbi F, Suntoke T, et al. Effects of genital ulcer disease and herpes simplex virus type 2 on the efficacy of male circumcision for HIV prevention: Analyses from the Rakai trials. PLoS Medicine. 2009;**6**(11):e1000187

[29] Weiss HA, Thomas SL, Munabi SK, Hayes RJ. Male circumcision and risk of syphilis, chancroid, and genital herpes: A systematic review and meta-analysis. Sexually Transmitted Infections. 2006;**82**(2):101-109 discussion 10

[30] Auvert B, Sobngwi-Tambekou J, Cutler E, Nieuwoudt M, Lissouba P, Puren A, et al. Effect of male circumcision on the prevalence of high-risk human papillomavirus in young men: Results of a randomized controlled trial conducted in Orange Farm, South Africa. The Journal of Infectious Diseases. 2009;**199**(1):14-19

[31] Tobian AA, Serwadda D, Quinn TC, Kigozi G, Gravitt PE, Laeyendecker O, et al. Male circumcision for the prevention of HSV-2 and HPV infections and syphilis. The New England Journal of Medicine. 2009;**360**(13):1298-1309

[32] Sobngwi-Tambekou J, Taljaard D, Nieuwoudt M, Lissouba P, Puren A, Auvert B. Male circumcision and *Neisseria gonorrhoeae, Chlamydia trachomatis* and *Trichomonas vaginalis*: Observations after a randomised controlled trial for HIV prevention. Sexually Transmitted Infections. 2009;**85**(2):116-120

[33] Gray RH, Kigozi G, Serwadda D, Makumbi F, Nalugoda F, Watya S, et al. The effects of male circumcision on female partners' genital tract symptoms and vaginal infections in a randomized trial in Rakai, Uganda. American Journal of Obstetrics and Gynecology. 2009;**200**(1):42.e1-42.e7

[34] Morrison BF. Risk factors and prevalence of penile cancer. The West Indian Medical Journal. 2014;**63**(6):559-560

[35] Larke NL, Thomas SL, dos Santos Silva I, Weiss HA. Male circumcision and penile cancer: A systematic review and meta-analysis. Cancer Causes & Control: CCC. 2011;**22**(8):1097-1110

[36] Tsen HF, Morgenstern H, Mack T, Peters RK. Risk factors for penile cancer: Results of a population-based case-control study in Los Angeles County (United States). Cancer Causes & Control: CCC. 2001;**12**(3):267-277

[37] McCance DJ, Kalache A, Ashdown K, Andrade L, Menezes F, Smith P, et al. Human papillomavirus types 16 and 18 in carcinomas of the penis from Brazil. International Journal of Cancer. 1986;**37**(1):55-59

[38] Castellsague X, Bosch FX, Munoz N, Meijer CJ, Shah KV, de Sanjose S, et al. Male circumcision, penile human papillomavirus infection, and cervical cancer in female partners. The New England Journal of Medicine. 2002;**346**(15):1105-1112

[39] Schoen EJ, Colby CJ, Ray GT. Newborn circumcision decreases incidence and costs of urinary tract infections during the first year of life. Pediatrics. 2000;**105**(4 Pt 1):789-793

[40] Hallett TB, Alsallaq RA, Baeten JM, Weiss H, Celum C, Gray R, et al. Will circumcision provide even more protection from HIV to women and men? New estimates of the population impact of circumcision interventions. Sexually Transmitted Infections. 2011;**87**(2):88-93

[41] Christakis DA, Harvey E, Zerr DM, Feudtner C, Wright JA, Connell FA. A trade-off analysis of routine newborn circumcision. Pediatrics. 2000;**105**(1 Pt 3):246-249

[42] Schoen EJ, Colby CJ, To TT. Cost analysis of neonatal circumcision in a large health maintenance organization. The Journal of Urology. 2006;**175**(3 Pt 1):1111-1115

[43] Kigozi G, Gray RH, Wawer MJ, Serwadda D, Makumbi F, Watya S, et al. The safety of adult male circumcision in HIV-infected and uninfected men in Rakai, Uganda. PLoS Medicine. 2008;**5**(6):e116

[44] Merkel R, Putzke H. After Cologne: Male circumcision and the law. Parental right, religious liberty or criminal assault? Journal of Medical Ethics. 2013;**39**(7):444-449

[45] Alahmad G, Dekkers W. Bodily integrity and male circumcision: An islamic perspective. *J ima*. 2012:**44**(1). DOI: 10.5915/44-1-7903

[46] Dekkers W, Hoffer C, Wils JP. Bodily integrity and male and female circumcision. Medicine, Health Care, and Philosophy. 2005;**8**(2):179-191

[47] Dekkers W. Routine (non-religious) neonatal circumcision and bodily integrity: A transatlantic dialogue. Kennedy Institute of Ethics Journal. 2009;**19**(2):125-146

[48] Benatar M, Benatar D. Between prophylaxis and child abuse: The ethics of neonatal male circumcision. The American Journal of Bioethics: AJOB. 2003;**3**(2):35-48

[49] Fadel P. Respect for bodily integrity: A Catholic perspective on circumcision in Catholic hospitals. The American Journal of Bioethics: AJOB. 2003;**3**(2):W9

[50] Benini F, Johnston CC, Faucher D, Aranda JV. Topical anesthesia during circumcision in newborn infants. Journal of the American Medical Association. 1993;**270**(7):850-853

[51] Taddio A, Katz J, Ilersich AL, Koren G. Effect of neonatal circumcision on pain response during subsequent routine vaccination. Lancet (London, England). 1997;**349**(9052):599-603

[52] Stevens B, Yamada J, Ohlsson A, Haliburton S, Shorkey A. Sucrose for analgesia in newborn infants undergoing painful procedures. The Cochrane Database of Systematic Reviews. 2016;**7**:Cd001069

[53] Taddio A, Ohlsson K, Ohlsson A. Lidocaine-prilocaine cream for analgesia during circumcision in newborn boys. Cochrane Database Syst Rev(2), Cd000496. 2000. DOI: 10.1002/14651858.cd000496

[54] Bronselaer GA, Schober JM, Meyer-Bahlburg HF, T'Sjoen G, Vlietinck R, Hoebeke PB. Male circumcision decreases penile sensitivity as measured in a large cohort. BJU International. 2013;**111**(5):820-827

[55] Morris BJ, Krieger JN. Does male circumcision affect sexual function, sensitivity, or satisfaction?—A systematic review. The Journal of Sexual Medicine. 2013;**10**(11):2644-2657

[56] Cox G, Krieger JN, Morris BJ. Histological correlates of penile sexual sensation: Does circumcision make a difference? Sexual Medicine. 2015;**3**(2):76-85

[57] Schneider JA, Michaels S, Gandham SR, McFadden R, Liao C, Yeldandi VV, et al. A protective effect of circumcision among receptive male sex partners of Indian men who have sex with men. AIDS and Behavior. 2012;**16**(2):350-359

[58] Qian HZ, Ruan Y, Liu Y, Milam DF, Spiegel HM, Yin L, et al. Lower HIV risk among circumcised men who have sex with men in China: Interaction with anal sex role in a cross-sectional study. Journal of Acquired Immune Deficiency Syndromes (1999). 2016;**71**(4):444-451

[59] Jameson DR, Celum CL, Manhart L, Menza TW, Golden MR. The association between lack of circumcision and HIV, HSV-2, and other sexually transmitted infections among men who have sex with men. Sexually Transmitted Diseases. 2010;**37**(3):147-152

[60] Doerner R, McKeown E, Nelson S, Anderson J, Low N, Elford J. Circumcision and HIV infection among men who have sex with men in Britain: The insertive sexual role. Archives of Sexual Behavior. 2013;**42**(7):1319-1326

[61] Sanchez J, Sal YRVG, Hughes JP, Baeten JM, Fuchs J, Buchbinder SP, et al. Male circumcision and risk of HIV acquisition among MSM. AIDS (London, England). 2011;**25**(4):519-523

[62] Wiysonge CS, Kongnyuy EJ, Shey M, Muula AS, Navti OB, Akl EA, Lo YR. Male circumcision for prevention of homosexual acquisition of HIV in men. Cochrane Database Syst Rev(6), Cd007496. 2011. DOI: 10.1002/14651858.CD007496.pub2

[63] Circumcision policy statement. Pediatrics. American Academy of Pediatrics Task Force on Circumcision. 2012;**130**(3):585-586

[64] ACOG Committee Opinion. Circumcision. Number 260, October 2001. Obstetrics and Gynecology. 2001;**98**(4):707-708

[65] Association TAU. Policy statement on circumcision. 2017

[66] Organization tWH. Training Package on Early Infant Male Circumcision under Local Anaesthesia 2012

[67] Bank TW. The World Bank in Thailand. 2017

[68] Programme UND. Human devlepment report 2016.199

[69] United Nations DoEaSA, Population Division. World Population Prospects: The 2017 Revision, custom data acquired via website. 2017

[70] Committee NA. Thailand AIDS response progress report 2015. 2015

[71] Kongsri S, Limwattananon S, Sirilak S, Prakongsai P, Tangcharoensathien V. Equity of access to and utilization of reproductive health services in Thailand: National Reproductive Health Survey data, 2006 and 2009. Reproductive Health Matters. 2011;**19**(37):86-97

[72] Lolekha R, Boonsuk S, Plipat T, Martin M, Tonputsa C, Punsuwan N, et al. Elimination of mother-to-child transmission of HIV—Thailand. MMWR Morbidity and Mortality Weekly Report. 2016;**65**(22):562-566

12

Endocrine Active Compounds Actions during Neonatal Period: Effect on the Ovary

Maria Slomczynska, Malgorzata Grzesiak and Katarzyna Knapczyk-Stwora

Abstract

Many female reproductive disorders observed during adulthood originate from the neonatal period, which is a critical stage toward the reproductive potency. Human and animal fertility are determined by the pool of primordial follicles that are established during fetal or neonatal life. The earliest stages of follicle development are under control of a variety of factors, including sex steroids. Neonatal period is a "critical developmental window" in which organisms are susceptible to the environmental chemicals that may affect the reproductive health. Endocrine active compounds (EACs) are found abundantly in the environment and interfere with sex steroids (predominantly androgens and estrogens) by either mimicking or blocking their functions. This review covers the current knowledge about the effects of selected EACs with androgenic (testosterone propionate), anti-androgenic (flutamide), estrogenic (diethylstilbestrol, bisphenol A, 4-tert-octylphenol, phtalates and genistein), anti-estrogenic (ICI 182,780 and parabens), or mixed activity (methoxychlor) on the ovary of neonates, focusing on their effects on the early stages of folliculogenesis. These chemicals have been shown to affect oocyte survival, follicle formation, and growth, as well as steroidogenic functions. The better cognition of mechanisms underlying the long-term consequences of the neonatal EACs exposure may in future lead to an understanding of human health risks and developing prevention strategies.

Keywords: endocrine active compounds, estrogens, anti-estrogens, androgens, anti-androgens, ovary, neonatal window

1. Introduction

Considerable evidence demonstrates that inappropriate steroid exposure during pre- and postnatal developmental periods may have long-term effects on the adult reproductive functions [1]. Female fertility is determined by the pool of primordial follicles within the ovary that is established during fetal or neonatal life. The earliest stages of follicle development are tightly coordinated by numerous factors, including steroids. Importantly, these fetal/neonatal periods are "critical developmental windows" in which organisms are susceptible to the environmental chemicals that may affect ovarian formation and disturb reproductive functions during adulthood, including conception rates, maintenance of pregnancy, and reproductive disorders [2]. Endocrine active compounds (EACs) comprise a wide variety of synthetic or natural chemicals found in the environment arising from anthropogenic, industrial, agricultural, and domestic sources. EACs may interfere with the natural regulation of endocrine system by either mimicking or blocking the function of endogenous hormones and also they may act directly on gene expression by means of epigenetic modifications [3]. This is of concern because women are exposed to EACs on a daily basis, and some EACs are known to target the ovary and cause reproductive health problems. However, the harmful effects of EACs during neonatal period may occur with exposure to much lower doses than those considered harmful to adults [4]. Although many disrupting chemicals are excluded from the everyday use since their dangerous properties have been described, they may persist in the environment for long periods of time. Furthermore, new products with similar properties are still introduced to the market. Therefore, these compounds have currently been one of the greatest concerns all over the world. To assess the effect of EACs on human ovarian and consequently reproductive functions, the animal models are extensively used in experimental studies.

In this chapter, we aim to point out a possible impact of androgens/estrogens excess or deficiency on neonatal ovary following EACs action. The effect of EACs with androgenic (testosterone propionate), anti-androgenic (flutamide), estrogenic (diethylstilbestrol, bisphenol A, 4-tert-octylphenol, phtalates and genistein), anti-estrogenic (ICI 182,780 and parabens), or mixed activity (methoxychlor) will be discussed.

2. Mechanism of steroids action

The action of androgens/estrogens, and their agonists or antagonists, depends on the presence of specific receptors in target cells. The types of receptors that are involved in the signal transduction decide on the signaling pathway. The effect of sex steroid hormones action within the cell may be genomic or nongenomic. A genomic response is usually induced by nuclear/cytoplasmic receptors, while nongenomic pathway is activated by membrane receptors, mostly G-protein-coupled receptor. It is now evident that there is crosstalk between nongenomic and genomic signaling pathways [5].

Steroid hormone receptors, which belong to the superfamily of nuclear receptors, are hormone-activated transcriptional factors. They are modular proteins consisting of C-terminal ligand-binding domain (LBD), highly conserved DNA-binding domain (DBD) with centrally located zinc fingers, and N-terminal domain [6]. Activation of these receptors is mediated by two transcriptional activating domains, AF-1 and AF-2. AF-1, characterized by a ligand-independent transcriptional activation, is localized in the N-terminal region of the receptor, while AF-2, activated by ligands, is localized within the LBD. The LBD and DBD of nuclear receptors are conserved regions, whereas the N-terminal domain is highly variable but important for full transcriptional activity [7]. The latter contains many sites for Ser/Thr phosphorylation, which may be involved in mediating cross-talk with other signaling pathways leading to modulation of AF-1 activity and interaction with coregulators [8].

Sex steroid hormones can freely diffuse across the plasma membrane and bind to their cognate receptors inducing dissociation from the heat-shock proteins. Ligand binding to LBD region causes conformational changes followed by the dimerization of receptors and its translocation into the nucleus. The dimer binds to the hormone response elements (HREs) typically located in the promoter of the target gene and leads to the recruitment of coregulators, either coactivators or corepressors [9]. However, some nuclear receptors (i.e., estrogen receptors, and ERs) are capable of binding to DNA sequence, lacking the classic HRE sequence. Such receptors associate with the components of the AP-1 transcription factor complex (i.e., c-Jun and c-Fos). Additionally, in the low steroids concentration, the ligand-independent signaling pathway occurs allowing the activation of receptors. This process depends on the growth factor receptors and involves MAPK/ERKs pathway, which enhances transcriptional activity through direct phosphorylation of steroid receptors [10]. These pathways are known as "genomic pathway" and are characterized by the regulation of the expression of specific sex steroid receptor-regulated genes [11].

Although steroids exert most of their biologic activity through direct or indirect genomic effects, there are several examples that do not fit to this regulatory scheme. This pathway known as "nongenomic" is much more rapid and involves receptors localized in the plasma membrane or in "lipid rafts" [12]. All sex steroid hormones may stimulate rapid effects in signal transduction pathway through the production of second messengers, ion channels transport, and protein kinase cascades. Rapid effects of androgens and estrogens have been reported in many cell types [13, 14]. Conventional steroid receptors located in the membrane trigger the signal transduction cascade by activation of the Src/Ras/Raf/MAPK/ERK1/2 pathway [15]. Furthermore, steroids may mediate rapid signaling by binding to transmembrane receptors unrelated to nuclear hormone receptors (usually, G protein-coupled receptor, GPCR) and to the modified forms of steroid receptor or to receptors for neurotransmitters. The involvement of the type of receptor may depend on the steroid and cell type [16]. GPCR activates a protein kinase cascade or acts at the level of secondary messengers such as PI3K/AKT/mTOR, PI3K/AKT/cAMP/Ca^{+2} or ERK-mediated pathways like PI3K/AKT/MAPK-ERK/Elk1 [17]. Among GPCR, there are GPR30 for estradiol, mPR for progesterone, and GPRC6A and ZIP9 for androgens [18–21]. All the abovementioned mechanisms of steroid action are presented in **Figure 1**.

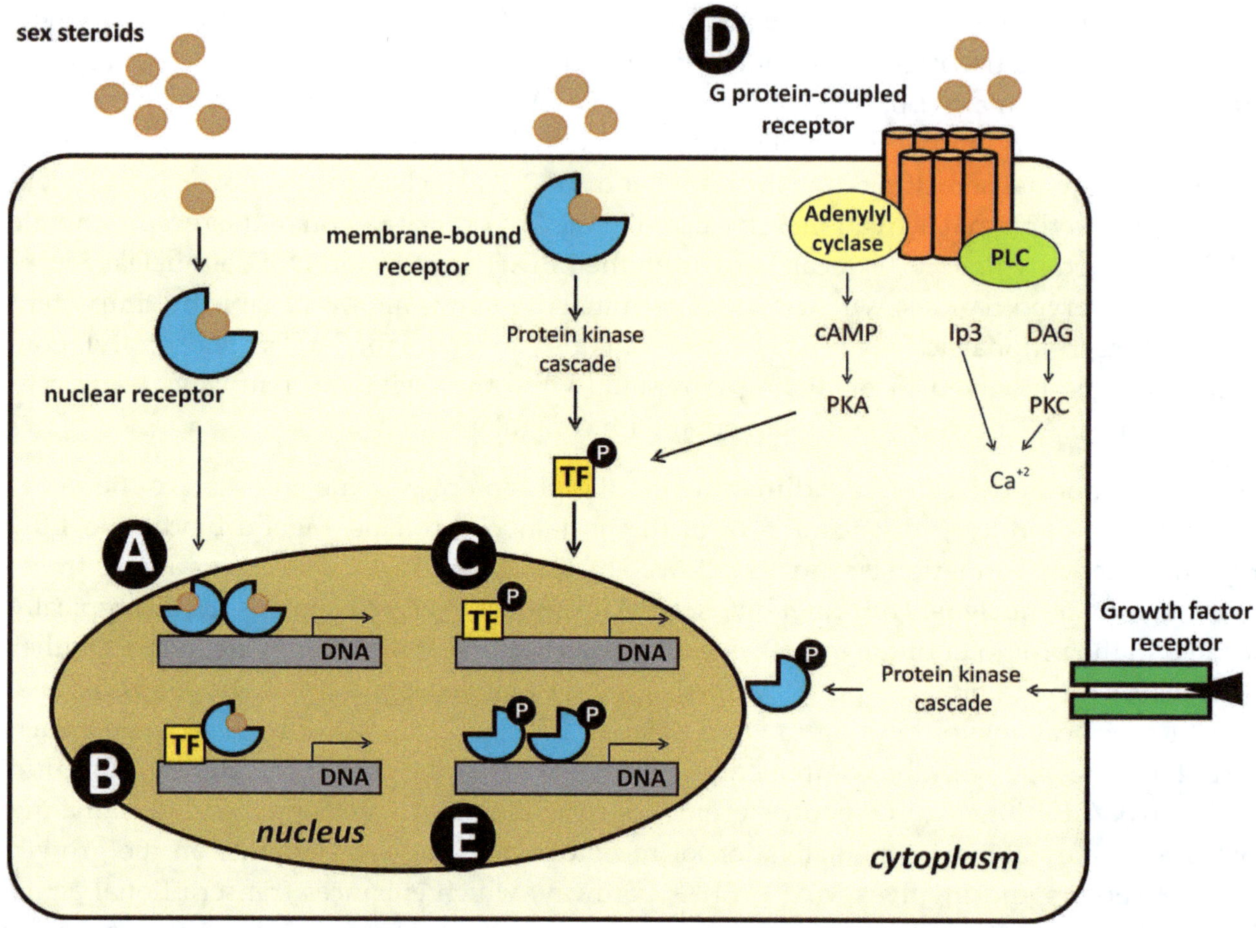

Figure 1. Molecular mechanism of the action of sex steroid hormone receptors. (**A**) Direct genomic effects. (**B**) Indirect genomic effects. (**C**) TF activation triggered by membrane receptor. (**D**) Nongenomic effects triggered by G-protein–coupled receptor. (**E**) Ligand-independent effects. TF, transcription factor; cAMP, cyclic AMP; PKA, protein kinase A; PLC, phospholipase C; IP3, inositol 1,4,5-triphosphate; DAG, diacylglycerol; PKC, protein kinase C. Based on Laurentino et al. [22].

3. The role of androgens and estrogens in the ovarian development

Primordial follicle assembly and the primordial-to-primary follicle transition are the major developmental events within the ovary [23]. The primordial follicle pool represents the total population of germ cells available during reproductive life and, therefore, determines the fertility potential of the female. In mammals, mitosis of oogonia and initiation of meiotic prophase I occur before birth, but the timing of oocyte meiotic arrest, follicle formation, and the initiation of follicle growth varies among species. During fetal ovarian development, primordial germ cells (PGSs) migrate from the endoderm of the yolk sac to the bipotential genital ridges. In mice (reviewed in Ref. [24]), which is a valuable animal model for studying embryogenesis, PGSs migrate into the undifferentiated gonad from around 8.5 day *post coitum* (dpc) to 11.5 dpc. The genital ridge is identical in both males and females and remains bipotential until sex determination (12.5 dpc). PGSs continue to proliferate mitotically during the migration and after arrival in the genital ridge until 12.5–13.5 dpc in mouse and 6th week of pregnancy in human. Then, at 13.5 dpc, in the mouse and between 8 and 13 weeks of gestation in human, meiosis is initiated, allowing oogonia to develop into oocytes that are arrested at the early diplotene phase of meiotic prophase I (reviewed in Ref. [25]). Oocytes initially develop as large, interconnected clusters of cells called oocytes nests. They are organized into long ovigerous cords surrounded by somatic or pregranulosa cells [24]. In rodents, oocyte nests break down in neonatal ovary that leads to the formation of primordial follicle. This is mediated by oocyte apoptosis starting at 16.5 dpc in mice. In addition, somatic cells can mediate nest breakdown by moving into the nest and intersperse between the remaining oocytes to form primordial follicles [26]. In the mouse ovary, the primordial follicles consist of an oocyte surrounded by a single layer of squamous pregranulosa cells that are formed fairly synchronously between 17.5 dpc and 4 postnatal day. Once assembled, some of the primordial follicles are immediately stimulated to growth, but most of them remain quiescent until selected follicles are gradually recruited into a growing follicle pool throughout reproductive life [27]. The recruitment of primordial follicles into growth (primordial-to-primary follicle transition) involves a change in the shape of the granulosa cells from squamous to cuboidal and the initiation of oocyte growth. The primordial-to-primary follicle transition is an irreversible process. Most of the growing follicles (99.9%) are destined to become atretic, and the rest will ovulate [28]. Around the end of the first postantal week, some secondary follicles are present in the mice ovary [29].

In contrast, in humans, ruminants, and pigs, follicle formation and the initiation of follicular growth are much less synchronous than in rodents and take place during fetal life. Although cattle and human have similar gestation lengths, follicle assembly in cattle was observed earlier (around 80 dpc) than in human (112–133 dpc). Besides, in bovine ovaries, the first primary and secondary follicles were observed around 140 and 210 dpc, respectively. No secondary follicles were observed in the fetal human ovary [30]. In pig, primordial follicle formation was observed between 70 and 90 dpc, while primordial to primary follicle transition was between 90 dpc and postnatal day 1 [31]. Interestingly, even antral follicles were present before birth in the sheep ovaries [32].

The early stages of folliculogenesis are believed to be gonadotropins-independent. All events related to early follicular development during fetal/neonatal period are mostly regulated by paracrine growth factors originating from the growing oocyte itself and from the somatic cells that surround it [33], and also by ovarian steroid hormones (i.e., progesterone, androgens, and estrogens). Although the pivotal role of androgens in the development of male reproductive organs is well understood, growing evidence supports the direct involvement of these hormones in female reproduction, including early follicular development [34]. The androgen receptor (AR) role in the female is implicated from the studies of various global and tissue-specific AR knockout (ARKO) mouse models. Granulosa cell-specific ARKO (GCARKO) mouse models have demonstrated that granulosa cells are important sites for androgen action and strongly suggested that the AR in these cells is an important regulator of androgen-mediated follicular growth and development. On the other hand, AR inactivation in the oocyte, as shown in the OoARKO female mouse model, appears to have no major overall effect on female fertility [35]. Fowler et al. [36] reported that the oocyte of the primordial follicles was able to synthesize androgens and that pregranulosa cells expressed AR in human fetal ovaries. Initiation of primordial follicle growth was stimulated in mouse, bovine, and primates ovaries by testosterone and dihydrotestosterone [37–39], while in sheep by dehydroepiandrosterone [40]. In general, androgens stimulate the primordial-to-primary follicle transition but impede the later stages of follicle development.

Studies using ERα knockout (αERKO) mice have demonstrated that the lack of ERα does not appear to affect folliculogenesis until the preantral stage of follicle development [41]. Similarly, in ERβ knockout (βERKO) mice, 17β-estradiol (E2) does not appear to be essential for the establishment of germ cell number or ovarian development [42]. However, Kezele and Skinner [43] have shown that both progesterone (P4) and E2 inhibit oocyte nest breakdown. It has been shown that fetal ovarian P4 and E2 concentrations decreased during the time as follicle assembly was initiated in the bovine ovary, while the maternal blood P4 and E2 levels were stable [44]. Recent work by Dutta et al. [45] also revealed that fetal mice produce their own steroid hormones to coordinate primordial follicle development. Notably, E2 promotes primordial follicle formation in hamster [46]. These data indicate that both P4 and E2 are important regulators of ovarian follicle assembly. Furthermore, E2 is likely to inhibit primordial-to-primary follicle transition, which was revealed in neonatal rat ovaries [43, 47]. In contrast, the lack of E2 in aromatase knockout (ArKO) mice was associated with decreased numbers of primordial and primary follicles [48]. Similarly, the primordial follicles number was reduced in estrogen-depleted fetal baboon ovaries [49]. These results indicate that although E2 is needed for early events in folliculogenesis, its excessive level inhibits these events. Abnormal control of primordial follicle assembly may affect the reproductive potential of the female and can lead to pathological conditions such as premature ovarian failure.

4. Effects of endocrine active compounds within the neonatal ovary

Many female reproductive disorders observed during adulthood originate from the neonatal period, which is a critical stage toward the reproductive potency. Consequently, it is important to study the effects of neonatal exposure to chemicals that mimic or antagonize the effects of estrogens and androgens to establish their role in ovarian function. Recent attention has been especially focused on environmental factors interfering with endogenous steroids action. There are synthetic and natural environmental compounds such as pesticides (i.e., dichlorodiphenyltrichloroethane (DDT); methoxychlor (MXC), vinclozolin, and atrazine); detergents and surfactants (4-tert-octylphenol, nonylphenol, and bisphenol A); plastics (phtalates); industrial compounds (polychlorinated biphenyl, PCB; 2,3,7,8-tetrachlorodibenzo-p-dioxin, TCDD); and fitoestrogens (genistein and coumestol) [4]. In the light of growing body of evidence that demonstrates the presence of EACs in the environment, understanding the mechanism of selected EACs action within neonatal ovaries provides a basic data for further research of the female reproductive potency. The susceptibility of target tissues is related to the stage of development, the exposure dose, and the individual immune status. Mammals are more sensitive to EACs during fetal and postnatal life than in adulthood. However, environmental influence during fetal and neonatal development may lead to adult onset pathology.

4.1. EACs with androgenic and anti-androgenic properties

Previous data on primates clearly showed the essential role of androgens in promoting early follicular growth [50]. These results were confirmed by *in vitro* study on bovine ovarian follicles, indicating that testosterone stimulated the primary-to-secondary follicle transition

[38]. Importantly, testosterone increased the number of secondary follicles with no impact of estradiol that suggested the direct effect of androgens without conversion to estrogens. Testosterone promotes the growth of bovine follicles *in vitro,* and its stimulatory effect was mediated through ARs in the follicular cells [38]. Thus, reprogramming of early folliculogenesis by androgens excess or deficiency seems to be crucial for understanding their adverse effects on female fertility.

Studies on sheep [51, 52] and primates [53] have shown that excess of androgens in fetal life resulted in reduced ovarian functions in adult life and may provide models for polycystic ovary syndrome (PCOS) in women. Research by Tyndall et al. [54] was undertaken to investigate the effects of different windows of testosterone propionate treatment during fetal or neonatal life in female rats to determine whether and when excess androgen exposure would cause disruption of adult reproductive functions. The findings from fetal exposure to testosterone propionate suggested the possibility of reducing the sensitivity threshold to neonatal androgens exposure in female animals. The results support the concept that androgen programming of adult female reproductive function occurs only during specific time windows in fetal and neonatal life with implications for the development of PCOS in women.

Neonatal androgenization by testosterone propionate induced early misprogramming of ovarian functions in the female rats [55]. The obtained results strongly suggested that transient neonatal hyperandrogenemia led to ovarian dysfunctions marked by altered steroidogenesis and folliculogenesis. Exposure to testosterone propionate resulted in the increase of primary and the decrease of antral follicle frequencies. Moreover, the higher proportion of atretic follicles and the lack of corpora lutea within the ovaries from testosterone propionate-treated rats were observed. Another research on rats revealed that exposure to excess of testosterone in neonatal period increased the LH and testosterone serum levels, the LH/FSH ratio, ovarian theca-interstitial area and expression of steroidogenesis-involved genes, and Lhr and Cyp17a1 in ovaries of adult animals [56]. These results provide some insight into the role of androgens on reproductive development and on the manifestations of clinical disorders such as PCOS.

Among EACs, there is a large group of chemicals exerting anti-androgenic effects and blocking endogenous androgens action. In our previous experiments, the androgen involvement in early stages of folliculogenesis was confirmed using *in vivo* animal model generated for studying androgen deficiency. We have utilized flutamide (2-methyl-N-[4-nitro-30-(trifluoromethyl)-phenyl] propamide), which is a nonsteroidal anti-androgen acting at the AR level and blocking androgen action. Flutamide promotes AR translocation to the nucleus and DNA binding, but nevertheless fails to initiate transcription, inhibiting the AR signaling pathway [57]. Although this is a pharmaceutical compound, it is regarded as a model anti-androgen in experimental studies [58].

In our recent research, flutamide (50 mg/kg body weight) was injected into pregnant gilts during gestational days 20–28 and 80–88 and into female piglets on postnatal days 2–10. We have found ovarian morphological changes indicating delayed folliculogenesis in neonatal pigs exposed *in utero* to flutamide [59]. Abnormal folliculogenesis was also seen in prepubertal pigs, following prenatal period of anti-androgen exposure [60], whereas in adult animals, only neonatal time of flutamide treatment exerted disturbances marked by altered luteinization and corpus luteum cyst formation [61]. Apart from morphological disturbances, the altered follicular functioning in adulthood was manifested by changes in production of steroids (estradiol and androgens) and gonadotropins (FSH and LH), as well as in expression of genes involved in proper ovarian functioning, including AR, FSHR, aromatase, connexin 43, β-catenin, and aquaporin 5 [61–63]. Furthermore, gestational or neonatal exposure to flutamide affected proliferation and apoptosis rates in large antral follicles of adult porcine ovary, which might influence the normal development of the follicles and pigs fertility as a consequence [64].

It seems that disturbed androgen action during gestational and neonatal periods by using flutamide led to reprogramming of the trajectory of ovarian development in pigs; however, neonatal window of exposure leads to long-term effects observed in adulthood.

4.2. EACs with estrogenic and anti-estrogenic properties

Compounds that mimic estrogens action through an interaction with ERs continue to receive considerable attention. One of them is 4-tert-octylphenol, which belongs to alkylphenol polyethoxylates derivative, which is a nonionic surfactant widely used in a variety of industrial applications [65]. It was demonstrated that pre- or postnatal exposure to 4-tert-octylphenol can advance the onset of puberty in rats [66] and pigs [67]. In addition, in a three-generation study, 4-tert-octylphenol given prenatally to sows induced some effects, including reduction in litter size, observed in the next generations [67]. Furthermore, 4-tert-octylphenol exposure during fetal and postnatal life accelerated the onset of puberty but did not disrupt FSH concentration and the dynamic of ovarian follicular growth in ewes [68]. On the other hand, research on rats revealed that neonatal administration to 4-tert-octylphenol altered hypothalamo-pituitary-ovarian axis resulting in atrophic and polycystic ovaries without corpora lutea [66]. In our most recent experiments using neonatal pigs treated with 4-tert-octylphenol, the advanced folliculogenesis has been shown. We assumed that these specific effects on folliculogenesis in neonatal pigs were characterized by changes in proliferation and apoptosis rates during initial follicular recruitment [69].

Both bisphenol A and diethylstilbestrol are another of the extensively studied EACs with estrogenic activity. Bisphenol A is a plasticizer used commonly in a wide range of consumer products such as food and drink containers, epoxy resins, plastics, baby bottles, thermal receipts, and dental sealants (reviewed in Ref. [70]). Zhou et al. [71] revealed that bisphenol A exposure significantly inhibited germ cell nests breakdown by altering the expression of key ovarian apoptotic genes in cultured neonatal mouse ovaries. Interestingly, exposure of neonates to estrogenic compounds like bisphenol A significantly increases the number of multiple oocyte follicles (MOFs) in adult mice ovaries. It was proposed that neonatal exposure to exogenous estrogens blocked cysts breakdown resulting in oocytes survival [72]. Apart from abovementioned influence of bisphenol A on oocyte nests, additional effects on the follicle development were found. Bisphenol A may interact with multiple factors produced by oocyte and granulosa cells to alter neonatal follicular dynamics. [73, 74]. It was shown that this compound reduced the primordial follicle pool by stimulating the initial recruitment in neonatal rats associated with an increased proliferation rate, which is likely mediated by an estrogenic pathway [75]. It could also decrease follicle activation in neonatal mice [76]. Additionally, the effect of neonatal exposure to bisphenol A on the reproductive axis was observed in adult rats, which may lead to the development of PCOS [77].

Diethylstilbestrol is a synthetic nonsteroidal estrogen. Studies on neonatal rodents injected with diethylstilbestrol demonstrated results similar to those of bisphenol A. Neonatal exposure to diethylstilbestrol of mice and hamster inhibited germ cell nest breakdown and induced MOFs formation, likely by interfering with the ERβ pathway and inhibiting programmed oocyte death and germ cell loss [78, 79]. Rodríguez et al. [75] used a relatively low concentration of diethylstilbestrol (20 μg/kg body weight) in the rat and found that primordial follicle activation was increased compared to studies of Karavan et al. [80] on mice, where the higher diethylstilbestrol concentration (100 μg/kg body weight) decreased the follicle activation. Both diethylstilbestrol and bisphenol A reduced follicle growth and development, resulting in the presence of more primordial follicles and fewer primary and secondary follicles in mouse neonatal ovary [80]. In prepubertal lambs treated with bisphenol A or diethylstilbestrol during neonatal period, the reduction of the primordial follicle pool and increased atresia was observed. That was surprising since nest breakdown in sheep is completed before birth. However, it seems that the reduction of the primordial follicle pool is due to stimulation of their initial recruitment and subsequent development until antral stage. These alterations may affect the ovarian function in the adulthood [81].

Genistein is a natural phytoestrogen with estrogenic activity found in soy products. The belief that estrogens can regulate nest breakdown is supported by a study of Jefferson et al. [82]. They have demonstrated exposure of neonatal mice to genistein, which inhibited the oocyte nests breakdown and increased oocyte survival. Moreover, ovaries from adult mice treated as neonates with genistein have an increased occurrence of MOFs, suggesting incomplete nests breakdown [83]. This indicates that cell survival/death pathways are altered following neonatal genistein treatment. The inhibition of oogonia/oocyte nests breakdown by EACs action was shown in the **Figure 2**.

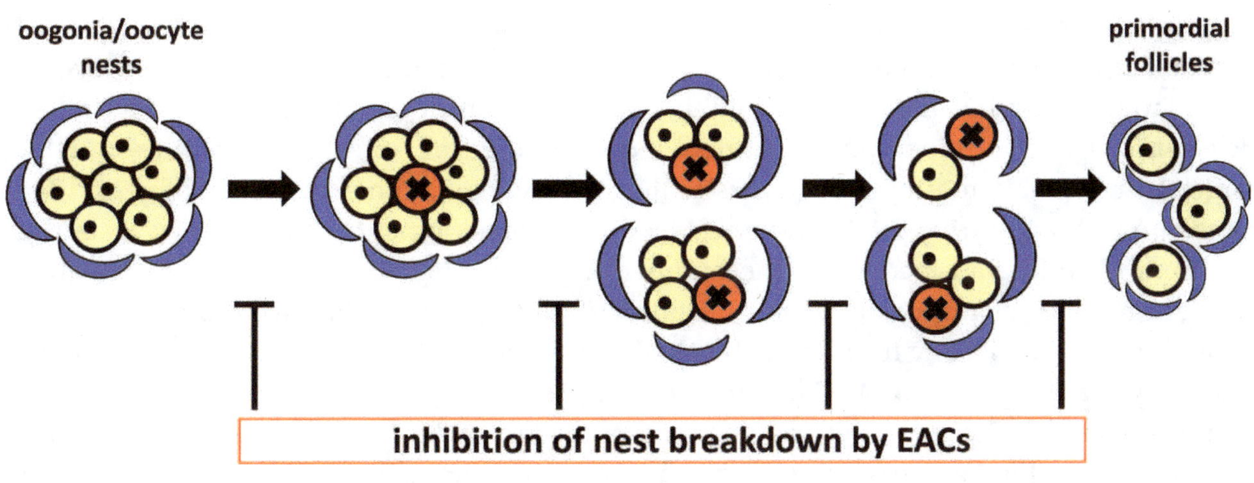

Figure 2. Schematic model of oogonia/oocyte nests breakdown and its inhibition by endocrine active compounds (EACs) with estrogenic activity (bisphenol A, diethylstilbestrol, and genistein).

Phthalates are commonly used as plasticizers in the manufacturing of flexible polyvinyl chloride products. Little information is available on the effects of phthalates on neonatal ovary. These compounds have been actually shown to affect germ cell nest breakdown and primordial follicle assembly in cultured newborn mouse ovaries [84]. In addition, early postnatal treatment with diethylhexyl phthalate accelerated folliculogenesis by decreasing the number of primordial follicles and increasing the number preantral and antral follicles in mice [85]. The decrease in primordial follicle pool indicated estrogenic action of these compounds.

ICI 182,780 is a widely used anti-estrogen that can bind to both ERα and ERβ with very high affinity and completely antagonize the effect of estrogens [86]. It was found that ICI 182,780 in combination with estradiol allowed oocytes cyst breakdown neonatal rat ovaries [87]. On the other hand, Wang and Roy [46] revealed that ICI 182,780 significantly increased apoptosis and caused a modest reduction in primordial follicle formation in neonatal hamster ovary. Likewise, ICI 182,780 accelerated primordial follicles formation from oocyte nests in the neonatal pig. However, the initial follicle recruitment marked by the number of growing was delayed [69].

The compounds that exert both estrogenic and anti-estrogenic properties are parabens, which are widely used as anti-microbial agents in the cosmetic and pharmaceutical industries. Parabens inhibited the early phase of folliculogenesis and steroidogenesis in the ovaries of neonatal rats [88]. Moreover, it appears that parabens through inhibition of transcriptional repressor Foxl2, regulated the levels of steroidogenic enzymes [88].

4.3. EACs with mixed properties

Methoxychlor (MXC) is an organochlorine pesticide metabolized predominantly to 1,1,1-trichloro-2-(4-hydroxyphenyl)-2-(4-methoxyphenyl) ethane (MOH) and the bisphenolic compound 1,1,1-trichloro-2,2-bis(4-hydroxyphenyl) ethane (HPTE) in the organism [89]. MXC along with its metabolites acts through ERs and possesses estrogenic, anti-estrogenic, and anti-androgenic activities depending on the receptor subtype [90]. In a variety of experimental studies, MXC administration in early pregnancy or during the prenatal and neonatal periods has been shown to cause adverse abnormalities in adulthood of female rats, such as reduced ovarian functions and ovulatory rates, as well as pregnancy outcome [1]. Uzumcu et al. [91] demonstrated that MXC administration during the primordial-to-primary follicle transition period in mice (postnatal days 3–10) inhibited follicular development and reduced antral follicle numbers. In addition, MXC treatment increased the level of AMH protein production, which in turn inhibited folliculogenesis within the ovary. Another research suggested that exposure to MXC during fetal and neonatal ovarian development led to adult ovarian dysfunction, including an increase in the number of preantral and early antral follicles and a reduced number of corpora lutea and female infertility in rats [92]. Furthermore, there are several reports suggesting the role of MXC in the induction of epigenetic modifications within the ovary. Rats exposed to MXC (20 or 100 μg/kg body weight) between embryonic day 19 and postnatal day 7 revealed altered methylation pattern in the promoter region of ERα that suppressed the ERα expression and caused ovarian dysfunction. Developmental exposure to MXC led to significant hypermethylation in the ERβ promoter regions, whereas the ERα promoter was unaffected [93].

5. Summary

The plausible link between EACs exposure during critical periods of early development and risk of chronic diseases in adulthood, including premature ovarian failure and PCOS, has been reported. The harmful effects of compounds with androgenic, anti-androgenic, estrogenic, and anti-estrogenic activities during neonatal window may occur with exposure to lower doses than those harmful for adults. These chemicals have been shown to target the ovary of neonates and adversely affect oocyte survival, follicle formation, and growth, as well as steroidogenic functions. There is a concern over EACs due to their common use and persistence within the modern living environment. The better cognition of mechanisms underlying the long-term consequences of the neonatal EACs exposure may in future lead to an understanding of human health risks and developing prevention strategies.

Acknowledgements

This work was supported by National Science Center, Poland, grant no. 2015/17/B/NZ9/01457 (to MS).

Author details

Maria Slomczynska[1], Malgorzata Grzesiak[2]* and Katarzyna Knapczyk-Stwora[1]

*Address all correspondence to: m.grzesiak@ur.krakow.pl

1 Department of Endocrinology, Institute of Zoology and Biomedical Research, Jagiellonian University, Krakow, Poland

2 Department of Animal Physiology and Endocrinology, University of Agriculture, Krakow, Poland

References

[1] Vaiserman A. Early-life exposure to endocrine disrupting chemicals and later-life health outcomes: An epigenetic bridge? Aging and Disease. 2014;**5**:419-429. DOI: 10.14336/AD.2014.0500419

[2] Woodruff TK, Walker CL. Fetal and early postnatal environmental exposures and reproductive health effects in the female. Fertility and Sterility. 2008;**89**:e47-e51. DOI: 10.1016/j.fertnstert.2007.12.029

[3] Uzumcu M, Zama AM, Oruc E. Epigenetic mechanisms in the actions of endocrine-disrupting chemicals: Gonadal effects and role in female reproduction. Reproduction in Domestic Animals. 2012;**47**:338-347. DOI: 10.1111/j.1439-0531.2012.02096.x

[4] Schug TT, Janesick A, Blumberg B, Heindel JJ. Endocrine disrupting chemicals and disease susceptibility. Journal of Steroid Biochemistry and Molecular Biology. 2011;**127**:204-215. DOI: 10.1016/j.jsbmb.2011.08.007

[5] Björnström L, Sjöberg M. Mechanisms of estrogen receptor signaling: Convergence of genomic and nongenomic actions on target genes. Molecular Endocrinology. 2005;**19**:833-842. DOI: 10.1210/me.2004–0486

[6] Beato M, Klug J. Steroid hormone receptors: An update. Human Reproduction Update. 2000;**6**:225-236. DOI: 10.1093/humupd/6.3.225

[7] Kumar R, Thompson EB. Transactivation functions of the N-terminal domains of nuclear hormone receptors: Protein folding and coactivator interactions. Molecular Endocrinology. 2003;**17**:1-10. DOI: 10.1210/me.2002–0258

[8] Rochette-Egly C. Nuclear receptors: Integration of multiple signalling pathways through phosphorylation. Cellular Signalling. 2003;**15**:355-366. DOI: 10.1016/S0898-6568(02)00115-8

[9] Khorasanizadeh S, Rastinejad F. Nuclear-receptor interactions on DNA-response elements. Trends in Biochemical Sciences. 2001;**26**:384-390. DOI: 10.1016/S0968-0004(01)01800-X

[10] Bunone G, Briand PA, Miksicek RJ, Picard D. Activation of the unliganded estrogen receptor by EGF involves the MAP kinase pathway and direct phosphorylation. EMBO Journal. 1996;**15**:2174-2183

[11] Picard D, Bunone G, Liu JW, Donzé O. Steroid-independent activation of steroid receptors in mammalian and yeast cells and in breast cancer. Biochemical Society Transactions. 1997;**25**:597-602. DOI: 10.1042/bst0250597

[12] Simons K, Toomre D. Lipid rafts and signal transduction. Nature Reviews Molecular Cell Biology. 2000;**1**:31-39. DOI: 10.1038/35036052

[13] Falkenstein E, Tillmann HC, Christ M, Feuring M, Wehling MC. Multiple actions of steroid hormones—A focus on rapid, nongenomic effects. Pharmacological Reviews. 2000;**52**:513-556

[14] Cato AC, Nestl A, Mink S. Rapid actions of steroid receptors in cellular signaling pathways. Sci STKE. 2002;**2002**:re9. DOI: 10.1126/stke.2002.138.re9

[15] Liao RS, Ma S, Miao L, Li R, Yin Y, Raj GV. Androgen receptor-mediated non-genomic regulation of prostate cancer cell proliferation. Translational Andrology and Urology. 2013;**2**:187-196. DOI: 10.3978/j.issn.2223-4683.2013.09.07

[16] Leitman DC, Paruthiyil S, Yuan C, Herber CB, Olshansky M, Tagliaferri M, Cohen I, Speed TP. Tissue-specific regulation of genes by estrogen receptors. Seminars in Reproductive Medicine. 2012;**30**:14-22. DOI: 10.1055/s-0031-1299593

[17] Revankar CM, Cimino DF, Sklar LA, Arterburn JB, Prossnitz ER. A transmembrane intracellular estrogen receptor mediates rapid cell signaling. Science. 2005;**307**:1625-1630. DOI: 10.1126/science.1106943

[18] Chevalier N, Paul-Bellon R, Camparo P, Michiels JF, Chevallier D, Fénichel P. Genetic variants of GPER/GPR30, a novel estrogen-related G protein receptor, are associated with human seminoma. International Journal of Molecular Sciences. 2014;**15**:1574-1789. DOI: 10.3390/ijms15011574

[19] Thomas P. Characteristics of membrane progestin receptor alpha (mPRalpha) and progesterone membrane receptor component 1 (PGMRC1) and their roles in mediating rapid progestin actions. Frontiers in Neuroendocrinology. 2008;**29**:292-312. DOI: 10.1016/j.yfrne.2008.01.001

[20] Pi M, Parrill AL, Quarles LD. GPRC6A mediates the non-genomic effects of steroids. Journal of Biological Chemistry. 2010;**285**:39953-39964. DOI: 10.1074/jbc.M110.158063

[21] Pascal LE, Wang Z. Unzipping androgen action through ZIP9: A novel membrane androgen receptor. Endocrinology. 2014;**155**:4120-4123. DOI: 10.1210/en.2014–1749

[22] Laurentino S, Pinto P, Correia S, Cavaco JE, Canário AVM, Socorro S. Structural variants of sex steroid hormone receptors in the testis: From molecular biology to physiological roles. OA Biotechnology. 2012;**1**:4

[23] McGee EA, Hsueh AJ. Initial and cyclic recruitment of ovarian follicles. Endocrine Reviews. 2000;**21**:200-214. DOI: 10.1210/edrv.21.2.0394

[24] Pepling ME. From primordial germ cell to primordial follicle: Mammalian female germ cell development. Genesis. 2006;**44**:622-632. DOI: 10.1002/dvg.20258

[25] Sarraj MA, Drummond AE. Mammalian foetal ovarian development: Consequences for health and disease. Reproduction. 2012;**143**:151-163. DOI: 10.1530/REP-11-0247

[26] Pepling ME, Spradling AC. Mouse ovarian germ cell cysts undergo programmed breakdown to form primordial follicles. Developmental Biology. 2001;**234**;339-351. DOI: 10.1006/dbio.2001.0269

[27] McLaughlin EA, McIver SC. Awakening the oocyte: Controlling primordial follicle development. Reproduction. 2009;**137**:1-11. DOI: 10.1530/REP-08-0118

[28] Hsueh AJ, Billig, H, Tsafriri A. Ovarian follicle atresia: A hormonally controlled apoptotic process. Endocrine Reviews. 1994;**15**:707-724. DOI: 10.1210/edrv-15-6-707

[29] Smith P, Wilhelm D, Rodgers RJ. Development of mammalian ovary. Journal of Endocrinology. 2014;**221**:R145-R161. DOI: 10.1530/JOE-14-0062

[30] Fortune JE, Yang MY, Allen JJ, Herrick SL. Triennial reproduction symposium: The ovarian follicular reserve in cattle: What regulates its formation and size? Journal of Animal Science. 2013;**91**:3041-3050. DOI: 10.2527/jas.2013–6233

[31] Ding W, Wang W, Zhou B, Zhang W, Huang P, Shi F, Taya K. Formation of primordial follicles and immunolocalization of PTEN, PKB and FOXO3A proteins in the ovaries of fetal and neonatal pigs. Journal of Reproduction and Development. 2010;**56**:162-168. DOI: 10.1262/jrd.09-094H

[32] McNatty KP, Smith P, Hudson NL, Heath DA, Tisdall DJ, O WS, Braw-Tal R. Development of the sheep ovary during fetal and early neonatal life and the effect of fecundity genes. Journal of Reproduction and Fertility. Supplement. 1995;**49**:123-135

[33] Eppig JJ, Wigglesworth K, Pendola FL. The mammalian oocyte orchestrates the rate of ovarian follicular development. Proceedings of the National Academy of Sciences of the United States of America. 2002;**99**:2890-2894. DOI: 10.1073/pnas.052658699

[34] Gervásio CG, Bernuci MP, Silva-de-Sá MF, Rosa-E-Silva AC. The role of androgen hormones in early follicular development. ISRN Obstetrics and Gynecology. 2014;**2014**:818010. DOI: 10.1155/2014/818010

[35] Chang C, Lee SO, Wang RS, Yeh S, Chang TM. Androgen receptor (AR) physiological roles in male and female reproductive systems: Lessons learned from AR-knockout mice lacking AR in selective cells. Biology of Reproduction. 2013;**89**:21. DOI: 10.1095/biolreprod.113.109132

[36] Fowler PA, Anderson RA, Saunders PT, Kinnell H, Mason JI, Evans DB, Bhattacharya S, Flannigan S, Franks S, Monteiro A, O'Shaughnessy PJ. Development of steroid signaling pathways during primordial follicle formation in the human fetal ovary. Journal of Clinical Endocrinology and Metabolism. 2011;**96**:1754-1762. DOI: 10.1210/jc.2010-2618

[37] Vendola K, Zhou J, Wang J, Famuyiwa OA, Bievre M, Bondy CA. Androgens promote oocyte insulin-like growth factor I expression and initiation of follicle development in the primate ovary. Biology of Reproduction. 1999;**61**:353-357. DOI: 10.1095/biolreprod61.2.353

[38] Yang MY, Fortune JE. Testosterone stimulates the primary to secondary follicle transition in bovine follicles in vitro. Biology of Reproduction. 2006;**75**:924-932. DOI: 10.1095/biolreprod.106.051813

[39] Yang JL, Zhang CP, Li L, Huang L, Ji SY, Lu CL, Fan CH, Cai H, Ren Y, Hu ZY, Gao F, Liu YX. Testosterone induces redistribution of forkhead box-3a and down-regulation of growth and differentiation factor 9 messenger ribonucleic acid expression at early stage of mouse folliculogenesis. Endocrinology. 2010;**151**:774-782. DOI: 10.1210/en.2009-0751

[40] Narkwichean A, Jayaprakasan K, Maalouf WE, Hernandez-Medrano JH, Pincott-Allen C, Campbell BK. Effects of dehydroepiandrosterone on in vivo ovine follicular development. Human Reproduction. 2014;**29**:146-154. DOI: 10.1093/humrep/det408

[41] Rosenfeld CS, Murray AA, Simmer G, Hufford MG, Smith MF, Spears N, Lubahn DB. Gonadotropin induction of ovulation and corpus luteum formation in young estrogen receptor-alpha knockout mice. Biology of Reproduction. 2000;**62**:599-605. DOI: 10.1095/biolreprod62.3.599

[42] Krege JH, Hodgin JB, Couse JF, Enmark E, Warner M, Mahler JF, Sar M, Korach KS, Gustafsson JA, Smithies O. Generation and reproductive phenotypes of mice lacking estrogen receptor beta. Proceedings of the National Academy of Sciences of the United States of America. 1998;**95**:15677-15682. DOI: 10.1073/pnas.95.26.15677

[43] Kezele P, Skinner MK. Regulation of ovarian primordial follicle assembly and development by estrogen and progesterone: Endocrine model of follicle assembly. Endocrinology. 2003;**144**:3329-3337. DOI: 10.1210/en.2002–0131

[44] Nilsson EE, Skinner MK. Progesterone regulation of primordial follicle assembly in bovine fetal ovaries. Molecular and Cellular Endocrinology. 2009;**313**:9-16. DOI: 10.1016/j.mce.2009.09.004

[45] Dutta S, Mark-Kappeler CJ, Hoyer PB and Pepling ME. The steroid hormone environment during primordial follicle formation in perinatal mouse ovaries. Biology of Reproduction. 2014;**91**:68:1-12. DOI: 10.1095/biolreprod.114.119214

[46] Wang C, Roy SK. Development of primordial follicles in the hamster: Role of estradiol-17beta. Endocrinology. 2007;**148**:1707-1716. DOI: 10.1210/en.2006-1193

[47] Ikeda Y, Nagai A, Ikeda MA, Hayashi S. Neonatal estrogen exposure inhibits steroidogenesis in the developing rat ovary. Developmental Dynamics. 2001;**221**:443-453. DOI: 10.1002/dvdy.1162

[48] Britt KL, Saunders PK, McPherson SJ, Misso ML, Simpson ER, Findlay JK. Estrogen actions on follicle formation and early follicle development. Biology of Reproduction. 2004;**71**:1712-1723. DOI: 10.1095/biolreprod.104.028175

[49] Zachos NC, Billiar RB, Albrecht ED, Pepe GJ. Developmental regulation of baboon fetal ovarian maturation by estrogen. Biology of Reproduction. 2002;**67**:1148-1156. DOI: 10.1095/biolreprod67.4.1148

[50] Vendola KA, Zhou J, Adesanya OO, Weil SJ, Bondy CA. Androgens stimulate early stages of follicular growth in the primate ovary. Journal of Clinical Investigation. 1998;**101**:2622-2629. DOI: 10.1172/JCI2081

[51] Steckler T, Manikkam M, Inskeep EK, Padmanabhan V. Developmental programming: Follicular persistence in prenatal testosterone-treated sheep is not programmed by androgenic actions of testosterone. Endocrinology. 2007;**148**:3532-3540. DOI: 10.1210/en.2007-0339

[52] Hogg K, McNeilly AS, Duncan WC. Prenatal androgen exposure leads to alterations in gene and protein expression in the ovine fetal ovary. Endocrinology. 2011;**152**:2048-2059. DOI: 10.1210/en.2010-1219

[53] Abbott DH, Dumesic DA, Franks S. Developmental origin of polycystic ovary syndrome—A hypothesis. Journal of Endocrinology. 2002;**174**:1-5. DOI: 10.1677/joe.0.1740001

[54] Tyndall V, Broyde M, Sharpe R, Welsh M, Drake AJ, McNeilly AS. Effect of androgen treatment during foetal and/or neonatal life on ovarian function in prepubertal and adult rats. Reproduction. 2012;**143**:21-33. DOI: 10.1530/REP-11-0239

[55] Ongaro L, Salvetti NR, Giovambattista A, Spinedi E, Ortega HH. Neonatal androgenization-induced early endocrine-metabolic and ovary misprogramming in the female rat. Life Sciences. 2015;**130**:66-72. DOI: 10.1016/j.lfs.2015.03.008

[56] Marcondes RR, Carvalho KC, Duarte DC, Garcia N, Amaral VC, Simões MJ, Lo Turco EG, Soares JM Jr, Baracat EC, Maciel GA. Differences in neonatal exposure to estradiol or testosterone on ovarian function and hormonal levels. General and Comparative Endocrinology. 2015;**212**:28-33. DOI: 10.1016/j.ygcen.2015.01.006

[57] Kemppainen JA, Lane MV, Sar M, Wilson EM. Androgen receptor phosphorylation, turnover, nuclear transport, and transcriptional activation. Specificity for steroids and antihormones. Journal of Biological Chemistry. 1992;**267**:968-974

[58] O'Connor JC, Cook JC, Slone TW, Makovec GT, Frame SR, Davis LG. An ongoing validation of a Tier I screening battery for detecting endocrine-active compounds (EACs). Toxicological Sciences. 1998;**46**:45-60. DOI: 10.1006/toxs.1998.2550

[59] Durlej M, Kopera I, Knapczyk-Stwora K, Hejmej A, Duda M, Koziorowski M, Slomczynska M, Bilinska B. Connexin 43 gene expression in male and female gonads of porcine offspring following in utero exposure to an anti-androgen, flutamide. Acta Histochemica. 2011;**113**:6-12. DOI: 10.1016/j.acthis.2009.07.001

[60] Kopera I, Durlej M, Hejmej A, Knapczyk-Stwora K, Duda M, Slomczynska M, Koziorowski M, Bilinska B. Effects of pre- and postnatal exposure to flutamide on connexin 43 expression in testes and ovaries of prepubertal pigs. European Journal of Histochemistry. 2010;**54**:e15. DOI: 10.4081/ejh.2010.e15

[61] Durlej M, Knapczyk-Stwora K, Duda M, Kopera-Sobota I, Hejmej A, Bilinska B, Slomczynska M. Prenatal and neonatal exposure to the antiandrogen flutamide alters connexin 43 gene expression in adult porcine ovary. Domestic Animal Endocrinology. 2011;**40**:19-29. DOI: 10.1016/j.domaniend.2010.08.003

[62] Grzesiak M, Knapczyk-Stwora K, Duda M, Slomczynska M. Elevated level of 17β-estradiol is associated with overexpression of FSHR, CYP19A1, and CTNNB1 genes in porcine ovarian follicles after prenatal and neonatal flutamide exposure. Theriogenology. 2012;**78**:2050-2060. DOI: 10.1016/j.theriogenology.2012.07.026

[63] Grzesiak M, Knapczyk-Stwora K, Luck MR, Mobasheri A, Slomczynska M. Effect of prenatal and neonatal anti-androgen flutamide treatment on aquaporin 5 expression in the adult porcine ovary. Reproduction in Domestic Animals. 2016;**51**:105-113. DOI: 10.1111/rda.12652

[64] Durlej M, Knapczyk-Stwora K, Slomczynska M. Prenatal and neonatal flutamide administration increases proliferation and reduces apoptosis in large antral follicles of adult pigs. Animal Reproduction Science. 2012;**132**:58-65. DOI: 10.1016/j.anireprosci.2012.04.001

[65] Giger W, Brunner PH, Schaffner C. 4-Nonylphenol in sewage sludge: Accumulation of toxic metabolites from nonionic surfactants. Science. 1984;**225**:623-625. DOI: 10.1126/science.6740328

[66] Katsuda S, Yoshida M, Watanabe G, Taya K, Maekawa A. Irreversible effects of neonatal exposure to p-tert-octylphenol on the reproductive tract in female rats. Toxicology and Applied Pharmacology. 2000;**165**:217-226. DOI: 10.1006/taap.2000.8940

[67] Bøgh IB, Christensen P, Dantzer V, Groot M, Thøfner IC, Rasmussen RK, Schmidt M, Greve T. Endocrine disrupting compounds: Effect of octylphenol on reproduction over three generations. Theriogenology. 2001;**55**:131-150. DOI: 10.1016/S0093-691X(00)00451-9

[68] Wright C, Evans AC, Evans NP, Duffy P, Fox J, Boland MP, Roche JF, Sweeney T. Effect of maternal exposure to the environmental estrogen, octylphenol, during fetal and/or postnatal life on onset of puberty, endocrine status, and ovarian follicular dynamics in ewe lambs. Biology of Reproduction. 2002;**67**:1734-1740. DOI: 10.1095/biolreprod.101.002006

[69] Slomczynska M, Knapczyk-Stwora K, Grzesiak M, Koziorowski M, Nowak S. Androgen and estrogen imbalance affects folliculogenesis in the neonatal porcine ovary influencing cell proliferation and apoptosis. In: Abstracts from the translational reproductive biology and clinical reproductive endocrinology conference held November 17-20, 2016. Journal of Assisted Reproduction and Genetics. 2016;**33**:1693-1708. DOI: 10.1007/s10815-016-0827-9

[70] Vandenberg LN, Hauser R, Marcus M, Olea N, Welshons WV. Human exposure to bisphenol A (BPA). Reproductive Toxicology. 2007;**24**:139-177. DOI: 10.1016/j.reprotox.2007.07.010

[71] Zhou C, Wang W, Peretz J, Flaws JA. Bisphenol A exposure inhibits germ cell nest breakdown by reducing apoptosis in cultured neonatal mouse ovaries. Reproductive Toxicology. 2015;**57**:87-99. DOI: 10.1016/j.reprotox.2015.05.012

[72] Suzuki A, Sugihara A, Uchida K, Sato T, Ohta Y, Katsu Y, Watanabe H, Iguchi T. Developmental effects of perinatal exposure to bisphenol-A and diethylstilbestrol on reproductive organs in female mice. Reproductive Toxicology. 2002;**16**:107-116. DOI: 10.1016/S0890-6238(02)00005-9

[73] Otsuka F, Shimasaki S. A negative feedback system between oocyte bone morphogenetic protein 15 and granulosa cell kit ligand: Its role in regulating granulosa cell mitosis. Proceedings of the National Academy of Sciences of the United States of America. 2002;**99**:8060-8065. DOI: 10.1073/pnas.122066899

[74] Hutt KJ, McLaughlin EA, Holland MK. Kit ligand and c-Kit have diverse roles during mammalian oogenesis and folliculogenesis. Molecular Human Reproduction. 2006;**12**:61–69. DOI: 10.1093/molehr/gal010

[75] Rodríguez HA, Santambrosio N, Santamaría CG, Muñoz-de-Toro M, Luque EH. Neonatal exposure to bisphenol A reduces the pool of primordial follicles in the rat ovary. Reproductive Toxicology. 2010;**30**:550-557. DOI: 10.1016/j.reprotox.2010.07.008

[76] Zhang HQ, Zhang XF, Zhang LJ, Chao HH, Pan B, Feng YM, Li L, Sun XF, Shen W. Fetal exposure to bisphenol A affects the primordial follicle formation by inhibiting the meiotic progression of oocytes. Molecular Biology Reports. 2012;**39**:5651-5657. DOI: 10.1007/s11033-011-1372-3

[77] Fernández M, Bourguignon N, Lux-Lantos V, Libertun C. Neonatal exposure to bisphenol a and reproductive and endocrine alterations resembling the polycystic ovarian

syndrome in adult rats. Environmental Health Perspectives. 2010;**118**:1217-1222. DOI: 10.1289/ehp.0901257

[78] Kim H, Nakajima T, Hayashi S, Chambon P, Watanabe H, Iguchi T, Sato T. Effects of diethylstilbestrol on programmed oocyte death and induction of polyovular follicles in neonatal mouse ovaries. Biology of Reproduction. 2009;**81**:1002-1009. DOI: 10.1095/biolreprod.108.070599

[79] Alwis ID, Maroni DM, Hendry IR, Roy SK, May JV, Leavitt WW, Hendry WJ. Neonatal diethylstilbestrol exposure disrupts female reproductive tract structure/function via both direct and indirect mechanisms in the hamster. Reproductive Toxicology. 2011;**32**:472-483. DOI: 10.1016/j.reprotox.2011.09.006

[80] Karavan JR, Pepling ME. Effects of estrogenic compounds on neonatal oocyte development. Reproductive Toxicology. 2012;**34**:51-56. DOI: 10.1016/j.reprotox.2012.02.005

[81] Rivera OE, Varayoud J, Rodríguez HA, Muñoz-de-Toro M, Luque EH. Neonatal exposure to bisphenol A or diethylstilbestrol alters the ovarian follicular dynamics in the lamb. Reproductive Toxicology. 2011;**32**:304-312. DOI: 10.1016/j.reprotox.2011.06.118

[82] Jefferson W, Newbold R, Padilla-Banks E, Pepling M. Neonatal genistein treatment alters ovarian differentiation in the mouse: Inhibition of oocyte nest breakdown and increased oocyte survival. Biology of Reproduction. 2006;**74**:161-168. DOI: 10.1095/biolreprod.105.045724

[83] Jefferson WN, Doerge D, Padilla-Banks E, Woodling KA, Kissling GE, Newbold R. Oral exposure to genistin, the glycosylated form of genistein, during neonatal life adversely affects the female reproductive system. Environmental Health Perspectives. 2009;**117**:1883-1889. DOI: 10.1289/ehp.0900923

[84] Zhang T, Li L, Qin XS, Zhou Y, Zhang XF, Wang LQ, De Felici M, Chen H, Qin GQ, Shen W. Di-(2-ethylhexyl)phthalate and bisphenol A exposure impairs mouse primordial follicle assembly in vitro. Environmental and Molecular Mutagenesis. 2014;**55**:343-353. DOI: 10.1002/em.21847

[85] Zhang XF, Zhang LJ, Li L, Feng YN, Chen B, Ma JM, Huynh E, Shi QH, De Felici M, Shen W. Diethylhexyl phthalate exposure impairs follicular development and affects oocyte maturation in the mouse. Environmental and Molecular Mutagenesis. 2013;**54**:354-361. DOI: 10.1002/em.21776

[86] Wakeling AE, Dukes M, Bowler J. A potent specific pure antiestrogen with clinical potential. Cancer Research. 1991;**51**:3867-3873

[87] Chen Y, Breen K, Pepling ME. Estrogen can signal through multiple pathways to regulate oocyte cyst breakdown and primordial follicle assembly in the neonatal mouse ovary. Journal of Endocrinology. 2009;**202**:407-417. DOI: 10.1677/JOE-09-0109

[88] Ahn HJ, An BS, Jung EM, Yang H, Choi KC, Jeung EB. Parabens inhibit the early phase of folliculogenesis and steroidogenesis in the ovaries of neonatal rats. Molecular Reproduction and Development. 2012;**79**:626-636. DOI: 10.1002/mrd.22070

[89] Patel S, Zhou C, Rattan S, Flaws JA. Effects of endocrine-disrupting chemicals on the ovary. Biology of Reproduction. 2015;**93**:1-9. DOI: 10.1095/biolreprod.115.130336

[90] Gaido KW, Maness SC, McDonnell DP, Dehal SS, Kupfer D, Safe S. Interaction of methoxychlor and related compounds with estrogen receptor α and β, and androgen receptor: Structure-activity studies. Molecular Pharmacology. 2000;**58**:852-858. DOI: 10.1124/mol.58.4.852

[91] Uzumcu M, Kuhn PE, Marano JE, Armenti AE, Passantino L. Early postnatal methoxychlor exposure inhibits folliculogenesis and stimulates anti-Mullerian hormone production in the rat ovary. Journal of Endocrinology. 2006;**191**:549-558. DOI: 10.1677/joe.1.06592

[92] Armenti AE, Zama AM, Passantino L, Uzumcu M. Developmental methoxychlor exposure affects multiple reproductive parameters and ovarian folliculogenesis and gene expression in adult rats. Toxicology and Applied Pharmacology. 2008;**233**:286-296. DOI: 10.1016/j.taap.2008.09.010

[93] Zama AM, Uzumcu M. Fetal and neonatal exposure to the endocrine disruptor methoxychlor causes epigenetic alterations in adult ovarian genes. Endocrinology. 2009;**150**:4681-4691. DOI: 10.1210/en.2009–0499

13

Pre- and Postnatal Surgery, Most Common Conditions, Diagnosis and Treatment

Carlos Baeza Herrera, Alin Villalobos Castillejos and Ricardo Cortés García

Abstract

The authors make a general but relevant description of the most common surgical problems occurring both in the human being that develops in the uterus and in the one that has already been born.

Keywords: prenatal surgery, postnatal surgery

1. Introduction

Congenital malformations, apart from the achievements in the prenatal care of women with high-risk pregnancies, are still a subject of great importance in our country. As Mexico is a developing country, due to various factors, an expeditious attention to newborns with malformations has not been achieved. An additional issue that affects the treatment of these children is the alarming increase in the prevalence of structural anomalies. Health statistics indicate that the birth rate is among the world's highest, which means that sometimes the state is incapable of providing the required assistance. Socioeconomic and educational factors are among those that have contributed to the increase in congenital malformations in the past 10 years, and the desired rate of recovery of these children has not been reached. Because of the above situation, specialists have had to refine their skills in elaborating the clinical diagnosis and instituting the appropriate therapeutic measures. In Mexico, neonatal surgery has become a specialty recognized by general pediatric surgery and by the Autonomous National University (UNAM).

2. Prenatal

Maternal-fetal medicine and intrauterine intervention in defects of the fetus, or unborn child, emerged and has evolved as a result of the technical advancements in medicine. The scope of these specialties is encouraging and promises advanced interventions with improved results. The refinement of ultrasound has made a great contribution to the field [1]. The use of ultrasound to visualize the fetus in its environment created a great interest to be able to identify malformations that could be corrected through intrauterine intervention. The most important antecedents of fetal surgery date back to the early 1960s, when Liley devised a technique for fetal transfusion [2]. In 1965, Adamson reported the first fetal surgery in humans, using a hysterotomy [3]. In this research line, experiments were carried out on lamb and monkey fetuses to perfect instruments and techniques, evaluate the results in these models and study their feasibility and reproducibility in humans.

The modern history of fetal surgery began at the University of California, San Francisco, with Michael Harrison. He first conceived his interest in intrauterine intervention for the treatment of congenital diaphragmatic hernia when he was an intern at Massachusetts General Hospital. Harrison's work continues today and is a valuable resource in the field [1–3]. In 1982, Harrison noted that diaphragmatic hernia, congenital hydronephrosis and hydrocephalus were defects which could be susceptible to prenatal treatment, as they were simple structural defects that prevented the normal fetal development of the structures involved. In that same year, the first open fetal surgery was performed at 21 weeks of gestation on a fetus with congenital hydronephrosis, which consisted of performing a hysterotomy to expose the lower abdomen of the fetus and place a double pigtail catheter to communicate the bladder with the amniotic cavity to promote the free flow of urine, thus relieving the obstruction causing the hydronephrosis [4]. The intervention was successful, and pregnancy continued for 14 weeks after intervention; however, at birth, the kidneys already showed irreversible damage, and it was clear that intervention had to be at an earlier stage of intrauterine life [5].

Neonatal surgery was not well known as a separate specialty of general pediatric surgery but has a history dating back to 1955 when P. Rickham, a pediatric surgeon from Switzerland, started a newborn surgery program in the city of Liverpool. Rickham's program began the systematization of neonatal care, especially for congenital anomalies. It was to be hoped that, having established a program of neonatal surgery, it would be recognized as a specialty. In spite of his prestige and worldwide fame, the specialty was not yet established. He published two editions of his classic book Neonatal Surgery, where in addition to the classically studied congenital defects, he narrated his experience operating on children with neurological conditions such as congenital hydrocephalus associated, or not, with pituitary-spinal malformations and musculoskeletal disorders such as club foot.

Neonatal surgery in the last third of the twentieth century has made remarkable advances in diagnostic resources. Postoperative management development has been especially important, with the implementation of ventilators and intravenous nutrition. In Mexico (specifically in the unit where the authors work), after years of managing hundreds of malformed newborns, a successful postgraduate project in neonatal surgery has been developed at the Universidad Nacional Autónoma de México, which is already being replicated in other institutions in Mexico and other Latin American countries.

2.1. Obstructive uropathy

Congenital hydronephrosis was the first condition to attract attention within the scope of prenatal interventions, especially in bladder outlet obstructions due to urethral valves [4]. Congenital obstruction of the lower urinary tract (bladder neck) comprises a set of conditions of which atresias and posterior urethral valve obstructions are representative. With an approximate incidence of 2.2 per 10,000 live births, it results in oligohydramnios, pulmonary hypoplasia and irreparable renal damage, with 45% mortality. The role of prenatal obstetric ultrasound is crucial as the defect can be detected in 85% of the cases. Ultrasonographic features suggestive of lower urinary tract obstruction are an enlarged fetal bladder and dilated proximal urethra with or without associated hydronephrosis. It has been observed that when the anomaly is present before 25 weeks of gestation and secondary oligohydramnios prevails for more than 14 days, this malformation is associated with neonatal mortality > 90%. The canalicular phase of lung development, crucial to the development of the human lung, occurs during 14–25 weeks of gestation. Morris et al. demonstrated that prenatal intervention to treat bladder obstruction by hydronephrosis using percutaneous or open bladder shunt by a vesico-amniotic shunt increases overall survival in neonates affected by this abnormality, however, the studies published in this regard are few [6].

2.2. Sacrococcygeal teratoma

Sacrococcygeal teratoma is the most common tumor in the newborn. This neoplasm arises between the base of the spine and the rectum and protrudes from inside of the pelvis outwards. The tumor is more frequent in females than in males (3:1), with an incidence of 1 per 40,000 births. The presentation may be grossly frank and is seen at birth. Type 1 has the best prognosis, as the tumor is predominantly external with a small pre-sacral component (**Figure 1**). The tumor corresponding to type 4 is invasive, deforming the pelvis and part of the abdomen. The risk of malignancy depends on two factors: the site and extent of the tumor and age at the time of diagnosis. The prenatal appearance of the sacrococcygeal teratoma on ultrasound is of a mixed solid lesion with a cystic component that arises from the sacrum, with hyperechogenic zones corresponding to calcifications. Recently, ultrafast fetal nuclear magnetic resonance imaging has been used to assess the vascular component of these neoplasms, as there is risk of fetal intrauterine hemorrhage with secondary anemia, hemodynamic decompensation due to the formation of arteriovenous fistulas, hydramnios, hydrops fetalis, placentomegaly and eventually, in severe cases, intrauterine death. The effect of the mass of a sacrococcygeal teratoma has been related to uterine distension, dystocia and tumor rupture at birth, as well as causing mirror syndrome and severe hypertensive states.

The hemodynamic effect of the coccygeal sacrum tumor can be evaluated with echocardiographic study, measuring the relationship between ventricular outflow and the diameter of the vena cava, descending aorta and umbilical vein. A poor prognosis is related to

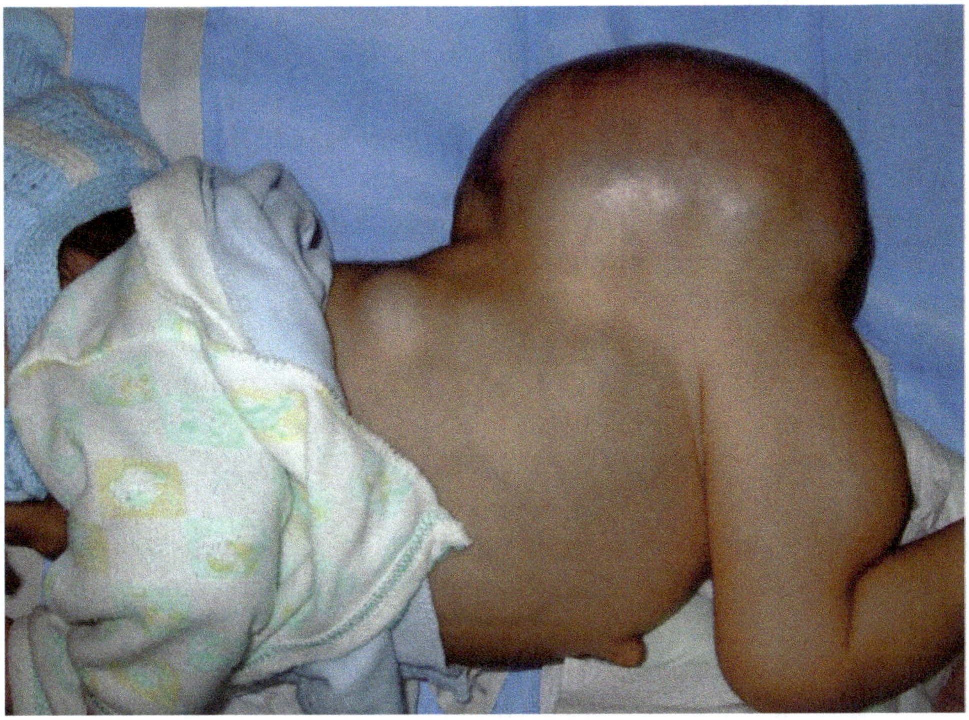

Figure 1. A giant sacrococcygeal teratoma in a newborn patient.

disproportionate tumor size (more than 150 cm per week is a very poor prognosis), high vascularity, predominantly solid component, placentomegaly, heart failure and concomitant maternal complications. The main objective of prenatal care is to identify the most reliable predictor of poor prognosis in fetuses with sacrococcygeal teratoma. The gestational age at the time of decompensation will determine the type of intervention; if it occurs after the 27th or 28th week of gestation, an emergency cesarean section or EXIT procedure (ex utero intrapartum treatment) will be chosen. If the hemodynamic imbalance is identified before week 27 in the cases of teratoma classes 1 and 2, open maternal-fetal surgery and partial resection of the tumor followed by definitive surgical intervention at birth should be chosen. There are other procedures that consist of disrupting tumor vascularity with dissimilar results, such as thermoregulation, radiofrequency ablation, alcohol sclerosis or laser ablation. The complications or side effects of these methods can result in extensive pelvic muscle damage, hemorrhage, nerve injury and hip dislocation [7].

2.3. Myelomeningocele

Within the congenital anomalies of the central nervous system, myelomeningocele is the most common variety of spina bifida and consists of the extrusion of the spinal tissue into a sac (meninges) occupied by cerebrospinal fluid. Its frequency is about 3.4 per 10,000 live births. Mortality is 10%, and survivors show varying degrees of disability depending on the height of the neural damage, including paralysis of the lower extremities and bladder and bowel dysfunction. In addition to exhibiting the anatomical neurological abnormalities characteristic of

Arnold-Chiari malformation.This anomaly is a generally congenital disease, consisting of an anatomical alteration of the base of the skull, which produces herniation of the cerebellum and brainstem through the foramen magnum to the cervical canal. This anomaly ultimately causes abnormal circulation of cerebrospinal fluid, culminating with hydrocephalus, central apnea, stridor and swallowing disorders. The embryonic pathophysiology of the defect is due to the combination of two strands or the two-hit model. The first effect consists of failure in the formation and closure of the neural tube, with an open defect, which exposes the neural elements to amniotic fluid (the second effect). It is important to note that in experimental models with fetal lambs, where an open neural defect was created and immediately surgically covered, effects on the lower extremities and on urinary continence and bowel movements were not observed. On the other hand, fetuses of lambs who underwent surgical repair of the myelomeningocele after 4 weeks of having experimentally created the defect showed good outcome after fetal intervention, urinary continence was maintained and preserved the neuromuscular function of their limbs, Which supports the hypothesis that prenatal intervention prevents neurological and associated confusion. Adzick in 2011 in a randomized clinical trial [8].

2.4. Pulmonary cystic adenomatoid malformation

Congenital pulmonary malformations have been divided for their study into those related to the bronchial tree: agenesis, aplasia and pulmonary hypoplasia and those of pulmonary parenchyma: congenital lung cystic adenomatoid disease, pulmonary sequestration, lobar emphysema and bronchogenic cyst. The high definition and quality provided by current sonographic studies have achieved better prenatal identification of the fetal lung lesions in the majority of cases detected on routine ultrasound between 18 and 20 weeks of gestation. These malformations have an incidence from 1 per 10,000 to 1 per 35,000 pregnancies. Sonographic study provides information on variables such as volume, location, arterial blood supply and venous drainage and consistency of the adenomatoid malformation, which can vary widely from solid (microcystic) to frankly cystic (macrocystic) [7].

Adenomatoid malformation, consisting of small cysts, generally grows unpredictably and causes compression on surrounding structures, as well as an effect of mass on the mediastinum, esophagus and lungs, causing pulmonary hypoplasia, obstruction of the vena cava, cardiac insufficiency, hydrops fetalis and polyhydramnios. As one method to identify serious cases, several investigators have proposed predictive indices and measures such as the cystic volume ratio (CVR), obtained by dividing the volume of the cystic lesion (length X width X height X 0.52) by the circumference of the head. In a retrospective study by Crombleholme, it was concluded that a CVR greater than 1.6 was associated with a 75% chance of developing hydrops fetalis, which justified prenatal intervention [7, 9]. In cases with a better prognosis, EXIT therapy is recommended, with resection of the mass before birth. Postnatal stabilization and thoracotomy are also acceptable. Macrocystic lesions may be prenatally decompressed by thoracentesis with a single needle or with drainage guided by amniotic thoracic ultrasound. At this time, microcystic lesions are not candidates for drainage and will require fetal surgery [10].

3. Postnatal

3.1. Esophageal atresia

Esophageal atresia is one of the most common congenital malformations and perhaps the most classic of structural abnormalities that exclusively involve the pediatric surgeon, as only a specialist can resolve the problem. Other specialists such as the urologist usually operate on an undescended testicle and a general surgeon on a pyloric stenosis, but even a thoracic surgeon would not attempt to correct an esophageal atresia. The frequency of the anomaly is one case per 3000 to 5000 births, predominately in males, and the prevalence may depend on the region or country being analyzed. How esophageal atresia occurs is unknown, but there are many theories, none of which has withstood the test of time. Esophageal atresia is usually accompanied by other defects, so acrostics are formed to list the components such as VACTERL, for vertebral, anorectal, cardiac, tracheo-esophageal, esophageal, renal and limb anomalies [11]. At times, it is sporadically associated with other defects of the digestive tract, such as duodenal atresia. In Mexico, the frequency measured in cases per year is between 12 and 16 cases a year in regional and specialty hospitals. The Moctezuma Pediatric Hospital, a specialty hospital of the Secretary of Health of Mexico City, sees the most cases per year [12].

3.1.1. Diagnosis

No specific biological teratogen is known, but the anomaly may be produced by the experimental administration of Adriamycin. More often than not, it is a sporadic malformation that does not obey genetic or hereditary patterns, although it is usually accompanied by trisomies such as 13 and 18 or those associated, without the atresia being the axis of clinical expression. It usually occurs in the products of conception of young women. Polyhydramnios can be found during the prenatal visit, which should be the most important warning sign [13, 14]. In pediatric surgery, it is said that sialorrhea in the newborn child is equivalent to an esophageal atresia until proven otherwise. If this is accompanied by cyanosis and asphyxia during feeding, the diagnosis is confirmed. Although it should be noted that it is currently the obligation of the obstetrician in the delivery room to make the clinical diagnosis of suspicion. In other words, waiting for the child to choke on ingested milk signifies malpractice and tardiness to integrate the diagnostic impression.

The routine introduction of a nelaton catheter into the stomach is a maneuver that should be performed in every delivery room. It is the most effective, advisable and efficient way for a child with esophageal atresia to achieve a good condition without additional risk during intervention. With the diagnosis confirmed, the next step is to inject 0.5 ml of water-soluble contrast medium for radiological study (**Figure 2**), which, in addition to highlighting the height of the atresia, will demonstrate a proximal fistula if it exists and for which a surgical procedure would be indicated [13]. When the defect is detected, a probe must be left in the proximal pouch so the saliva is prevented from spilling over into the respiratory tract. The tube should be constructed as a trap so as to provide continuous suction without pinching the esophageal mucosa and avoid blockage. This is achieved by introducing a thin probe through the counter-aperture in the middle third of a larger probe. The thicker probe should be very close to the bottom of the pouch, and the thinner probe will serve to continuously instill saline solution to keep the system efficient.

From the clinical point of view, esophageal atresia has been divided into four varieties and classified into letters or numbers. The system with letters is the most used: type A, two blind pouches, but no fistula; type B, two segments with the upper one connected to the airway; type C, two segments with the distal esophagus in the airway; and type D, both segments that contain a fistulous path. Radiological studies, in addition to revealing the aforementioned findings, may show a cardiac silhouette that suggests right aortic arch cardiopathy, as the presence of some skeletal malformations such as hemi-vertebra or spina bifida can be detected. The prognosis may be definitive when an area of pulmonary consolidation is identified. The presence of air in the digestive tract indicates the existence of the most frequent variety, an atresia type C or D. The absence of air in the digestive tract identifies variety A or B. Once the diagnosis has been confirmed, studies to reduce the risk to the child should be made. Thus, when a condition that has a high risk for esophageal atresia is detected, such as hydrocephalus or obstruction of the urinary tract, it should be given priority [15].

3.1.2. Treatment

The management of esophageal atresia requires zeal and closeness to the patient as with few other anomalies. In no other condition is it so important for the pediatric surgeon to be aware that the suction device works and the child's vital signs and laboratory values have been restored. Antibiotics are essential. In ideal conditions, an end-to-end esophageal anastomosis

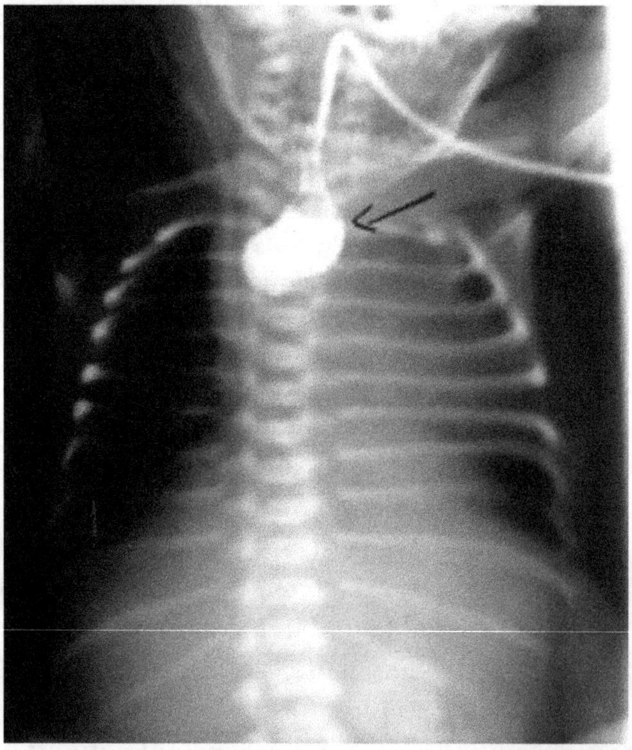

Figure 2. Simple thoracic X-ray, revealing the fundus of the proximal sac contrasted with a water-soluble medium. This is an esophageal atresia type A.

should be performed by right thoracotomy, regardless of whether it is in one or more anatomical planes. It is important that it is done with fine, inert material and the placement of the stitches is firm and their number and location are correct. Ideally, it should be done outside the pleural space, but if it is not feasible, a pleural tube should be placed and removed on the day of the esophagogram to prove that there is no dehiscence and/or refistulization. In approximately a week, they may begin oral feeding; meanwhile, they must be maintained intravenously.

Prognostic criteria can identify those who are included in the favorable group and those who will survive. The best-known criteria have to do with the weight of the product of conception, the presence of other malformations and if bronchial aspiration pneumonia is present. Based on these criteria, those classified as risk type A are those weighing more than 2500 grams, lacking significant malformations and without pneumonia, and more than 90% of these cases survive. Mortality is 50% or more in the opposite, high-risk conditions. Complications, which can be classified as immediate and mediate, are frequent. In the former, it is the dehiscence of the anastomosis, which always has a reserved prognosis, and during late onset, it is the pathological gastro-esophageal reflux [15].

3.2. Duodenal atresia

Atresia of the duodenum is the congenital obliteration of any portion of the small intestine, which lies between the most distal pylorus and the most proximal part of the ligament of Treitz. This is a very common malformation and almost a permanent occupant of neonatal intensive care units, as one case appears for every three to five thousand births [16]. It almost always appears as a sporadic condition but may be part of some chromosomopathies such as trisomy 21. It has been assumed that it appears between 5 and 12 weeks of gestation. The most accepted theory is that of Tandler. Known as recanalization, it consists of the appearance of the concentric histolysis phenomena due to the invasion of vacuoles into the solid cord, an essential characteristic of the duodenum in the embryonic stage, to the degree that the invasion converts the cord in its definitive form, into a tube [17]. Other theories, such as ischemia may have a basis, especially in segment atresia accompanied by a loss of duodenal continuity with or without intermediate fibrous cord.

Anatomically, duodenal atresia has been divided into two forms: the proximal and distal to the ampulla of Vater and divided into three forms clinically—when it appears as a septum or as "wind sock," when there is an interruption of continuity and when these segments are joined by a thin fibrous cord. Regarding the wind sock variety, it should be emphasized that duodenal blockage does not appear at the transition site of the dilated proximal segment and the thin distal segment but that the membrane always emerges a few millimeters above the narrow area.

3.2.1. Diagnosis

Duodenal atresia usually appears early in pregnancy, accompanied by polyhydramnios. When performing sonographic screenings in prenatal consultation, the presence of polyhydramnios should alert the specialist to look for data suggesting blockage of the digestive tract, such as atresia of the duodenum or of other distal structures. Once the product has been born, the correlation can be made by gastric lavage with a catheter as a routine measure and obtaining 20–25 ml of transparent or biliary fluid, which indirectly evidences alterations in the dynamics of the movement of amniotic fluid. If the mongoloid facies resulting from trisomy is added as relevant data, the suspicion of a duodenal block is strengthened. On inspection, there is an increase in volume of the upper abdomen, the skin is taut and shiny and there is early vomiting. Depending on the level of the blockage, the expelled liquid will be yellow, thick and abundant if the blockage is below the ampulla of Vater and the vomitus will be transparent if the obstruction is proximal to the main bile duct outlet. Due to alterations in the enterohepatic circulation, this anomaly is almost always accompanied by jaundice, which disappears as soon as the problem is resolved through surgical intervention. If several days elapse before identifying the anomaly, from the clinical viewpoint, there are usually hydroelectrolytic alterations, exacerbation of jaundice and signs of a systemic inflammatory response. Regarding radiology, simple radiography of the abdomen in an upright position is sufficient, as air is the best contrast medium in those cases. When children have a tube inserted in the stomach, 15–20 ml of air should be injected at the time of the study in order to maintain the contrast. Observing the image of the "double bubble" (**Figure 3**), it is a certainty that the duodenum is totally or partially blocked, and there is a presupposition of the existence of defects such as annular pancreas, malrotation, presence of a narrow angle mesenteric artery and the preduodenal portal vein. However, the presence of the facies, umbilical hernia and macroglossia are usually diagnostically determinant factors so that before the surgical intervention, with a good degree of certainty, it is assumed that the baby suffers from duodenal atresia. No endoscopy or introduction of liquid contrast material is necessary.

3.2.2. Treatment

In our country, this type of patient usually arrives in a serious condition. Vomiting is early, and in less than 24 h, there is an important loss of fluids and electrolytes, so the patient must be immediately transferred to an intensive care unit, where a gastric tube must be installed to allow the exit of all the liquid that is lodged in the stomach in utero, a quantity much superior to the normal gastric capacity. Antibiotics should always be used, as there is often respiratory infection aggravated by microaspirations. Once the gastric tube has been installed and the patients' condition improved, the patient must be transferred to the operating room where, depending on the findings, the intervention of choice will be instituted. If confronted with an atresia without loss of duodenal continuity (variety I), a slight concentric depression should be located on the surface of the duodenum. That indicates the point where the obstructive diaphragm is inserted. Once this reference is placed, a horizontal incision is made on the depression, the septum is removed, the mucosa is sutured with a continuous line of absorbable fine material and the duodenal wall is repaired vertically. This method is known as the Heinecke-Mikulicz technique. If, on the contrary, atresia shows separation of segments, then it must be resolved through two types of access: through a minimally invasive procedure consisting of the introduction of very thin laparoscopy tubes and laparotomy [17]. In both methods, the surgical technique will be the duodenal-duodenal diamond-shaped anastomosis, proposed by Kimura et al. [18], which consists of joining both blind segments, making a horizontal incision in the proximal and a vertical one in the distal so that when anastomosis is terminated, intercommunication is wide enough for the intestinal flow.

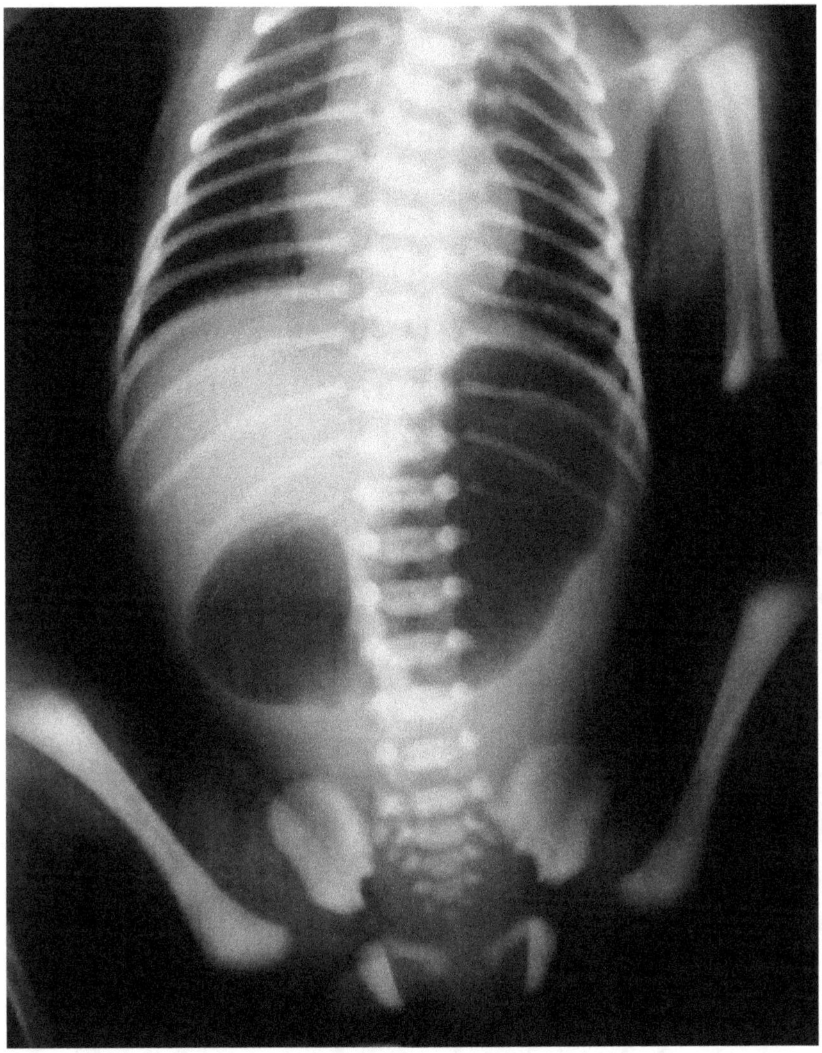

Figure 3. Simple abdomino-thoracic radiological study showing great gastric dilation and obstruction of the second portion of the duodenum.

The original report of the diamond anastomosis technique says that the oral feeding route in the postoperative period could be initiated in the first 5–7 days; however, in our experience [19], the waiting period for tolerance of fluid intake can be extended up to 4 weeks, which means that those children must undergo intravenous nutrition for at least 15 days. We believe that duodenal dilatation resulting from the receipt of large amounts of fluid results in alterations in emptying movements, which is corrected spontaneously but later in postnatal life. An additional problem is that these infants suffer from recurrent nosocomial infections due to their prolonged hospital stay and the use of a catheter, which makes their recovery more difficult. Management also includes a gastric probe that protects the anastomosis, the use of antimicrobials and analgesics.

3.3. Jejunoileal atresia

The small intestine is a complex and vital organ. Jejunoileal atresia accounts for almost one-third of all cases of intestinal obstruction in the neonatal period.

The pathogenesis of jejunoileal atresia is still controversial. In the middle of the last century, it was proposed that the atresia was due to a failure in recanalization; however, Louw and Barnard, through experimental studies, showed that this anomaly occurs as a consequence of an ischemic phenomenon that culminates with segments of mesenteric ischemia and in atresia. Subsequently it was shown that abdominal catastrophic events in utero were responsible and that the most common conditions were invagination, perforation, volvulus, strangulation by an internal hernia or thromboembolism. The spectrum of atresia depends on the extent, severity and duration of the ischemia, since the mucosa and submucosa are more susceptible. An incidence from 1 to 5 per 10,000 live births has been estimated. It affects both sexes equally. It affects both the jejunum and the ileum similarly. Compared to duodenal atresia, associated anomalies are less frequent. Multiple intestinal atresias can be an autosomal recessive disorder, more commonly seen in combination with some degree of immunodeficiency and in Canadians. Mutations have been observed in the TTC7A protein, important for the development and function of the intestinal epithelium. This mutation has also been associated with early presentation of inflammatory bowel disease [20].

Based on their anatomical characteristics, four types of atresias have been described. Type I is an intramural membrane of mucosa and submucosa that is continued with a cord, with no mesenteric defect. In Type II, there is intestinal discontinuity but no mesenteric defect. Type III has two subtypes; in suwbtype IIIA, continuity of the intestine is interrupted and there is also a V-shaped defect of the mesentery. In subtype IIIB, there is a lack of continuity of the intestine and it is wrapped around the superior mesenteric artery, giving the appearance of a Christmas tree or apple peel. Type IV consists of a segment with multiple atresias that resemble a string of sausages. We have designated a type V, which consists of a combination of atresias types I, II and IIIA present in the same intestinal segment [21].

3.3.1. Diagnosis

The typical presentation is that of a newborn on the first or second day of life with biliary vomiting, a history of polyhydramnios and abdominal distension, which will be more severe the more distal the obstruction. The most serious form of presentation is intestinal perforation. The diagnosis can be made prenatally through the use of ultrasonography. Findings suggesting atresia, in nearly one-third of cases, include dilated bowel and polyhydramnios. If there is strong suspicion, fetal magnetic resonance usually determines the diagnosis. Once the product of conception is born and suspected, simple vertical and horizontal x-rays of the abdomen should be taken. When a jejunal atresia is present, X-ray will show multiple hydroaerial levels (**Figure 4**) and the "triple bubble" sign. The presence of calcifications suggests the catastrophe and may be present in about 12% of cases. In that scenario, confirmation of atresia is obtained by colonic enema, when a microcolon is observed [21, 22].

3.3.2. Treatment

Once the diagnosis has been made, a gastric tube is placed to empty the proximal digestive tract, the hydroelectrolytic alterations are corrected, antibiotic management is added and a central venous catheter is installed. The operation can be performed by an open or a laparoscopic approach, in order to resect the proximal atresic bulbous segment and perform a primary anastomosis with the distal segment. A precautionary transoperative routine measure is the instillation of saline solution to the distal intestine in order to rule out the presence of other obstacles [22, 23].

Mortality is related to prematurity, associated anomalies, infections and short bowel syndrome. Postoperative complications that may occur are leakage, stenosis of the anastomosis site and short bowel, if there was extensive bowel resection. Food intolerance may be a mediate complication. Success is rated by the time of initiation of enteral feeding, postsurgical complications and the duration of feeding with total parenteral nutrition. The prognosis of neonates with jejunoileal atresia is very good, with a survival rate greater than 90%.

3.4. Necrotizing enterocolitis

Necrotizing enterocolitis (NEC) is one of the leading causes of death of gastrointestinal origin in the preterm infant. It is a devastating disease, and at present, it can be considered as part of a spectrum of diseases acquired in the neonatal period characterized by necrosis of the ileum and/or colon. The incidence is 1–5 per 1000 newborns [24]. In multicenter studies, it has been

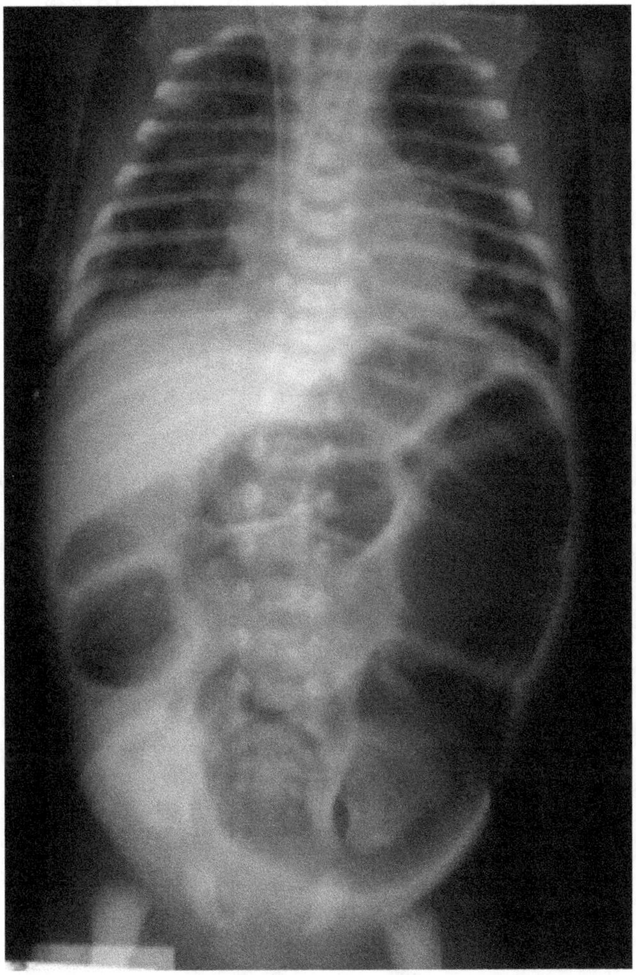

Figure 4. Simple abdomino-thoracic radiological study in horizontal position showing a great dilatation of the small intestine. Note the pelvic opacity.

estimated that NEC is present in 7–13% of neonates younger than 33 weeks of gestation and weighing less than 1000 g. Mortality is almost 50%, mainly in those requiring surgical treatment. The majority of cases occur in premature babies and a lower percentage in term births [24].

The intestinal epithelium of premature infants is predisposed to have an exaggerated inflammatory response to bacterial colonization, allowing destruction of the mucosa and damage to mesenteric perfusion. This inadequate inflammatory response triggers the emergence of TLR4 (toll-like receptor 4), a response receptor found in the premature gut epithelium that recognizes the lipopolysaccharides of membranes of Gram-negative bacteria. This regulation of the signaling pathway includes nuclear factor kappa beta 1 and IL-1 receptors. Other important risk factors that have been implicated in its development include intestinal immaturity, inadequate bacterial colonization of the intestine, asphyxia, anemia, presence of congenital defects such as gastroschisis and persistent ductus arteriosus, use of medications such as indomethacin, low birth weight, Apgar score of five or less, use of mechanical ventilation, feeding with milk formula and, more recently, the presence of an exaggerated inflammatory response [24, 25].

3.4.1. Diagnosis

The typical newborn with NEC is a premature infant who suddenly develops food intolerance, bloating, bloody stools and signs of sepsis (changes in heart rate, breathing, temperature and blood pressure). An important consideration in the diagnosis of NEC is gestational age and age of presentation. In other words, preterm infants born at 27 weeks of gestation are at greater risk, and symptoms occur at 4–5 weeks of life, compared to term infants. This may be because preterm infants have later colonization of the digestive tract, a prolonged hospital stay and have had broad-spectrum antibiotics used [25].

Bell's classification is widely used to classify the diseases: stage I is non-specific, and stage II is characterized by abdominal distension, wall edema, thrombocytopenia and metabolic acidosis. Radiologically intestinal and hepatic pneumatosis is usually observed. In stage III, signs and symptoms of stage II plus hypotension are present, signs of peritonitis, metabolic acidemia and shock are present. Radiologically, there is pneumoperitoneum (free air in the cavity) as an unequivocal sign of intestinal perforation (**Figure 5**) [25].

Currently, certain biomarkers have been valued in the diagnosis of NEC, which include C-reactive protein and pro-inflammatory cytokines (IL-6, IL-8, TNF-α). In addition, organ-specific markers can indicate damage to the enterocyte as proteins bound to intestinal fatty acids, hepatic, fecal calprotectin and claudin-3. It has been mentioned that the use of Doppler ultrasound is a useful tool to avoid unnecessary surgical operations, since it can verify perfusion of the intestinal wall and eventually identify necrotic intestinal segments before perforation occurs, a benefit that is not obtained with simple radiological studies [26].

3.4.2. Treatment

The initial treatment of patients with necrotizing enterocolitis includes fasting with gastric drainage, broad spectrum antibiotics, intravenous fluids according to the requirements and

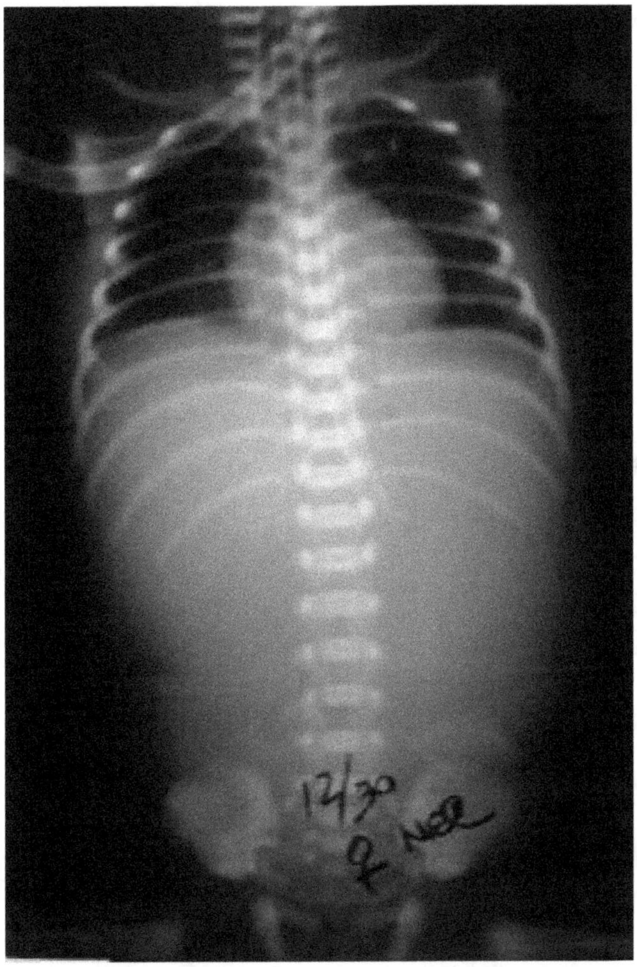

Figure 5. Abdomino-thoracic radiography with total abdominal opacity known as "frosted glass sign," showing enterocolitis in its extreme stage.

water balances, correction of metabolic alterations and adequate management of acid-base imbalances, and inotropic support will be used when there is Clear signs of hypoperfusion.Mortality may range from 15 to 63% according to the revised series. Surgery is necessary in more than 50% of the cases, and the objective is to result in the least mutilation possible. Peritoneal drainage without laparotomy may be sufficient and has been reserved almost exclusively for those infants weighing less than 750 g or in those with increased intra-abdominal pressure and compromised ventilation. A laparotomy will be required in 74% of cases. In a typical scenario, there are two alternatives, to perform a primary anastomosis or an enterostomy. In our experience, a primary anastomosis should be performed, particularly if the patient's condition is good and the extirpation of the diseased bowel was extensive (**Figure 6**).

The prognosis of children affected by NEC is characterized by a morbidity of 20–50%; but in developing countries, this percentage is higher, and recurrence after the first event (4–10%), retarded growth (10%), bowel stenosis, mainly of the colon (12–35%), short bowel syndrome (20–35%), neurodevelopmental disorders (30–50%) and stoma complications (50%) are emphasized. The mortality ranges from 15 to 63% according to the series studied [27].

3.5. Neonatal hirschsprung disease

Hirschsprung disease (HD) or congenital agangliosis is a disease of unknown origin, first described in 1888, but it took 60 years for researchers in the field to find the first surgical measure that was more or less effective. This condition is relatively frequent, with one case for every 5000 births and with greater prevalence in males. This abnormality is characterized by the absence of enteric ganglion cells in the distal portion of the colon and, depending on the level of arrest of the neuronal migration, it has been classified as classic, when the ganglionic absence reaches up to 80% in the rectosigmoids and 17% involving sigmoids, splenic angle and transverse colon. The long segment is all forms that go beyond the blind pouch, and total colonic agangliosis is called total agangliosis coli and that which extends from the pectinate line to the duodenum is very rare [28].

Normally, the enteric ganglion cells, which emerge from the neural crest, must innervate from proximal segments of the digestive tract to the terminal colon, and this phenomenon takes place between 5 and 12 weeks of gestation. These cells are responsible for the mobility, not only of the small intestine but also particularly of the colon, which when absent makes the propulsive movements ineffective and the distal intestine function as a deposit. Regarding the etiology and pathogenesis of the disease, many studies have been done; however, conclusions have not been clear. It has been assumed that it appears as a consequence of defects in differentiation due to environmental changes, but there are also studies suggesting that it occurs due to an ectopic expression of class II antigens [29]. Likewise, the influence that genes could have on the disease has been speculated, and it has been found that when the extension is greater,

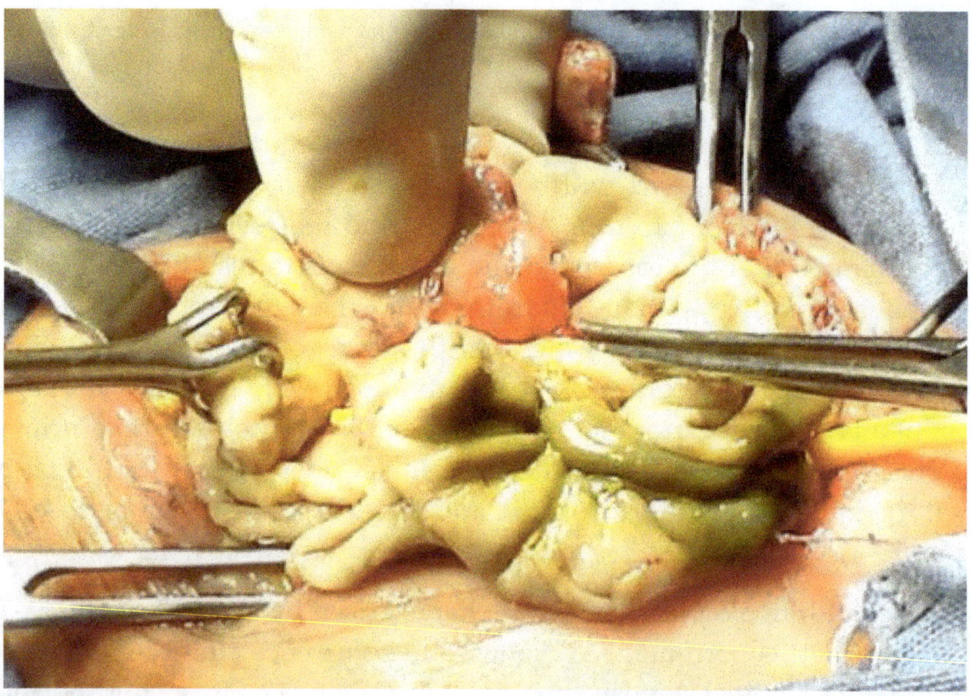

Figure 6. A transoperative image of the previous case. The contrast of the necrotic intestinal tissue with the normal appearance of the proximal (arrow).

the hereditary tendency increases. Thus, when agangliosis is total, the family tendency may be up to 50%, and if it is in the entire colon, the tendency descends to 15–21%. In relation to chromosomal phenomena, segregation studies have shown that Hirschsprung's disease is a genetic condition transmitted as autosomal dominant, autosomal recessive and polygenic forms. In one karyotype, an autosomal dominant gene was found to cause the disease in the chromosomes 10q11.2. [30]. At the experimental level, it has been found that agangliosis has been able to be reproduced in chicken embryos by extirpation of a segment of intestine, which stopped the neuronal migration [31]. In relation to genetic interference, it is known that the offspring of a woman suffering from the condition is 360 times more likely to transmit the disease than the normal population. The most important constant is that the greater the extension of the aganglionar segment, the greater the risk of inheriting the condition. The conditions that usually accompany HD are neonatal appendicitis [32] and those it shares embryological origin with, such as Wardenburg syndrome, neuroblastoma, pheochromocytoma and Ondine's disease.

3.5.1. Diagnosis

Although HD can occur in non-newborn infants [33], it usually manifests and is frequently identified in the first days of postnatal life. An antecedent of delay in the first meconium emission is useful information, a fact that is usually present in more than 90% of the cases. In the case of a neonate who emits his first evacuation after 48 h of postnatal life and with the passage of days suffers constipation, it must be assumed that the cause is congenital agangliosis. Vomiting and abdominal distention are also typical, causing discomfort that can be improved with the application of a suppository or a probe. After showing improvement, they relapse. They are only able to be well for a few days and then suffer from the same picture. There is usually diarrhea, which is almost unequivocally a manifestation of enterocolitis, the most frequent complication of the condition. Radiological study, according to the majority of the authors, is very useful in more than 80% of the cases. A vertical study is recommended, and several findings can be highly suggestive: hydroaerial levels, edema of the intestinal wall, total pelvic opacity and intestinal dilatation. With these data, the next step is to perform the colonic enema (**Figure 7**), which should be done with water-soluble material, without previous enemas and with the introduction of a nelaton tube no more than 1 cm deep and manually gently inject the contrast medium, while obtaining an x-ray in the lateral position. Images such as jagged rectal wall, a transition zone between a contracted narrow distal portion and a proximal dilatation are highly suggestive. A late study is very useful at 24–48 h. The golden rule for making the diagnosis is undoubtedly rectal biopsy. Performed during or prior to the operation, it will reveal the absence of ganglion cells. Manometry is often useful, especially in older children. One should be very careful to not transgress the normally aganglionar area (a distance from the pectinate line of 10 mm) when performing the biopsy as it leads to false-positive interpretation.

3.5.2. Treatment

Non-surgical management is important prior to any procedure, since some of the parameters of the metabolic state of the neonate must be restored. Once the diagnosis is established, a transrectal catheter should be introduced if the patient is very distended and uncomfortable.

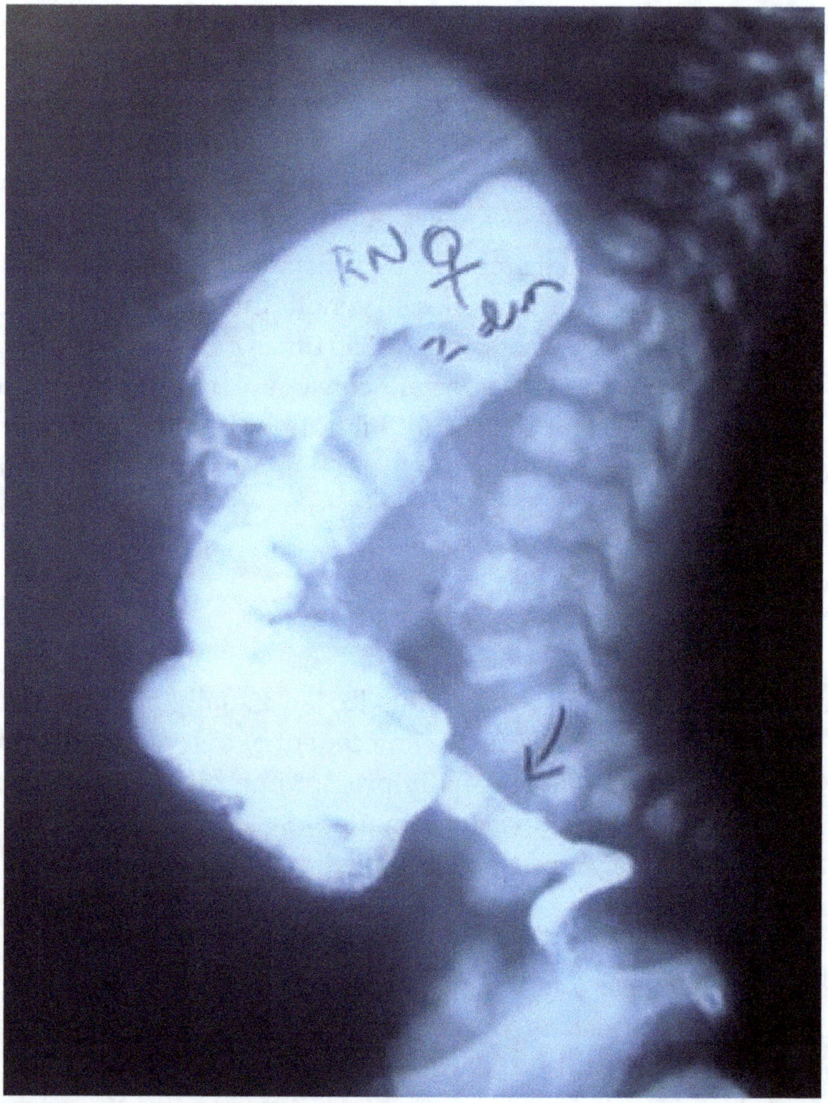

Figure 7. The colon shown by enema in lateral position. The spastic area is indicated by an arrow, which is equivalent to the aganglionic segment.

Antimicrobials are indicated as well as intravenous solutions suitable for the patient's age and condition. De la Torre and Ortega [34, 35] have proposed the surgical method of choice in these children, which should ideally be done during the first week of life and in a single operation, that is, without protective colostomy, in order to avoid the disadvantages of bacterial colonization. Unfortunately, this operation requires several requirements so that it can be implemented and three are the most important are to have a confirmed diagnosis within a few days of postnatal life, not to have an aganglionosis coli and to have a reliable pathologist, as much of the success of the procedure depends on them. It is widely demonstrated that at that age and with those requirements met, success is assured in more than 80% of the cases. The classic operations, Swenson, Duhamel and Soave, are left for later. The complications are diverse and include among the mediate complications, stenosis and fecal incontinence, and among the immediate ones, toxic enterocolitis, which is the one most responsible for death. It appears almost indistinctly as a violent infectious diarrheal syndrome, which immediately aggravates the condition of the baby, requiring a neonatal intensive care unit for correction, since the risk of death is very high.

3.6. Gastroschisis

Gastroschisis is a congenital defect of the abdominal wall consisting of evisceration of the midgut and other intra-abdominal organs, such as the stomach, through a small defect of 2–8 cm usually located to the right of the umbilical cord and in direct contact with the amniotic fluid, which gives them the characteristic serous aspect. It occurs between 5 and 10 weeks of gestation and can be identified in utero from week 20. The pathogenesis is still uncertain, with multiple theories. However, it is mentioned that it can be the result of a hemorrhage or thrombosis, which causes an alteration of the flow during the closing process of the wall, causing the exposure of the intra-abdominal organs. A significant increase in global prevalence has been observed in recent decades and ranges from 3 to 20 per 10,000 live births. This may be due to epigenetic changes [36, 37].

Multiple risk factors are mentioned: such as a mother younger than 20 years old or an adolescent, intake of certain medications such as acetylsalicylic acid, pseudoephedrine or ibuprofen, use of drugs, alcohol and tobacco, use of hormonal contraceptives, anemia, exposure to aromatic hydrocarbons, urinary tract infection and, in recent years, the intake of omega-6 fatty acids and alterations in lipid metabolism and pro-inflammatory cytokine substrates [38, 39].

Often the form of presentation of gastroschisis is sporadic and simple, that is, without major or minor malformations, but in a small percentage of cases, it may be part of other syndromes or chromosomal alterations, as well as other conditions such as skeletal dysplasias, Hirschsprung's disease, hydrocephalus and heart disease [40].

3.6.1. Diagnosis

Once the product is born, by either delivery or cesarean section, a preterm newborn between 35 and 37 weeks of gestation with low weight for gestational age is usually identified. In most cases, basic resuscitation is performed, and with respect to the local management of the defect, it is essential to immediately cover the exposed organs with a sterile, non-adherent, resistant, flexible and soft material to reduce loss of fluids and exposure of the peritoneal serosa to the environment. Avoid covering the exposed organs with gauze or compresses [41]. The most severe form of this malformation is a variety called "closed gastroschisis" (**Figure 8**), through the apparently integral abdominal wall, or with an millimetric orifice to the right of the umbilical cord, there is a black or green structure, turgid or fibrous, pediculate and mobile, of a soft consistency, 2–5 cm in length corresponding to the terminal ileum, cecum, cecal appendix and obliterated right colon. This segment is anchored to a fine fibrovascular network that, like a mesentery, keeps it irrigated. There is also intestinal malrotation and an umbilical membrane that is directed proximally toward a very dilated segment that sometimes ends in jejunal atresia variety IIIA. The other end of the digestive tract corresponds to the left colon, which is also obliterated. This occurs between 4.5 and 9% in cases of gastroschisis. There is always almost total absence of the jejunum and ileum [42]. Another variety is evanescent gut. In these cases, the gastroschisis is identified prenatally and at the moment of birth the abdominal wall is integrated; however, the patient presents intestinal occlusion data that requires an exploratory laparotomy that finds jejunal atresia with no more than 20 cm of small intestine and left colon. These children, in our experience, have a fatal outcome.

3.6.2. Treatment

It is important to initiate large amounts of intravenous fluids, electrolytes and antibiotics (**Figure 9**), place a 10–14 gauge Fr. orogastric probe, perform an evacuation enema with a warm solution at 10 ml/kg, avoid hypothermia, correct the acid-base state and, if necessary, provide ventilatory support. Regarding surgical treatment, there are two options: in the case of non-complex gastroschisis, the first alternative is umbilicoplasty, the introduction of exposed organs into the abdominal cavity without enlarging the defect, suturing the aponeurosis and skin and preserving the umbilical cord, preferably in the first 24 h of extrauterine life. We recommend that it should be attempted in all cases. However, success depends on whether there is viscero-abdominal disproportion, and therefore, it would not be possible to introduce all the intestinal loops or if there is compartmental syndrome. If so, a gradual, delayed closure is preferred between 6 and 10 days, covering it with a PVC membrane or a prefabricated silo. In a comparative study of the two surgical techniques, we found no difference, except that with umbilicoplasty, in-hospital stay time and that the days that the patients required mechanical ventilation and total parenteral nutrition were shorter than with delayed closure [6]. The complex varieties of gastroschisis always require a laparotomy, removal of the necrosed segment or atresia and a primary anastomosis between the residual and viable segments [42].

The prognosis in non-complex cases is generally good with a survival rate greater than 90%; however, in developing countries, mortality may be up to 60% of cases. The main complications are related to prematurity, sepsis, ischemia and intestinal perforation, renal insufficiency or multiple organ dysfunction as well as difficulties for enteral feeding. The prognosis in closed gastroschisis and evanescent intestine is fatal, and both varieties lead to short bowel syndrome, cholestasis, liver failure, sepsis and death.

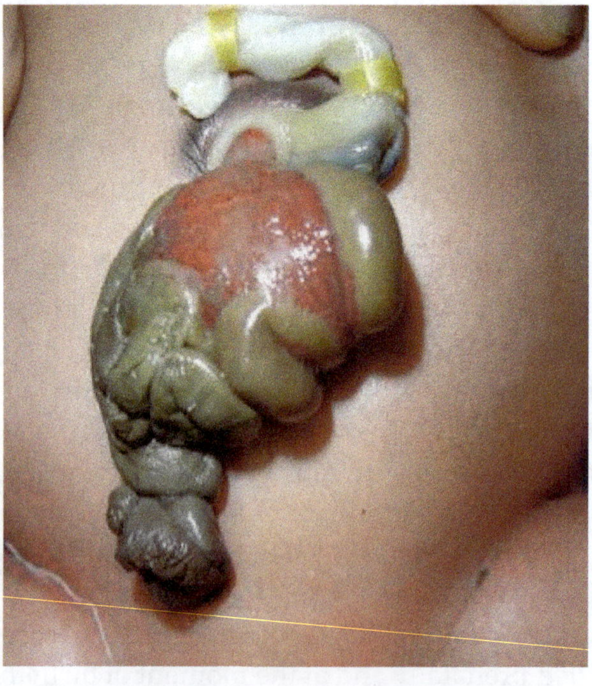

Figure 8. The clinical aspect of a "closed gastroschisis" in which should be noted the absence of parietal defect, necrosis of the middle intestine and normal aspect of the distal colon, what we call "Antenatal-Paraumbilical-Intestinal-Strangulation" (APIS).

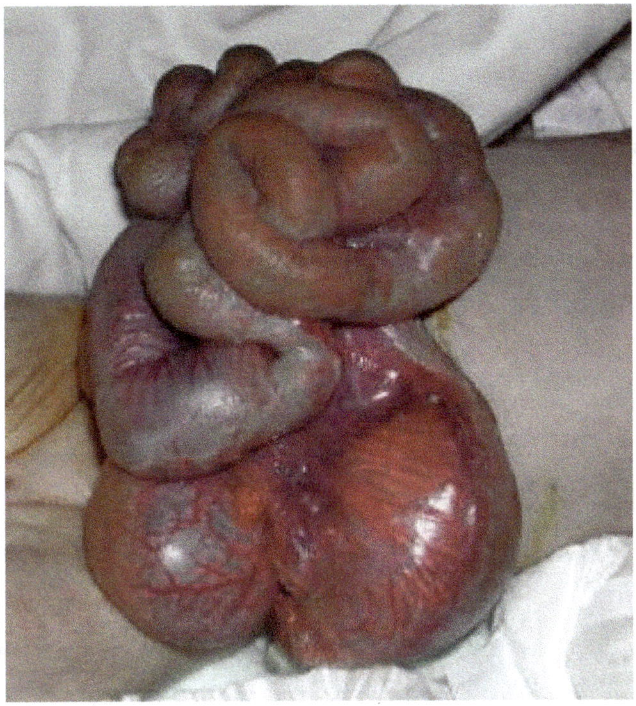

Figure 9. A clinical picture immediately after birth, in which evisceration of the stomach, a good part of the middle intestine and a small portion of the colon can be observed. There is no great serositis because the defect occurred late in gestation.

Acknowledgements

To Douglas C. Nance for his valuable and timely help in translating this chapter.

Author details

Carlos Baeza Herrera[1,2,3], Alin Villalobos Castillejos[4,5,6]* and Ricardo Cortés García[7,8]

*Address all correspondence to: sicaru00@yahoo.com.mx

1 Universidad Nacional Autónoma de México (UNAM), Mexico

2 Guadalupe Victoria General Hospital, Texcoco, Mexico

3 National Academy of Medicine of México and Mexican Academy of Surgery, Mexico

4 Department of Pediatric Surgery, Guadalupe Victoria General Hospital, Texcoco, México

5 Regional Specialty Hospital of Ixtapaluca, México

6 Masters of Science program, UNAM, México

7 Moctezuma Pediatric Hospital, UNAM, México

8 Hospital of Gynecology and Obstetrics number, "Luis Castelazo Ayala" Mexican Social Security Institute, México

References

[1] Bruner JP. In their footsteps: A brief history of maternal-fetal surgery. Clinics in Perinatology. 2003;**30**:439-447

[2] Deprest JA, Flake AW, Gratacos E, Ville Y, Hecherk, et al. The making of fetal surgery. Prenatal Diagnosis. 2010;**30**:653-667

[3] Wenstrom KD, Carr SR. Fetal surgery principles, indications, and evidence. Obstetrics and Gynecology. 2014;**124**:817-835

[4] Jancelewicz T, Harrison MR. A history of fetal surgery. Clinics in Perinatology. 2009;**36**: 227-236

[5] Harrison MR, Golbus MS, Filly RA. Management of the fetus with a correctable congenital defect. Journal of the American Medical Association. 1981;**246**:774-777

[6] Morris RK, Malin GL, Khan KS, Kilby MD. Systematic review of the effectiveness of antenatal intervention for the treatment of congenital lower urinary tract obstruction. British Journal of Obstetrics and Gynaecology. 2010;**117**:382-390

[7] Partridje EA, Flake AW. Maternal-fetal surgery for structural malformations. Best practice and research. Clinical Obstetrics and Gynecology. 2012;**26**:669-682

[8] Adzick NS, Thom EA, Spong CY, Brock JW, Burrows PK, et al. A randomized trial of prenatal versus postnatal repair of myelomeningocele. The New England Journal of Medicine. 2011;**364**:993-1004

[9] Crombleholme TM, Coleman B, Hedrick H, et al. Cystic adenomatoid malformation volume ratio predicts outcome in prenatally diagnosed cystic adenomatoid malformation of the lung. Journal of Pediatric Surgery. 2002;**37**:331-338

[10] Adzick NS. Open fetal surgery for life-threatening fetal anomalies. Seminars in Fetal and Neonatal Medicine. 2010;**15**:1-8

[11] Salinas TVM, Perez GN, Perez GG. Clinical, cytogenetic, environmental and inheritance findings in Mexican neonates with VACTERL association. Indian Journal of Pediatrics. 2015;**82**:84-88

[12] Baeza HC, Lopez CJ, Atzin FJL, Sanjuan FH. Esophageal atresia: A second level hospital experience. Cirugía y Cirujanos. 2005;**73**:259-262

[13] Brosens E, Ploeg M, Van Veber Y, Koopmans A, et al. Clinical and etiological heterogeneity in patients with tracheoesophageal malformations. The European Journal of Medical Genetics. 2014;**57**:440-452

[14] Smigiel R, Lebioda A, Blaszczynski M, Korecka K, et al. Alternations in genes expression of pathway signaling in esophageal tissue with atresia: Results of expression microarray profiling. Diseases of the Esophagus. 2015;**28**:229-233

[15] Beasley SW. Esophageal atresia and tracheoesophageal fistula. In: Oldham KT, Colombani PM, Foglia RP, editors. Surgery of Infants and Children. Philadelphia: Lippincott Raven; 1997. pp. 1021-1033

[16] Quintero RF, Woo JS, Bomberg EM, Wallace WD, et al. Duodenal atresia in 17q12 microdeletion including HNF1B: A new associated malformation in this syndrome. American Journal of Medical Genetics Part A. 2015;**164A**:3076-3082

[17] Baeza HC, Suarez EC, Guido RO, Vidrio PF. Sindrome de oclusion intestinal alta. In: Baeza HC, editor. Temas selectos de cirugia neonatal. Mexico: Alfil; 2011. pp. 3313-3337

[18] Kimura K, Mukohara N, Nishijima E. Diamond-shaped anastomosis for duodenal atresia: An experience with 44 patients over 15 years. Journal of Pediatric Surgery. 1990;**25**: 977-981

[19] Baeza HC, Salinas MJ, Salinas MG, Montero UCA, Lopez CJ. Congenital duodenal obstruction: Two comparative corrective methods. Revista de Gastroenterologia de Mexico. 2009;**74**:1-5

[20] Grant M, Kennedy A, Cochran W. Small bowel congenital anomalies: A review and update. Current Gastroenterology Reports. 2016;**18**(4):16

[21] Baeza HC, Cortes GR, Gonzalez MT. Atresia ileoyeyunal. In: Baeza HC, editor. Temas selectos de cirugia neonatal. Mexico: Alfil; 2011. pp. 387-406

[22] Bing L, Shun Lin X, Wei Bing C. Laparoscope-assisted intestinal lengthening using an anterior flap in jejunal atresia. Pediatric Surgery International. 2015;**31**:1183-1187

[23] Devi S, Meeta S, Nita K. Histomorphological features of intestinal atresia and its clinical correlation. Journal of Clinical and Diagnostic Research. 2015;**9**(11):26-29

[24] Niño DF, Sodhi C, Hackman DJ. Necrotizing enterocolitis: New insights into pathogenesis and mechanisms. Nature Reviews Gastroenterology and Hepatology. 2016;**13**:590-600

[25] Downrad C. Treatment of necrotizing enterocolitis: An American Pediatric Surgical Association Outcomes and Clinical Trials Committee systematic review. Journal of Pediatric Surgery. 2012;**47**:2111-2122

[26] Cuna A, Sampah V. Genetic alterations in necrotizing enterocwolitis. Seminars in Perinatology. 2016;**6**:342-349

[27] Nigel J, Simon E, Agostino P. Necrotizing enterocolitis: Prevention, treatment and outcome. Journal of Pediatric Surgery. 2013;**48**:2359-2367

[28] Kamagata S, Donahoe PK. The effect of fibronectin on cholinergic differentiation of the fetal colon. Journal of Pediatric Surgery. 1985;**20**(4):307-314

[29] Kobayashi H, Hirakawa H, Puri P. Overexpression of intercellular adhesion molecule-1 (ICAM-1) and MHC class II antigen on hypertrophic nerve trunks suggests an immunopathologic response in Hirschsprung's disease. Journal of Pediatric Surgery. 1995;**30**(12): 1680-1683

[30] Lyonett S, Bolino A, Pelet A, et al. A gene for Hirschsprung's disease maps to the proximal long arm of chromosome 10. Nature Genetics. 1993;**4**:346-350

[31] Meijers JH, Tibboel D, van der Kamp AW, van Haperen-Heuts IC, Molenaar JC. A model for aganglionosis in the chicken embryo. Journal of Pediatric Surgery. 1989;**24**(6):557-561

[32] Baeza HC, Lopez MP, Vidal MJM, Cruz VM, Velasco SL. Hirschsprung's disease and appendicitis: A rare association. Acta Pediátrica de México. 2016;**37**:159-164

[33] Baeza HC, Herrera DVP, Garcia CLM, Cortes RHH, Sanjuan FH. Hirschsprung's disease in older children. Revista de Gastroenterologia de Mexico. 2002;**67**:241-244

[34] De la Torre ML, Ortega SJA. Transanal endorectal pull-through for Hirschsprung's disease. Journal of Pediatric Surgery. 1998;**33**:1283-1286

[35] Elhalaby EA, Hashish A, Elbarbary MM, Soliman HA, Wishahy MK, et al. Transanal one-stage endorectal pull-through for Hirschsprung's disease: A multicenter study. Journal of Pediatric Surgery. 2004;**39**(3):345-351

[36] Davenport M, Haugen S, Greenough A. Closed gastroschisis: Antenatal and postnatal features. Journal of Pediatric Surgery. 2001;**36**:1834-1837

[37] Lubinsky M. A vascular and thrombotic model of gastroschisis. American Journal of Medical Genetics Part A. 2014;**164A**:915-917

[38] Weiss LA, Chambers CD, Gonzalez V, Hagey LR, Jones KL. The omega-6 fatty acid linoleic is associated with risk of gastroschisis: A novel dietary risk factor. American Journal of Medical Genetics Part A. 2012;**158**:803-807

[39] Jones KL, Weiss LA, Hagey LR, Gonzalez V, Benirschke K, Chambers CD. Altered lipid metabolism in gastroschisis. A novel hypothesis. American Journal of Medical Genetics Part A. 2013;**161A**(8):1860-1865

[40] Robledo AM, Bobadilla ML, Mellin SEL, Corona RA, Perez MJJ, Cardenas RV, Corona RJR. Prevalence and risk factors for gastroschisis in a public hospital from west Mexico. Congenital Anomalies. 2015;**55**(2):73-80

[41] Baeza HC, Cortes GR, Cano SMC, Garcia CLM. Gastrosquisis. Su tratamiento en un estudio comparativo. Acta Pediátrica de México. 2011;**32**:266-272

[42] Baeza HC, Arcos AA, Suarez EC, Garcia CLM. Gastrosquisis cerrada. Informe de cuatro casos. Propuesta de una nueva designacion. Acta Pediátrica de México. 2009;**30**:317-321

14

Reducing Early Neonatal Mortality in Nigeria—The Solution

Hippolite O. Amadi and Mohammed B. Kawuwa

Abstract

The West African nation of Nigeria seems to have run out of ideas on how their neonatal mortality rate may be lowered. This situation has become dare as the country could not make any significant progress even with the great supports of the last 10 years of Millennium Development Goal. Presently, one in every two deceased child under 5 years of age in Nigeria is a neonate. Literature reveals that most of these deceased neonates are classified preterm or low birthweight, of which nearly four in five must die within first 7 days. This clearly identified the categories and stages of highest mortality; however, it is disappointing that the authorities of the Nigerian health care system have for too long been unable to devise a solution for the neonates. Probably, inadequacy of climatic and cultural compatibilities might partly be responsible for the failure of their current conventional ideas and technologies—these being predominantly imported. Yet, there seems to be lack of interest in some home-grown unconventional ideas that have achieved the needed reduction at few centers. In this chapter, we present the unconventional approaches and encourage across-the-nation translation of the applications to achieve accelerated end to this situation.

Keywords: neonate, Nigeria, neonatal mortality, innovative technique, thermal distress

1. Introduction

Neonatology in the West African sub region, especially in Nigeria, will remain in a state of "scientific comma" until a decisive solution is found to reverse her high neonatal mortality that has continued to be the highest in the world. The solutions required might not necessarily be conventional, as practiced in developed countries of the world, since such imported scientific methods and systems have failed to completely eliminate or drastically reduce the mortality rates. These certified foreign solutions have been probably rendered ineffective within the Nigerian practice due to complications of poor infrastructure, climate, and above all poor work ethics and cultural inadequacies. The effective solution might not necessarily be the "state-of-the-art" procedures that are applied in the United States of America, United Kingdom, and Europe as Nigerian practitioners continue their endless importation of all kinds of relevant and irrelevant ideas but without the necessary infrastructural base to effectively operate these. This country requires a new breed of scientists and neonatologists that can believe in themselves, look inwards, and apply research methods to develop culturally compatible neonatal solutions using easy-to-acquire and locally available materials.

The Nigeria neonatal record is among the worst in the world. There is no evidence to suggest that more neonates are surviving in Nigeria today as compared to 10 years ago, even with the very celebrated millennium development goal (MDG) campaign. Presently, neonatal contribution to mortality rate below 5 years of age in Nigeria has risen in the last 10 years from 40 to nearly 50% despite the huge expenditure of MDG in Nigeria on importation of ideas and systems [1]. The big questions before anyone who might attempt to solve the high neonatal mortality in Nigeria are:

1. What is *really* the primary factor(s) behind the failure to achieve improved overall neonatal survival in Nigeria?
2. Up to 18 morbidity factors contribute to neonatal deaths in Nigeria but are these contributing equally?
3. Is it needful to save time and resources from some factors and dedicate these to synthesize absolute solutions just for one factor or few that could bring about huge impact, and what could this one factor be?
4. Are there any cluster point(s) of highest mortality that might require in-depth investigation within the spectrum of neonatal life-span of 28 days from birth?
5. How may any locally grown "appropriate technological" solution be integrated into Nigeria's health care system; how may this be applicable both at the tertiary and primary health care levels and be made available to the hardest-to-reach neonates across the hinterlands of the country?

In this chapter, our research group of a team of young Nigerian neonatologists and technologists will discuss our vast experiences and progressive syntheses of ingenious local-content ideas that have drastically reduced the neonatal mortality rate at pockets of neonatal centers across Nigeria; thus, achieving an average facility-based mortality rate of 33/1000 presenting neonates as compared to the national average of 248/1000. We shall discuss the various applications that have restored hope to neonates within our practice—including the handy-approach and initial-setpoint-algorithm (ISA) techniques—and how all the applications have contributed to achieve nearly 100% facility-based survival of premature and low birthweight neonates (including 600-g birthweight) within their first 7 days of life.

2. Many are dying

In 2016, an estimated average of 248 neonates out of 1000 presenting at special care baby units (SCBUs) in Nigeria died. Most of these babies reportedly died of various causes during their first 1 week of life. These data were extracted from a collection of independent outcome publications during the 47th national conference of Paediatrics Association of Nigeria (PANCONF) in January 2016. It is a common practice in Nigeria that SCBUs try to use this annual conference to showcase their discoveries, best practices, and outcomes. Therefore, data that were presented could be taken to be what they considered the most impressive or the best of what the centers were prepared to let others know about. The beauty of the content of the proceeding of the PANCONF 2016 on this subject was that the seven coincidental reports came from centers spread equally across the entire country. This includes:

(1) Yariman Bakura Specialist Hospital (YBSH) Gusau in the North-west [2]

(2) University of Abuja Teaching Hospital (UATH) Gwagwalada in the North-central/middle-belt [3]

(3) Lagos State University Teaching Hospital (LASUTH) Ikeja in the South-west [4]

(4) Stella Obasanjo Specialist Hospital (SOSH) Benin-city in the Mid-west [5]

(5) University of Port Harcourt Teaching Hospital (UPTH) in the South-south [6]

(6) Federal Medical Centre (FMC) Owerri in the South-east [7]

(7) Federal Medical Centre (FMC) Asaba in the South-south [8]

It is worthy of note that six of these independent outcomes came from data sets that were generated based on the conventional techniques of newborn care in Nigeria. This resulted in a national mortality average of 248/1000 [2–6, 8]. However, two of these independent centers presented outcome data that had been influenced by their adoption and practice of the various unconventional methods that were developed through the collaborative research of Neonatal Concerns for Africa [9]. In-between these two institutions, the average neonatal mortality crashed below 34/1000 [3, 7]. This translates to a national average reduction of facility-based mortality by a whopping 86%.

Previous publications on conventional practices within the last 10 years have reported facility-based averages such as 254/1000 and 250/1000 [9, 10]. These figures are quite similar to the present 248/1000; hence, this raises the question of why the custodians of neonatal health in Nigeria have been unable to articulate decisive solutions for such a national emergency situation. The scientists seem far too busy with other things than to own the blame, put on their thinking caps, and synthesize an affordable and sustainable home-grown solution to save their neonates. Instead, the over-dependence on unsustainable importation of foreign technologies and ideas have left the Nigerian health care professionals so scientifically lazy that the neonates are still far away from their hope for survival. It was expected that the high publicity and available funds during the last 10 years of the millennium development goals

(MDG) would have empowered a great success. Since this was an unfortunate failure for the neonatal sector at the national level, Nigeria could restore hopes by a humble study of what constituted the pockets of successes recorded by some few centers that adopted unconventional techniques.

3. Change is compulsorily needed

Neonatal health care professionals in West Africa, especially Nigeria, need to understand that the world expects them to apply whatever science they can manage to deliver a drastic reduction in the neonatal mortality rates as it has been known for the last 10 years. It ought to be a challenge to the health care providers in this country that no significant improvements have been achieved, even after ten years of accelerated campaigning and spending—from the 2007 demographic data of the World Health Organization (WHO) to that of Nigeria's Federal Ministry of Health (FMoH) of 2010, to that of UNICEF's 2012, and perhaps up to the indices of 2017 (**Figure 1**) [1, 11–14].

The question that remained unanswered is whether there are any more untried ideas left for the Nigeria's FMoH and the other custodians of neonatal health in Nigeria that can help lower their well-known horrible indices, including:

(a) Neonatal deaths accounting for nearly 50% of all deaths of children under 5 years of age [1, 15]

(b) Nearly 80% of all deceased neonates dying within their first 1 week of life [14, 16]

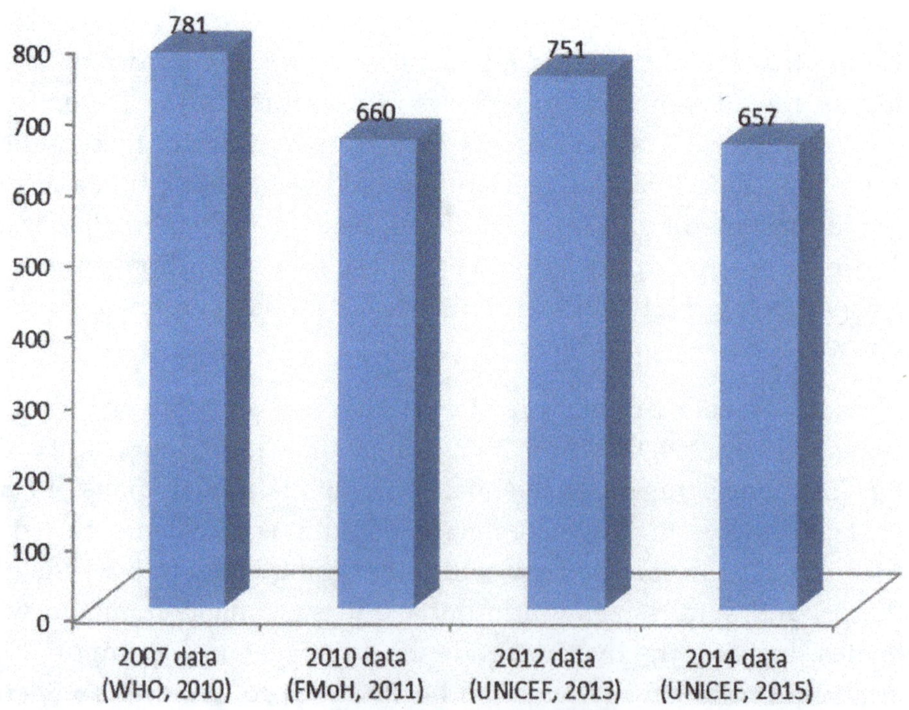

Figure 1. Daily newborn mortality over last 8 years of MDG.

This showed that most deceased neonates died before their 7th postnatal day, beyond which most surviving neonates would successfully go home alive. We hypothesize that after the first quarter of neonatal life, i.e., 7 of 28 days, most Nigerian neonates are strong enough to contribute their minimal quotas in resisting and fighting their various debilitating morbidities, howbeit, within a conducive and stable physiological state. The first few days after birth are their greatest period of need for external life support systems and procedures. Inadequate support and procedures during this period would normally be associated with such high rate of death as reported in Nigeria. The most vulnerable of the neonates is the premature ones who may necessarily require knowledgeable support for survival. Nigerian authors have shown that mortality for very preterm and extremely low birthweight neonates at some hospital centers can be quite high, even as high as 933/1000 [17–20]. It is our opinion that the current Nigerian conventional facility-based practices during early neonatal life is inadequate or fundamentally faulty. Our resonating questions remain: Has Nigeria got any other ideas for preventing such high rate of early neonatal deaths that has not yet been tried since the last 10 years as these are urgently needed? Is it time for the FMoH and the establishments to come out openly to accept the failure? Is it time to have compassion on the neonates and search for other sustainable, and perhaps, unconventional methods as have been demonstrated in few pockets of Nigerian centers? The time cannot be any sooner than now.

4. Wholesale importation is unsustainable

It is always attractive to import latest technologies for application in Nigeria. However, poor infrastructural development makes such applications unsustainable. Modern medical equipment is quite expensive and unaffordable to many medical institutions that must look after the neonates. However, the procurement of these systems is not necessarily the main problem. Sadly, the age long pattern at these mostly government-owned referral centers is such that after many years of impoverished neonatal outcomes and political harassments, the government manages to provide appropriate funds to purchase only few of the required equipment. However, no sooner this is done, the center goes back into comatose due to inability to maintain the systems. The efficiency of a system or procedure can often depend on factors relating to infrastructural base, climate, peoples' culture, work attitude, manpower, maintenance supply chain, etc. It is essential that these factors are carefully considered, or else a wholesale adoption of a foreign idea may not yield same result as expected. Nigeria's 100% reliance on importation of needed technologies and ideas are unsustainable due to these factors. The best options forward are either adaptation or synthesis of own solutions.

5. Adaption requires scientific thinking

Most of Nigeria's neonatal systems, techniques, and procedures are imported from the United Kingdom, Europe, or America where these are well-proven to be very effective, reliable, and sustainable. Unfortunately, similar outcomes would depend on the abilities of the importing country to adapt the application within their own variables of culture, climate, and infrastructure. This requires some scientific thinking. There may be a need to understand the basic physics of the application in order to know the aspect of the application that needs tweaking; and how best to do this to make the application reliably operable in the setting. The Nigerian scientific and research community must be alive, active, and confident to create such intermediate technologies. We think that a quicker success could be made if technologies are tweaked to fit the Nigerian weather and culture rather than the more difficult route of "tweaking culture for a piece of imported technology". This challenge is both for the Nigerian government but much more for the Universities, research institutions, and their Professors.

6. Syntheses of unconventional techniques

Our hypothesis created the drive to search for the possible factor that could be secretly at work or that might provide a huge positive impact for the neonates if isolated. The search began with a nationally circulated questionnaire that identified lack of functional incubators as a major factor militating against neonatal survival in Nigeria [17]. However, advancing consistently with various careful comparative investigations, our research can presently reveal a strong association of "thermoneutral instability", hiding behind a host of co-morbid conditions that had been said to be responsible for high rate of neonatal mortality in Nigeria [15]. Consistent thermal stability within body temperatures of 36.5–37.4°C is essential for the neonate's physiological wellness to fight disabling conditions, maintain positive progress, and for survival. Lack of thermal stability leaves the neonates so moribund that the other presenting co-morbid factors become excessively too powerful for the neonates in their fights for survival. Hence, unbroken provision of neonatal thermoneutral environment—without excuses of unfavorable weather, climate, cultural, and work attitudes—could be the one-factor game-changer that has eluded neonatal practice in Nigeria.

We developed and tested applications as we investigated various phenomena that were very evident in the Nigerian setting. Methods that applied locally available materials were more easily sustainable, affordable, and maintainable. We opted for these, thereby introducing applications, procedures, and advocacies at various times as published in Ref. [9]. We hence created a package of stand-alone activities that supplemented each other to produce the reported great outcomes at Special Care Baby Units of the Federal Medical Centre Owerri and University of Abuja Teaching Hospital in 2016 [3, 7]. These applications were:

6.1. The Recycled incubator technology (RIT)

In a period of economic recession such as Nigeria is currently experiencing, neonatal incubators are increasingly unaffordable due to skyrocketing foreign exchange. Dysfunctional and broken-down incubators litter the hospitals, yet the preterm babies are arriving in their thousands every day. We developed some techniques that Nigeria could use to re-engineer and activate these dysfunctional systems, offering up to 10 fresh years of life-expectancy at costs that are less than 20% of selling price of modern incubators. Recycled incubator technology (RIT) has worked very well for our collaborating hospitals centers, ensuring consistent availability of over 15 functional incubators at all times. This grants them an outstanding position when compared with the other government centers that hide behind lack of funds to deny the neonates of this vital system. Any Nigerian hospital with any available casing of broken-down incubator does not actually have excuses to give in support of their denial and neglect for this basic neonatal need. The RIT upgrading or conversion is affordable and does not necessarily require special government subvention as many of our collaborating centers fund this from their internally generated revenue. This simple unconventional technology of the RIT is saving huge amount of lives in Nigeria without huge spending; hence, the Nigerian government and the custodians of neonatal health in Nigerian should pay attention.

6.2. The failure-preventive audit culture (FAC)

One wonders why routine maintenance of these items of neonatal equipment in Nigeria is so neglected. Neonatal systems such as the incubator, as a life support machine, works nonstop, day-in and day-out, yet the conventional Nigerian practice does not involve a compulsory regular maintenance by qualified personnel. Regular professional maintenance of neonatal systems, even in their countries of manufacture, is a routine never to be compromised. Yet anyone wonders why there are so many broken-down systems at Nigerian centers where machines are run continuously without servicing until they are destroyed. The systems at our centers are always functionally available because the hospitals run a six monthly mandatory failure-preventive audit culture (FAC) for the incubators. Similar assiduous care must be made compulsory at all SCBUs operating in Nigeria. Suffice to mention that many of the incubators are homes for the microbes that infect the dying neonates as a result of lack of routine technical cleaning and decontamination. As this is an unlawful life-threatening exposure of a neonate to harmful environment, the seriousness of the Nigerian government should be measured by their willingness to prosecute defaulting professionals and institutions.

6.3. The power banking system (PBS)

The widespread exposure of the neonate to hypothermia even when functional incubators are available can be due to epileptic power supply or outright power failures that last hours unending. The incubator becomes useless when there is no power to run it. Grid power failure can even last for days in Nigeria such that a standby fossil fuel generator becomes inadequate and unsustainable to provide uninterrupted incubator care. Nigeria is yet to provide a decisive solution for her inability to deliver uninterrupted grid power to the nation. Many centers rely on this limitation to offer excuses for the high neonatal mortality. In our few centers, however, the incubators run uninterrupted by the application of our power banking system (PBS) initiative. We used batteries to store up power from the grid and generators whenever these were available. This was in addition to trickling recharging of the batteries using photovoltaic cells mounted on the rooftops, especially when there was failure of both grid and fossil generator powers that lasted longer than necessary.

6.4. Evening-fever syndrome (EFS) antidote

The Nigerian climate can get excessively hot with a higher temperature of up to 47°C in some cities during the dry season [21, 22]. Preterm neonates are often unable to regulate their body temperatures downward from the high room temperatures in excess of 38°C. This leads to periodic fever that sets in during late afternoons and abates later in the evening, long after sunset. This phenomenon of evening-fever syndrome (EFS) was investigated leading to the proposal of a weather-resilient building technique for neonatal nurseries in Nigeria [22, 23]. We discovered that the periodic hyperthermia due to EFS, often misdiagnosed as a disease process, has the consequences of neonatal thermal distress that drastically slowed down baby's response to treatment. It was hence essential that all our nurseries were renovated or properly relocated within the hospital complexes so as to eliminate or minimize this phenomenon. Neonates in our centers were hence kept within allowable physiological temperatures even when climatic ambient temperatures soared higher above 45°C.

6.5. SCBU nurses retention advocacy

One obnoxious common practice in Nigerian tertiary hospitals is the periodic reshuffling of nurses around various departments of the hospital irrespective of specialities. This practice has such huge negative impact on neonatal outcome that some managers have refused to pay attention to. The practice might be useful in adult wards, some may argue, but this is definitely counterproductive in the special care baby units. It takes much longer than 1 year to transform a general nursing practitioner into one with enough skills to effectively manage the neonates. Learning on the job comes along with its own consequences of blunders that are often committed, some leading to neonatal deaths. However, just as some of these, on-the-job trainees are about to become useful, they are asked to move on while a new bunch of starters are brought in to continue with the devastation. This practice of replacing trained and knowledgeable nurses with learners and starters might sound unbelievable to readers of this article from developed nations; however, this is really one of those practices that have quietly contributed to huge numbers of preventable neonatal deaths in Nigeria. The parochial views of the nursing establishments in Nigeria, including such arguments as "any qualified nurse could work in any department of the hospital", are so powerful that nursing managers seem to have completely lost their senses of reasoning to protect these poor neonates. The management of our few hospital centers has standing rules, after many advocacies, to limit this nurses' reshufflings within only 10% of the entire SCBUs nursing crew. This posting is, however, forbidden to affect the best of the crew members. The challenge here is that members of the SCBU crew are so overworked that many often seek to be posted away. So to minimize this, special incentives other than what all nurses received were given to SCBU crew members in appreciation. This allowed incentives and privileges are still hotly contested in some of our hospitals by supporters of other greedy nurses who would not even want to work at the SCBUs themselves.

6.6. Breathing/apnoea monitors

Lack of adequate number of nursing staff in Nigerian hospitals is an age-long problem that has remained unsolved. This has a huge negative impact on neonatal outcome at Nigerian newborn centers. Hospital managements quickly agree with the need for more staff whenever confronted. However, they easily argue their ways through with the use of Government's endless embargo on employment. This problem is as bad as having only two nurses to look after 38 neonates during a work-shift in one of Nigeria's busy University Teaching Hospital where this corresponding author once worked as a visiting consultant. How on earth would anyone explain what happens to four neonates that could be undergoing apnoeic attack simultaneously during such a shift? Sure, many of them died from the apnoeic attacks without ever being noticed - most of these from easily preventable causes. Yet, the nursing managements would not reason that the SCBUs needed more nurses relative to the other adult and adolescent wards. The use of affordable simple devices for neonatal chest and body movements monitoring hence became inevitable to use in our centers. Our standard practice of the use of only incubators and cots with installed apnoea monitors for all critically ill neonates and all other premature neonates—especially during their first-seven-days (F7D) of life—must, hence, never be compromised. By this practice, nurses were easily alerted as soon as such neonates go into apnoeic mode. The job of keeping such neonate alive, awaiting proper intervention, becomes the job of any available staff and not just the overworked nurses. For our centers, the apnoea monitor has become the inevitable "third eye" of our nurses to frustrate neonatal "sudden death syndrome" until proper intervention is administered to correct the underlying fault.

6.7. The handy approach

Careful examination of various plots of neonatal body temperature against lifetime, especially during the first few days of life, revealed a startling consistent physiological inadequacy. We created a "regional band" on the graphs, representing the physiological safe-zone temperatures of 36.5–37.4°C (**Figure 2**). This enabled easy assessment of how well the neonates had been assisted to maintain this safezone temperature that is essentially required for thermoneutrality, and hence neonatal survival. We investigated this in many hospitals across the regions of Nigeria—from the South to the North—and we concluded that this was a national problem [9]. It was however more disturbing that the nonphysiological temperature profile also emerged from some neonates that could be seen to have undergone incubator care.

We began to investigate this and quickly discover the complete absence of any standard protocol or algorithm for achieving neonatal normotherm in the Nigerian practice. This led to the synthesis of the handy-approach algorithm, developed as a set of rules that could guide the normalization of a deviating neonatal body temperature back to its safezone temperatures [21]. Ability to use this application became compulsory, and, a necessary requirement for all the nursing and clinical staff of the SCBUs within our neonatal research network (**Figure 3**). Subsequently, a validation study was carried out. This showed that the technique led to greatly improved neonatal temperature profiles and also for better overall outcome [9]. The handy approach is an easy-to-handle tool that practitioners at the rest of Nigeria's SCBU should study for the sake of the multitudes of Nigerian neonates under their care.

6.8. The ISA

The initial set-point algorithm (ISA) was developed as a supplementary temperature control protocol to maximize the impact of the handy approach. This targets a quick attainment of normotherm at the onset of incubator intervention (**Figure 4**). This effectively removes the

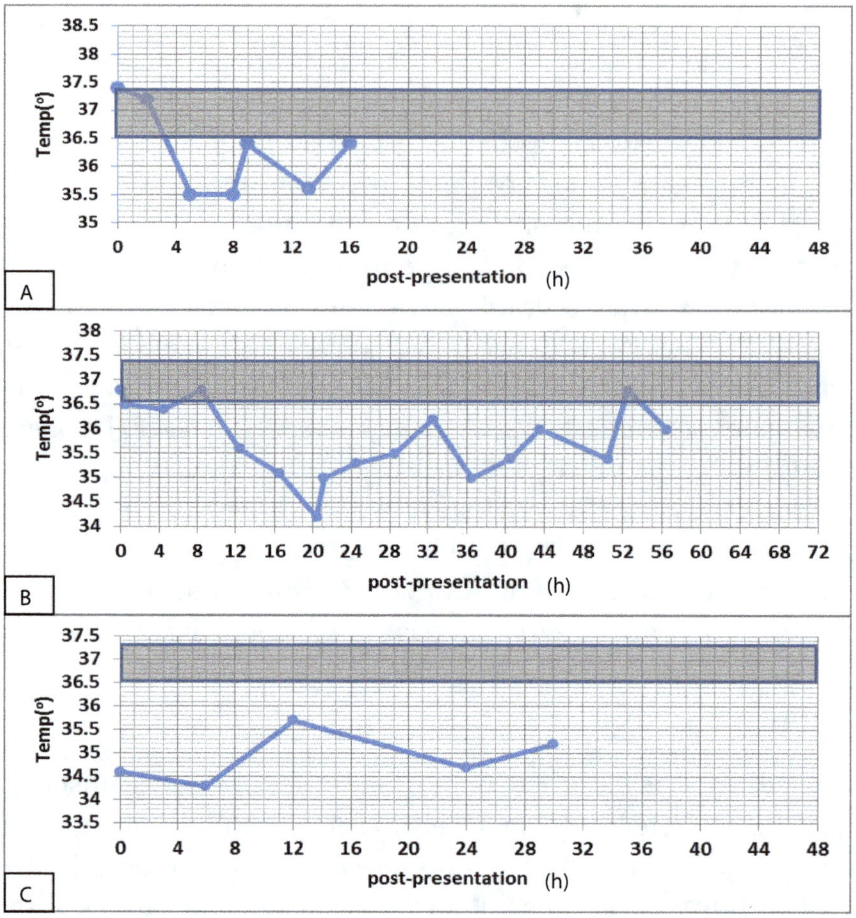

Figure 2. Temperature—Lifetime plot revealing safezone band. (Plots of deceased incubator-nursed neonates from 3 different regional teaching hospitals in Nigeria, A—south: BW = 2000 g admitted 16/01/2013; B—middlebelt: BW = 1580 g admitted 17/11/2012; C—north: BW = 600 g admitted 02/08/2012).

often long postnatal exposure of neonates to temperatures outside the safezone, as this has been argued to inflict a lasting damage that trails some of them to death within their first week of life [15]. The ISA was such a powerful tool that might have coincidentally led to the reduction of F7D contribution to mortality, from 71 to 0%, in a set of studied neonatal cohorts at the University of Abuja Teaching Hospital Nigeria [15]. The devastating postnatal thermal shock described in the research was widespread across Nigerian centers and explained the reason behind the WHO figure of 79% for the mortalities happening before the seventh postnatal day; this figure has never changed between the 2008 and 2013 demographic survey reports [14]. ISA application enabled clinicians at our center to achieve neonatal normotherm in an average of 28 min as compared to conventional average outcome of 12 h and 24 min. The thermal devastation of almost 12½ h long in a hostile environment is unbearable for the poor neonates, especially the preterms, as they are coming from the well-regulated comforts of the womb [15]. Thus, the ISA has been demonstrated to be an effective tool for the care of preterm neonates and a dependable response to this problem. Having also been scientifically validated and peer-reviewed, this has remained a compulsory tool to apply while admitting premature neonates at many of our centers. This has led to drastic overall reduction in the mortality of premature neonates at these few centers; figures falling from 63 to 7% at

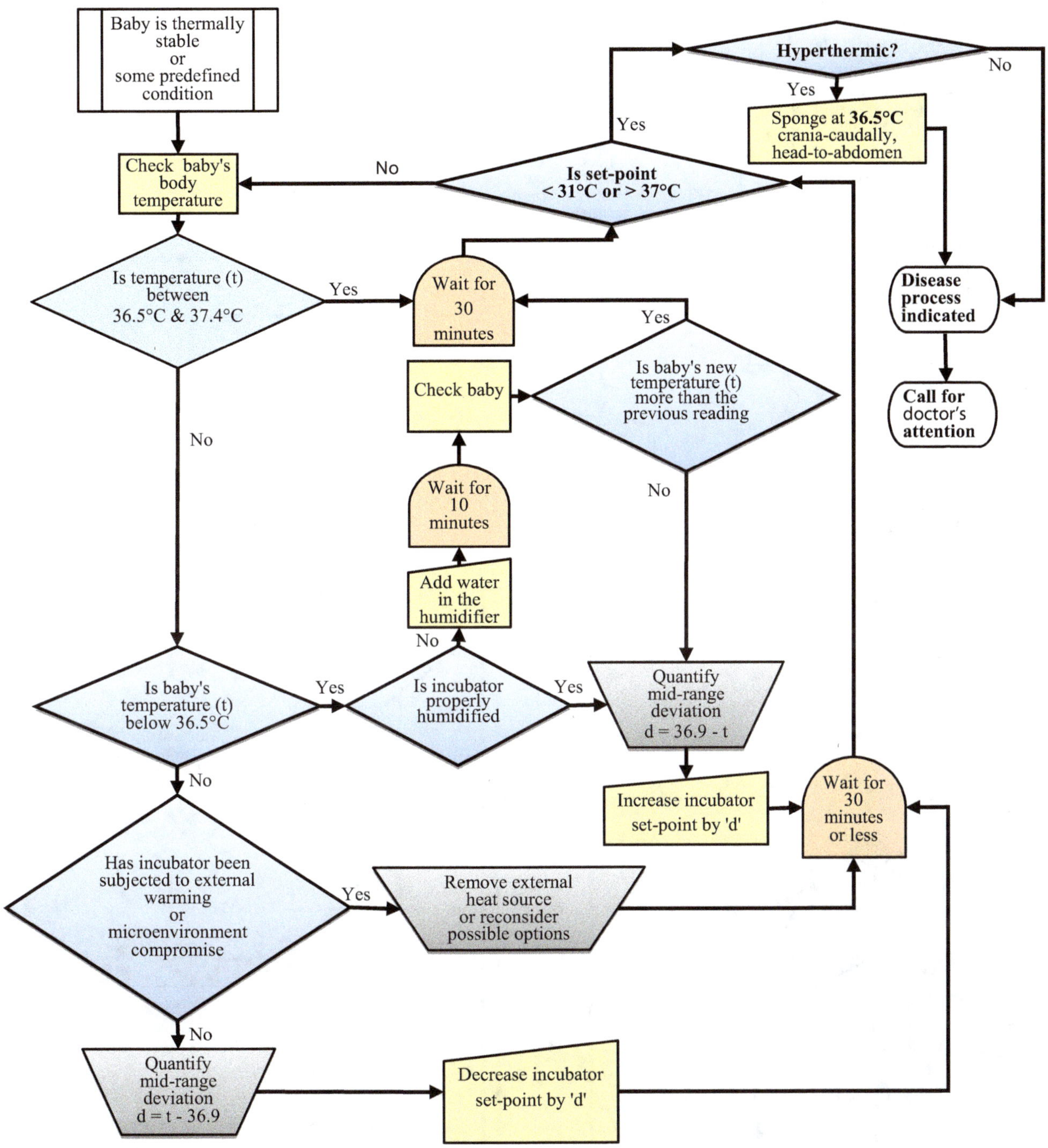

Figure 3. The handy approach. Modified from Amadi [21].

the University of Abuja Teaching Hospital, Gwagwalada Nigeria, for example. The ISA is an unconventional step, all Nigerian and West African centers might have to adopt if they must lower their high facility-based mortality rate of premature neonates. In addition to this excellent overall outcomes with the handy-approach and ISA procedures developed, the Federal Medical Centre (FMC) Owerri Nigeria, became the hospital that nursed the tinniest baby ever to survive in a Nigerian hospital with the use of these applications—baby "Majesty," as they nicknamed her, was born after 26 weeks GA weighing 550 g and went home after 83 days of nursing care on the 26th of April 2015 (**Figure 4**).

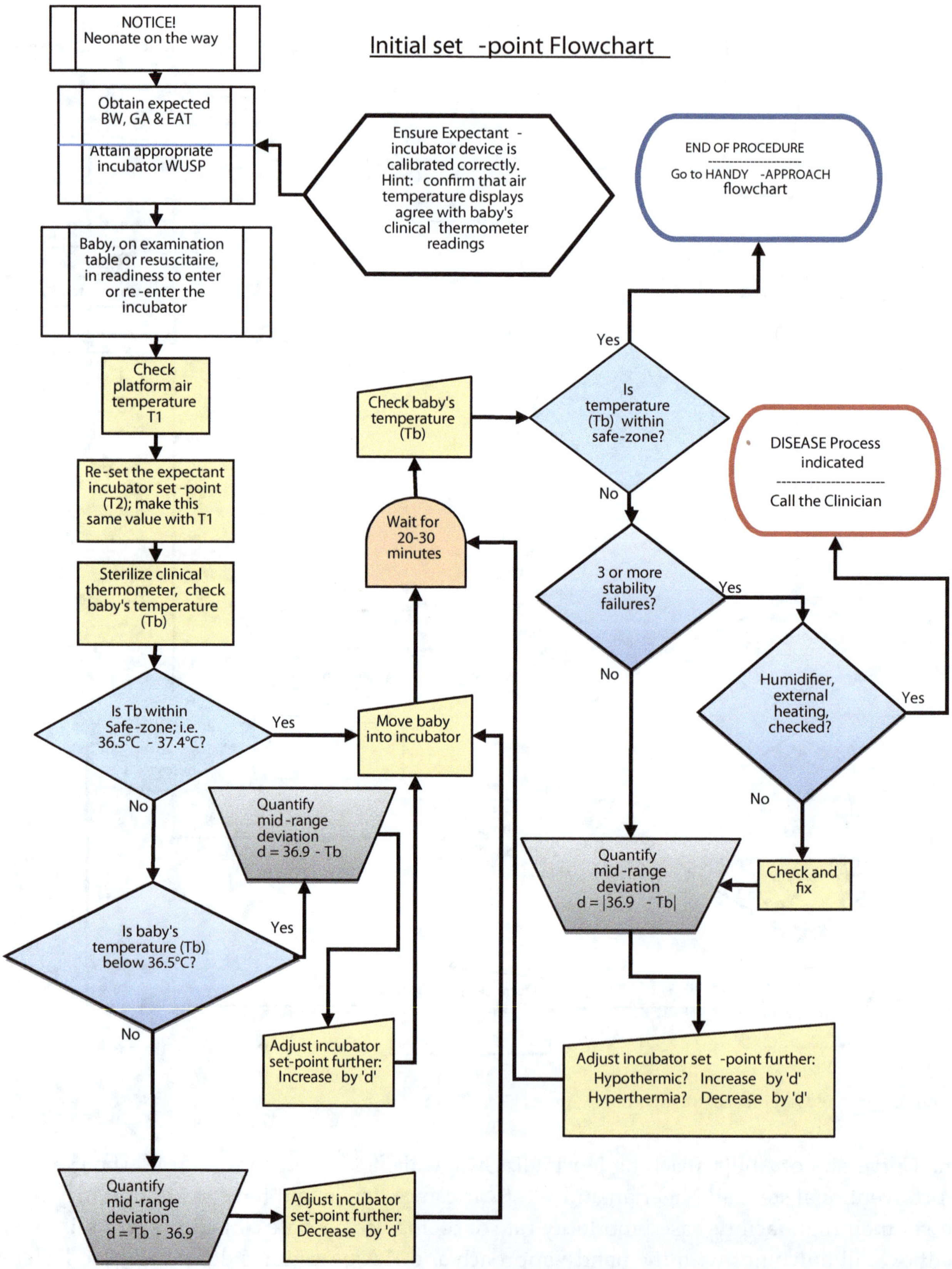

Figure 4. The ISA flowchart. Modified from Amadi et al. [15].

6.9. Pediatrics incubation technique (PIT) courses

Within the limits of our research findings, we can strongly affirm that poor thermal control is largely to blame for the high rate of mortality of premature neonates in Nigeria, especially during the first few days of life. It therefore became essential that the theories and etiology of neonatal thermal shock was well-understood and communicated to would be and practicing neonatal nurses and doctors. These were the roles expected of the pediatrics incubation technique (PIT) courses that were introduced very early in this research group. The PIT courses isolate the Nigerian peculiar climate, weather, culture, and financial dispositions, relating these factors to the neonatal need of adequate warmth for survival. The courses were used to teach practitioners on the best incubator practices within the Nigerian tropical contexts. In Nigeria, being a technologically dependent country in medical devices including incubators, the PIT discusses the tweaks that are appropriately necessary in order to get the best out of these foreign systems. The courses are elective at the Pediatrics Departments of our partner hospitals; however, it is mandatory for the SCBU staff of our centers. There is the desire for zero tolerance to the devastating effect of early neonatal thermal shock at our centers. Therefore, all staff of some of our SCBUs are required to achieve a minimum grade of "Merit" (65% or above) at both PIT level-1 and PIT level-2 courses to guarantee a good career progress at the centers.

7. Conclusions and recommendations

The Nigerian neonatal records are among the worst in the world. This has remained high for far too long, and there seems to be no fresh ideas—those that had not been previously tried or any immediate sustainable solutions from the government, health institutions, or the academia. In our work, we have carefully investigated the mortalities and struggles of the early days of premature neonates in Nigeria and can conclude that this is more than a "nightmare" for them. In the course of our various investigations and publications, we have identified that thermal inadequacies is one factor that must be tackled and decisively resolved before the Nigerian neonates that can be liberated.

We have synthesized unconventional solutions, tried, and validated these using rigorous methodologies to generate our often multicenter- and center-controlled data. The various comparative analyses against conventional techniques in Nigeria have also revealed that our unconventional approaches have succeeded where these failed irrespective of disabling policies and social factors at work. In a center-controlled cohorts study that tested a package of the developed unconventional techniques on extremely premature neonates (**Figure 5**), overall mortality rate (NNMR) fell from 63/100 for conventional techniques to 7/100; the fraction of neonates that would not see their seventh day after birth (f7dMR) fell from 51/100 to 0; and the fraction of the deceased neonates that died before the seventh day (f7d-in-NNM) in the conventional technique cohorts was quite similar to the World Health Organization demographic figure for this [15]. It is still a puzzle that the Nigerian health authorities and their corporate institutions have turned a blind eye to a package of methods so reliable; thereby

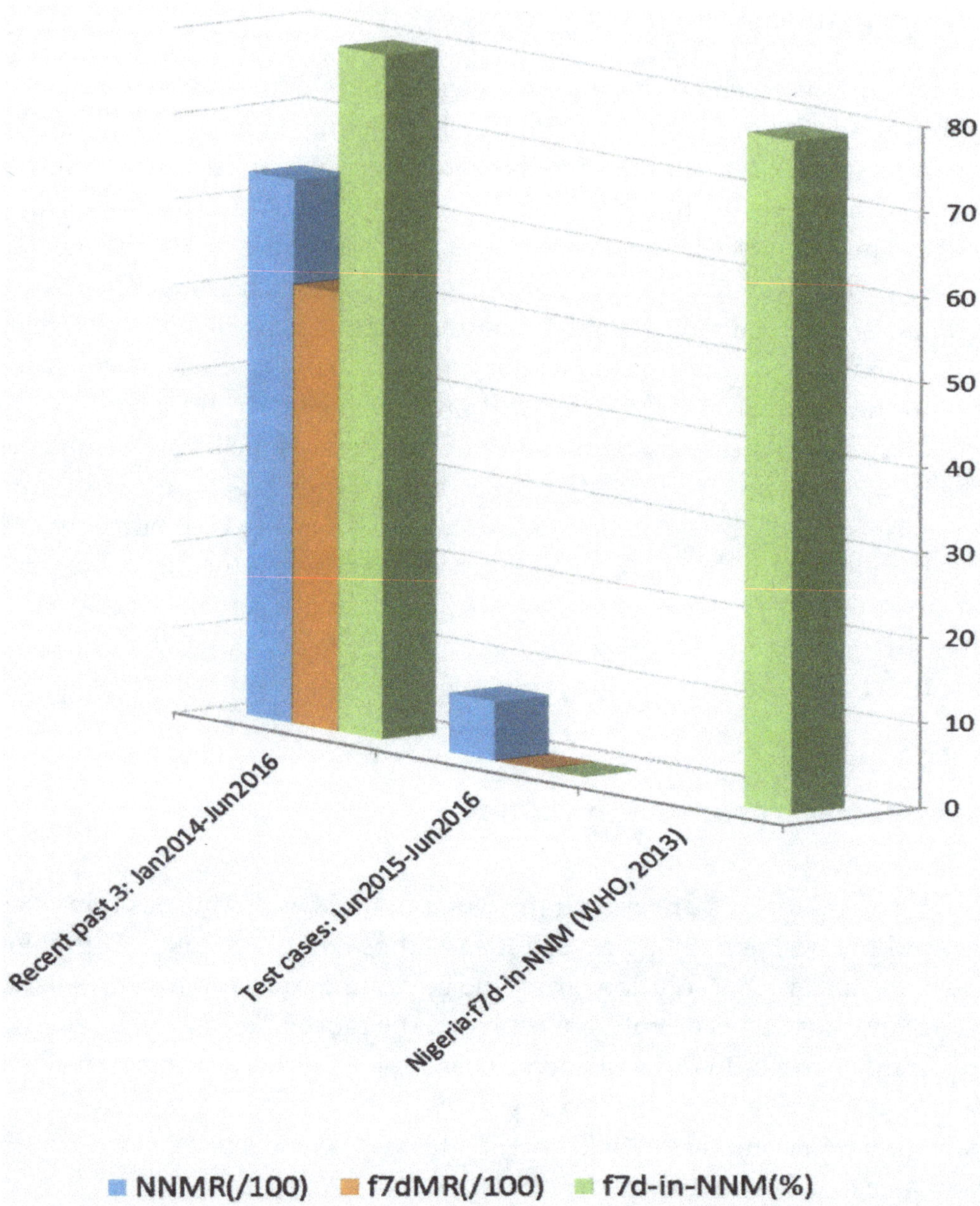

Figure 5. Comparative outcome of a centre-controlled cohort study of ELBW neonates managed with conventional techniques in "recent past" as against unconventional techniques on "test cases"; modified from Amadi et al. [15].

being uncompassionate as thousands of these neonates are sent to their untimely graves. If a set of techniques could so-smash the W.H.O.'s "f7d-in-NNM" demographic figure of 79% for Nigeria, literally eradicating this on a cohort of extremely premature neonates, what are they still waiting for before translating this idea into their national practice?

In the face of ever dwindling and crashing Nigerian economy, we think that our unconventional techniques as presented in our various publications have a great role to play if Nigeria must emancipate from this age long neonatal situation. The use of these affordable systems and ideas are recommended to replace the insatiable crave for unsustainable importation of ideas and technologies that are not consistent with the Nigerian climate, weather, and infrastructural development.

Acknowledgements

We wish to thank all members of our neonatal research network across Nigeria. We will particularly mention Professor JC Azubuike, Professor OA Mokuolu, Dr EK Olateju, Professor A Osibogun, Dr P Alabi, and Professor SA Kuranga. Everyone has worked hard to enable us unravel "temperature" as the hidden factor that had destroyed our neonates, especially the premature ones. We thank Neonatal Concerns for Africa and Polchazum Engineering Limited, subsidiaries of the Mastermind Group Nigeria, for being the primary funders of these investigations. We also appreciate the kind supports received from the Hornchurch Baptist Church Essex United Kingdom and the Bioengineering Department of Imperial College London United Kingdom.

Conflicts of interest

Both authors declare no conflicts of interests concerning this publication.

Author details

Hippolite O. Amadi[1,2,4*] and Mohammed B. Kawuwa[3,4]

*Address all correspondence to: h.amadi@imperial.ac.uk

1 Bioengineering Department, Imperial College London, United Kingdom

2 College of Medicine, Imo State University, Owerri, Nigeria

3 Department of Obstetrics and Gynaecology, University of Maiduguri, Nigeria

4 Federal Medical Centre, Nguru, Yobe State, Nigeria

References

[1] UNICEF, WHO, World Bank, UN Pop Div. Levels and Trends in Child Mortality Report 2015 [Internet]. 2015 [Updated: 2015]. [Accessed: 02-02-2017]

[2] Garba BI. Prevalence, risk factors and outcome of preterms at a specialist hospital in Gusau, Nigeria. In: Alikor EA, editor. 47th Annual Conference of the Paediatrics Association of Nigeria; 19-23 January 2016; Port Harcourt Nigeria. Port Harcourt; 2016. p. 25

[3] Adesina TC, Olateju EK, Okechukwu AA, Alabi P, Amadi HO. The impact of an initial set-point prediction tool for prompt attainment of stability during neonatal incubator care—A comparative study. In: Alikor EA, editor. 47th Annual conference of the Paediatrics Association of Nigeria; 19-23 January 2016; Port Harcourt Nigeria; 2016. p. 35

[4] Animasahun AB, Ubuane OP, Gbelee O, Njokanma F. A two-year review of outcome of neonatal admissions at the children emergency room of the Lagos State University Teaching Hospital Ikeja. In: Alikor EA, editor. 47th Annual conference of the Paediatrics Association of Nigeria; 19-23 January 2016; Port Harcourt Nigeria. Port Harcourt; 2016; p. 27

[5] Mbarie IA, Blessing I, Iyoha A. Morbidity profile and outcome of newborns admitted into the neonatal unit of a secondary health care centre in Benin City. In: Alikor EA, editor. 47th Annual conference of the Paediatrics Association of Nigeria; 19-23 January 2016; Port Harcourt Nigeria. Port Harcourt; 2016. p. 29

[6] Obikwu U, Okagua J, Opara PI, Eneh AU. Morbidity and mortality patterns of admission into the special care baby unit of University of Port Harcourt Teaching Hospital. In: Alikor EA, editor. 47th Annual Conference of the Paediatrics Association of Nigeria; 19-23 January 2016; Port Harcourt Nigeria; 2016. p. 50

[7] Emerenini FC, Ezeofor TC. Outcome of newborn admissions in the special care baby unit of Federal Medical Centre Owerri. In: Alikor EA, editor. 47th Annual Conference of the Paediatrics Association of Nigeria; 19-23 January 2016; Port Harcourt Nigeria; 2016. p. 38

[8] Nwankwo O, Uche C, Okolo AA. Burden of severe birth asphyxia at Federal Medical Centre Asaba—Lessons and proposal for alleviation. In: Alikor EA, editor. 47th Annual Conference of the Paediatrics Association of Nigeria; 19-23 January 2016; Port Harcourt Nigeria. Port Harcourt; 2016. p. 36

[9] Amadi HO, Osibogun A, Olateju EK, Kawuwa MB, Uwakwem AC, Ibekwe MU, Alabi P, Ezeaka VC, Eleshin DG, Ibadin MO. Challenges and frugal remedies for lowering facility based neonatal mortality—A comparative study. International Journal of Pediatrics. 2014;**2014**:986716

[10] Amadi HO, Azubuike JC, Etawo US, Offiong UR, Ezeaka C, Eyinade O, Adimora GN, Osibogun AO, Ibeziako N, Iroha EO, Dutse AI, Chukwu CO, Okpere EE, Kawuwa MB, El-Nafaty AU, Kuranga SA, Mokuolu OA. The impact of recycled neonatal incubators in Nigeria: A 6-year follow-up study. International Journal of Pediatrics. 2010;**2010**:269293. DOI: 10.1155/2010/269293

[11] WHO, UNICEF. Progress Towards Millennium Development Goals 4 and 5 – Countdown to 2015 Decade Report. [Internet]. 2010 [Updated: 2010]. Available from: http://whqlibdoc.who.int/publications/2010/9789241599573_eng.pdf [Accessed: 02-02-2017]

[12] Federal Ministry of Health Nigeria, Save the Children, Jhpiego. Saving Newborn Lives in Nigeria: Newborn Health in the Context of the Integrated Maternal, Newborn and Child Health Strategy, 2nd edition [Internet]. 2011 [Updated: 2011]. Available from: http://resourcecentre.savethechildren.se/content/library/documents/nigeria-newborn-health-report-context-integrated-maternal-newborn-and-chil. [Accessed: 12-08-2016]

[13] UNICEF. Statistics at a Glance – Nigeria [Internet]. 2013. Available from: https://www.unicef.org/infobycountry/nigeria_statistics.html?p=printme [Accessed: 02-02-2017]

[14] MCA, World Health Organisation. Maternal and Perinatal Health Profile of Nigeria, Africa Region. Maternal and Perinatal Country Profile [Internet]. 2014 [Updated: 2014]. Available from: http://www.who.int/maternal_child_adolescent/epidemiology/profiles/maternal/nga.pdf [Accessed: 02-02-2017

[15] Amadi HO, Adesina TC, Olateju EK, Omokaro S, Okechukwu AA, Alabi P, Haruna AS. Validation of a novel technique that minimises early neonatal deaths – A comparative study. Journal of Paediatrics and Neonatal Care. 2017;**6**(1):00232

[16] Orobaton N. Selected findings: The mother–newborn dyad: Community-based distribution of misoprostol and chlorhexidine in Sokoto State, Nigeria [Internet]. 2014 [Updated: 2014]. Available from: http://wordpress.sph.harvard.edu/mhtf-2/wp-content/uploads/sites/32/2014/09/NOSA.Harvard-MHTF.SEPT2014.pdf [Accessed: 02-02-2017]

[17] Amadi HO, Mokuolu OA, Adimora GN, Pam SD, Etawo US, Ohadugha CO, Adesiyun OO. Digitally recycled incubators: Better economic alternatives to modern systems in low-income countries. Annals of Tropical Paediatrics. 2007;**27**:207-214

[18] Okechukwu AA, Achonwa A. Morbidity and mortality patterns of admissions into the special care baby unit of University of Abuja Teaching Hospital, Gwagwalada Nigeria. Nigeria Journal of Clinical Practice. 2009;**12**:389-394

[19] Onalo R, Olateju EK. A four-year retrospective review of very low birth weight babies seen at the University of Abuja Teaching Hospital Nigeria. Nigerian Postgraduate Medical Journal. 2015;**22**:93-99

[20] Ogunlesi TA. Factors influencing the survival of newborn babies weighing <1.5 kg in Sagamu, Nigeria. Archives of Gynecology and Obstetrics. 2011;**284**:1351-1357

[21] Amadi HO. Neonatal thermoneutrality in a tropical climate. In: Rodriguez-Morales AJ, editor. Current Topics in Tropical Medicine. 1st ed. Intech: Rijeka Croatia; 2012. pp. 513-544. Available from: http://www.intechopen.com/books/current-topics-in-tropical-medicine/neonatal-thermoneutrality [Accessed: 02-02-2017]

[22] Amadi HO, Mohammed IL, Kawuwa MB, Oyedokun A, Mohammed H. Synthesis and validation of a weatherproof nursery design that eliminates tropical evening-fever-syndrome in neonates. International Journal of Paediatrics. 2014;**2014**:986760. DOI: 10.1155/2014/986760

[23] Amadi HO, Mokuolu AO, Obasa T. The effect of high sunlight intensity on the neonatal incubator functionality. Journal of Neonatal Nursing. 2013;**19**:122-128

Permissions

All chapters in this book were first published in STNC, by InTech Open; hereby published with permission under the Creative Commons Attribution License or equivalent. Every chapter published in this book has been scrutinized by our experts. Their significance has been extensively debated. The topics covered herein carry significant findings which will fuel the growth of the discipline. They may even be implemented as practical applications or may be referred to as a beginning point for another development.

The contributors of this book come from diverse backgrounds, making this book a truly international effort. This book will bring forth new frontiers with its revolutionizing research information and detailed analysis of the nascent developments around the world.

We would like to thank all the contributing authors for lending their expertise to make the book truly unique. They have played a crucial role in the development of this book. Without their invaluable contributions this book wouldn't have been possible. They have made vital efforts to compile up to date information on the varied aspects of this subject to make this book a valuable addition to the collection of many professionals and students.

This book was conceptualized with the vision of imparting up-to-date information and advanced data in this field. To ensure the same, a matchless editorial board was set up. Every individual on the board went through rigorous rounds of assessment to prove their worth. After which they invested a large part of their time researching and compiling the most relevant data for our readers.

The editorial board has been involved in producing this book since its inception. They have spent rigorous hours researching and exploring the diverse topics which have resulted in the successful publishing of this book. They have passed on their knowledge of decades through this book. To expedite this challenging task, the publisher supported the team at every step. A small team of assistant editors was also appointed to further simplify the editing procedure and attain best results for the readers.

Apart from the editorial board, the designing team has also invested a significant amount of their time in understanding the subject and creating the most relevant covers. They scrutinized every image to scout for the most suitable representation of the subject and create an appropriate cover for the book.

The publishing team has been an ardent support to the editorial, designing and production team. Their endless efforts to recruit the best for this project, has resulted in the accomplishment of this book. They are a veteran in the field of academics and their pool of knowledge is as vast as their experience in printing. Their expertise and guidance has proved useful at every step. Their uncompromising quality standards have made this book an exceptional effort. Their encouragement from time to time has been an inspiration for everyone.

The publisher and the editorial board hope that this book will prove to be a valuable piece of knowledge for researchers, students, practitioners and scholars across the globe.

List of Contributors

Lidia Decembrino and Mauro Stronati
Neonatal Intensive Care Unit, Fondazione IRCCS Policlinico San Matteo, Pavia, Italy

Nunzia Decembrino
Pediatric Oncohaematologic Unit, Fondazione IRCCS Policlinico San Matteo, Pavia, Italy

Wissam Shalish and Guilherme Mendes Sant' Anna
Department of Pediatrics, McGill University Health Center, Montreal Children's Hospital, Montreal, Canada

Adauto Dutra Moraes Barbosa, Israel Figueiredo Júnior and Gláucia Macedo de Lima
Fondazione IRCCS Policlinico San Matteo, Pavia, Italy

Petja Fister
Department of Neonatology, University Children's Hospital, University Medical Centre Ljubljana, Ljubljana, Slovenia

Štefan Grosek
Department of Pediatric Surgery and Intensive Therapy, Surgical Service, University Medical Centre Ljubljana, Ljubljana, Slovenia
Department of Pediatrics, Medical Faculty, University of Ljubljana, Ljubljana, Slovenia

Štefan Grosek
Department of Pediatric Surgery and Intensive Therapy, Surgical Service, University Medical Centre Ljubljana, Ljubljana, Slovenia
Department of Pediatrics, Medical Faculty, University of Ljubljana, Ljubljana, Slovenia

Petja Fister
Department of Neonatology, University Children's Hospital, University Medical Centre Ljubljana, Ljubljana, Slovenia

Rejane P. Neves, Carolina M. da Silva, André F.G. Leal and Henrique J. Neves
Department of Mycology, Centre of Biosciences, Federal University of Pernambuco (UFPE),Recife, Brazil

Ana Maria R. de Carvalho Parahym and Danielle P.C. Macêdo
Department of Pharmaceutical Sciences, Center for Health Sciences, UFPE, Recife, BrazilKriengkrai Srithanaviboonchai
Faculty of Medicine, Chiang Mai University, Chiang Mai, Thailand
Research Institute for Health Sciences, Chiang Mai University, Chiang Mai, Thailand

Teja Škodič Zakšek, Anita Jug Došler, Ana Polona Mivšek and Petra Petročnik
Faculty of Health Sciences, University of Ljubljana, Ljubljana, Slovenia

Reginaldo G. Lima-Neto
Department of Tropical Medicine, Center for Health Sciences, UFPE, Recife, Brazil

Petja Fister
Department of Neonatology, University Children's Hospital, University Medical Center Ljubljana, Ljubljana, Slovenia

Štefan Grosek
Department of Pediatric Surgery and Intensive Therapy, Surgical Service, University
Medical Center Ljubljana, Ljubljana, Slovenia
Department of Pediatrics, Medical Faculty, University of Ljubljana, Ljubljana, Slovenia

Koichi Miyake, Noriko Miyake and Takashi Shimada
Department of Biochemistry and Molecular Biology, Division of Gene Therapy Research Center for Advanced Medical Technology, Nippon Medical School, Japan

Esra Caliskan
Department of Anesthesiology and Reanimation, Baskent University Faculty of Medicine, Ankara, Turkey

Maria Slomczynska and Katarzyna Knapczyk-Stwora
Department of Endocrinology, Institute of Zoology and Biomedical Research, Jagiellonian University, Krakow, Poland

Malgorzata Grzesiak
Department of Animal Physiology and Endocrinology, University of Agriculture, Krakow, Poland

Carlos Baeza Herrera
Universidad Nacional Autónoma de México (UNAM), Mexico
Guadalupe Victoria General Hospital, Texcoco, Mexico
National Academy of Medicine of México and Mexican Academy of Surgery, Mexico

Alin Villalobos Castillejos
Department of Pediatric Surgery, Guadalupe Victoria General Hospital, Texcoco, México
Regional Specialty Hospital of Ixtapaluca, México
Masters of Science program, UNAM, México

Ricardo Cortés García
Moctezuma Pediatric Hospital, UNAM, México
Hospital of Gynecology and Obstetrics number, "Luis Castelazo Ayala" Mexican SocialSecurity Institute, México

Hippolite O. Amadi
Bioengineering Department, Imperial College London, United Kingdom
College of Medicine, Imo State University, Owerri, Nigeria
Federal Medical Centre, Nguru, Yobe State, Nigeria

Mohammed B. Kawuwa
Department of Obstetrics and Gynaecology, University of Maiduguri, Nigeria
Federal Medical Centre, Nguru, Yobe State, Nigeria

Index

A

Adenosine Triphosphate, 33, 36, 57

Adjuvant Therapies, 16

Analgesia, 75-76, 80, 88-90, 105, 158, 166-168, 179, 189

Androgens, 191-198, 204-205

Anesthetic Management, 152-154, 158-160, 165-166

Antenatal Steroids, 67, 69, 72, 78

Antibiotics, 1, 3, 5-7, 11, 59, 65, 67-69, 71, 79-81, 84, 117, 216, 218, 222, 228

Antifungal Therapy, 6, 113, 117-119, 123

Asphyxia, 38, 46, 131, 142, 156, 215, 222, 248

Avascular Necrosis, 7

B

Blood Gases, 15, 17

Blood Pressure, 52, 67-68, 75-77, 80, 91-92, 115, 126-130, 133-135, 139, 141, 155, 157, 161, 222

Bone Scintigraphy, 4

Breast Milk, 44, 59, 61, 89, 159

Breastfeeding, 40-41, 50-52, 54-65, 75, 88-89

Bronchopulmonary Dysplasia, 12, 16, 28, 67, 95, 102, 111-112, 159

C

Cardiac Muscle, 33, 57

Catecholamines, 33, 55, 57, 98

Cerebral Palsy, 16, 69, 82, 116

Child's Immune System, 60-61

Colostrum, 59-61, 73

D

Diazoxide, 42-44, 46

Dopamine, 53, 55-56, 92, 141

E

Endocrine Active Compounds, 191-192, 196, 199

Epinephrine, 35, 55, 77, 136

Estrogen, 53, 193, 196, 199-200, 202-205, 207-209

Exendin, 44-45

Extra-uterine Life, 96-98

F

Fetal Growth, 32-33

Fungal Infections, 113-116, 118-122, 125

G

Gastroschisis, 222, 227-228, 232

Gestational Age, 13, 17, 32, 34-35, 92, 97-100, 107, 116, 120, 163, 213, 222, 227

Gluconeogenesis, 33, 38-40, 42, 57, 163

Glycogenolysis, 33, 57, 135

Growth Hormone, 33, 35, 42-44, 57

H

Healthy Birth Practice, 50, 53, 62

Hyaline Membrane, 97, 100, 109, 159

Hyperinsulinemia, 31, 34-35, 37, 39

Hypoglycemia, 31-49, 57, 61, 68, 70, 73, 156, 158-159

Hypophosphatasia, 143, 147, 149-151

I

Intensive Care, 8, 12-13, 25, 29, 46, 65, 67-68, 82, 84, 90, 96, 98, 113-115, 117, 121-127, 129, 131, 135, 138-141, 143, 158, 167, 217-218, 226

L

Labor, 51-52, 54-55, 69, 79, 81, 153, 177

Laryngeal Mask Airway, 160, 162, 168

M

Mechanical Ventilation, 12, 14, 25, 28-29, 79, 88, 90, 105, 112, 117, 222, 228

Meningitis, 9, 61, 74

Metachromatic Leukodystrophy, 143-145, 150

Methylxanthines, 27, 79, 94, 101-102, 110

þÿ M i c r o o r g a n i s m s , 1

Molecular Mechanisms, 31

N

Neonatal Osteomyelitis, 1, 8-11

Neonates, 1-7, 10, 12-16, 19-20, 24, 26-30, 32, 34-35, 37-39, 41-42, 45, 48-49, 69, 76, 82-94, 145-146, 151-158, 177, 191, 201, 212, 221-222, 230, 233-243, 245-247, 249

Neonatology, 12-13, 17, 25-27, 45, 80-82, 85, 94-95, 97, 108-111, 138-142, 152, 166-167, 233

Newborn, 2-3, 8-10, 41, 45-54, 56-57, 59-65, 68-75, 78-80, 98, 100, 108-109, 111-112, 116-117, 127, 134, 141, 144, 163, 178, 186, 188-189, 200, 215, 220, 222, 225, 227, 240,

Nonopioid, 76

O

Octreotide, 43

Ovary, 191-192, 194-201, 203-209

Oxygenation, 13, 17, 24-25, 71, 77, 79-80, 96, 98, 104-107, 110, 126-128, 135-136, 142, 156

Oxytocin, 53-56, 60, 64

P

Pain Management, 68, 74-75, 88-89
Pancreatic Beta Cells, 35-36, 42
Patent Ductus Arteriosus, 67-68, 80, 93-94, 96, 102, 117
Pathogenesis, 31, 34, 220, 224, 227, 231
Perfusion, 5, 67-68, 77-80, 96-98, 107, 126-128, 130, 133-136, 141-142, 161, 164, 222
Perioperative Evaluation, 152
Placenta, 33, 39, 50, 57-58, 96, 98
Postnatal Surgery, 210
Postoperative Care, 152-153, 158
Prenatal Care, 68, 80, 210, 213
Probiotics, 59
Prolactin, 53-55
Prophylactic Caffeine, 17
Pulse Oximetry, 13-14, 135, 161

R

Respiratory Distress, 15, 27, 38-39, 67-68, 80-81, 85, 96-99, 107-112, 117, 126, 138-139, 142
Respiratory Distress Syndrome, 15, 27, 39, 67-68, 81, 85, 108-112, 117, 126, 138
Respiratory Support, 12-13, 15-16, 25-26, 78-80, 83, 96, 98, 101-104, 106-107, 111

S

Sepsis, 2-3, 18-19, 38-39, 69-71, 73, 77, 79-80, 84, 113, 115-119, 122-125, 158-159, 222, 228
Septic Arthritis, 1-3, 6-11
Sirolimus, 43-44, 48
Skin-to-skin Contact, 50, 52-54, 59-60, 62-65
Surfactant, 12, 15, 17, 20, 27, 29, 39, 78, 96-98, 100, 102-104, 106-107, 110-111, 130, 139, 198

T

Thermoregulation, 50, 52, 56, 67, 137, 154, 167, 213

www.ingramcontent.com/pod-product-compliance
Lightning Source LLC
LaVergne TN
LVHW080927210926
848485LV00004B/747